Enhancing Surgical Performance

A Primer in Non-Technical Skills

EDITED BY

Rhona Flin
University of Aberdeen
School of Psychology, King's College
Aberdeen, United Kingdom

George G. Youngson
Aberdeen University Medical School
Royal Aberdeen Children's Hospital
Aberdeen, United Kingdom

Steven Yule
Harvard Medical School
Brigham and Women's Hospital
Neil and Elise Wallace STRATUS Center for Medical Simulation
Boston, Massachusetts, USA

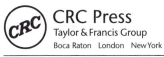

CRC Press
Taylor & Francis Group
Boca Raton   London   New York

CRC Press is an imprint of the
Taylor & Francis Group, an **informa** business

D0323076

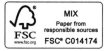

CRC Press
Taylor & Francis Group
6000 Broken Sound Parkway NW, Suite 300
Boca Raton, FL 33487-2742

© 2016 by Taylor & Francis Group, LLC
CRC Press is an imprint of Taylor & Francis Group, an Informa business

No claim to original U.S. Government works

Printed on acid-free paper
Version Date: 20150616

International Standard Book Number-13: 978-1-4822-4632-2 (Paperback)

Visit the Taylor & Francis Web site at
http://www.taylorandfrancis.com

and the CRC Press Web site at
http://www.crcpress.com

Contents

PART III   IMPLEMENTATION AND IMPROVEMENT   **153**

9   Training methods for non-technical skills   155
      Steven Yule, Nikki Maran, Akira Tsuburaya and Ajit K Sachdeva
      9.1   Introduction   155
      9.2   Training design and development for non-technical skills   156
      9.3   Evaluation   157
             9.3.1   Kirkpatrick's levels of evaluation   158
      9.4   Integrating non-technical skills training into surgical training   159
             9.4.1   Technical skills training curricula   160
             9.4.2   Non-technical skills training curricula   160
      9.5   Training modalities   161
             9.5.1   Simulation training for individual surgeons   161
             9.5.2   Simulation training for surgical teams   162
             9.5.3   Classroom teaching   163
             9.5.4   Coaching   164
      9.6   Practical matters and future possibilities   165
      References   166
10   Assessing non-technical skills in the operating room   169
      Simon Paterson-Brown, Stephen Tobin and Steven Yule
      10.1   Introduction   169
      10.2   Emergence of non-technical skills assessment   170
      10.3   Principles of assessment   171
      10.4   Behavioural marker systems   174
             10.4.1   What are behavioural marker systems and why assess non-technical skills? 174
             10.4.2   How to use behaviour assessment tools and the accuracy of assessments 176
             10.4.3   Who should be an observer?   176
      10.5   Practical issues and problems with behavioural marker systems   176
      10.6   Current methods for assessing surgeons   177
             10.6.1   In-training assessment: Australasia   177
             10.6.2   Procedure-based assessments   178
             10.6.3   Multi-source feedback   179
             10.6.4   Workplace-based assessment in non-technical skills   179
             10.6.5   Dealing with poor performance   179
             10.6.6   Degradation and remediation of skills   180
             10.6.7   Age and surgical performance   180
      10.7   Summary   180
      Acknowledgement   180
      References   180
11   What next? Development of non-technical skills   185
      George G Youngson and Thoralf M Sundt III
      11.1   Acquisition: education in patient safety and non-technical skills   186
             11.1.1   Workplace-based acquisition   186
             11.1.2   Patient safety in medical school curricula   187
             11.1.3   Methods of undergraduate teaching   187
      11.2   Using, developing and enhancing non-technical skills   188
             11.2.1   How others do it   188
             11.2.2   Who is qualified to teach and assess?   188

Preface

When I took the first stumbling steps on the ladder of my profession, there was so much to learn. What others did looked easy until I tried. The acquisition of the essential knowledge and hand–eye co-ordination seemed to take so long, and I have to admit that even after 20 years it still occasionally deserts me. But with constant repetition my skills have developed, and often even I'm surprised by my apparently effortless achievement of good results.

But I am also haunted by a spectre. Reading about incidents to colleagues, it became apparent early on that what seemed to cause career-limiting problems, even injury and death, wasn't a failing of just hand–eye co-ordination, or lack of reading, but something harder to define. After we've gained our initial experience, we still make small slips; but we're also good enough to counter those, and they rarely cause a problem. What seemed to be causing issues though was something bigger, as if the whole system we worked in could conspire to create problems so complex that our apparent effortless skill could deliver us to disaster without us even knowing until it was too late.

As I read through the history books, it became obvious that the old way of ensuring results – knowledge of everything – simply couldn't be relied on. Technical experts still got caught out, and death and maiming followed. I, and my colleagues, needed re-skilling. Our hand–eye co-ordination was still important and our knowledge still critical; but on their own, they wouldn't deliver us a conscience-free retirement, or for that matter an easy working day.

The evidence base behind this new set of non-technical skills is clear. My personal testimony is that I simply can't imagine how my colleagues of old survived without them. In reality, many didn't. I first started teaching the concepts behind this book in 1998. Since then, it has become an essential component of the skill set of those who choose to work in my profession; indeed, you won't get into my profession now without the willingness to embrace these skills. The public wouldn't have it any other way and neither would my colleagues.

In 1993, I nearly lost my life at the hands of an experienced instructor pilot who was technically gifted, with fine hand–eye co-ordination. Very poor situational awareness and decision making almost delivered disaster only averted by luck, pure luck. Twelve years later, it was my wife in the hands of a technically skilled and very experienced clinical team. Her last moments were unconscious witness to a team whose situational awareness, decision making, leadership and teamworking all failed them. But they'd never heard of non-technical skills; they were educated by the old school, where technical mastery gave you everything. Their re-education, in approximately 35 minutes, will live with them forever.

If I was to choose three people to write this book, it would have been Rhona Flin, George Youngson and Steve Yule. They are world-leading experts, balanced by pragmatism and real-world experience. You are in good hands.

Martin Bromiley
Airline pilot
Chair, Clinical Human Factors Group

Acknowledgements

The editors thank Irfan Ahmed, Adrianna Crowell-Kuhnberg, Mark Flitter, Rachel Lennon, Carol Anne Moulton, Dara O'Keeffe, Renzo Pessotto, Zahid Raza, Dianali Rivera-Morales, John Scott, Sharon Teitelbaum and Jennifer Yule for their advice and contributions. They particularly acknowledge the assistance of Wendy Booth in preparing the final manuscript.

The material from *The Non-Technical Skills for Surgeons (NOTSS) System Handbook* is reproduced with the permission of the University of Aberdeen, Scotland, and the Royal College of Surgeons of Edinburgh.

Contributors

Sonal Arora, Patient Safety Translational Research Centre, Imperial College, London, United Kingdom, is an academic clinical lecturer and colorectal surgical registrar. She leads the research team within the Simulated Operating Theatre at St Mary's Hospital. Her PhD in simulation and patient safety focuses on the use of innovations in training and assessment to enhance surgical performance and quality of care. Her research interests include assessment and training in non-technical skills, workplace-based learning, surgical stress and interventions to optimize patient safety. Sonal holds the Surgical Education Research Fellowship (awarded by the Association of Surgical Education, United States) and is also a clinical adviser to the World Health Organization.

Augusto Azuara-Blanco is a clinical professor of ophthalmology and an honorary consultant ophthalmologist, Queen's University, Belfast, United Kingdom. His academic career and research interests focus on improving patient care and investigating the efficacy, efficiency and safety of new developments for glaucoma (e.g. interventions, diagnostic tests and models of eye care). He is the chief investigator of an international multi-centre randomized controlled trial comparing primary lens extraction versus laser iridotomy in patients with PACG without cataract (EAGLE study, https://viis.abdn.ac.uk/HSRU/eagle/) and a United Kingdom–based multi-centre glaucoma diagnostic study evaluating automated imaging technologies (GATE, https://w3.abdn.ac.uk/hsru/gate/). He was the chair of the UK & Eire Glaucoma Society in 2012 and is a member of the Scientific Committee of the Royal College of Ophthalmologists and an examiner for the Royal College of Surgeons of Edinburgh. He was the lead of the CCRN-NIHR (Scotland, 2010–2012). He received the American Academy of Ophthalmology achievement award in 2008.

Rhona Flin holds the chair of applied psychology and is the director of the Industrial Psychology Research Centre at the University of Aberdeen, Scotland. She was involved in the NOTECHS project to develop a non-technical skills rating tool for pilots, and she supervised the ANTS, NOTSS, SPLINTS and ANTS-AP projects. She led the Scottish Patient Safety Research Network (2007–2012). She was awarded the Roger Green Medal for Human Factors in Aerospace (Royal Aeronautical Society) and the John Bruce Medal for Behavioural Science in Surgery (Royal College of Surgeons Edinburgh). Her current research is on non-technical skills, surgeons' intra-operative decision making and senior managers' safety leadership. She was a member of the Surgical Never Events Task Group (National Health Service England, 2013) and is a member of the Safety Advisory Committee, Military Aviation Authority and Ministry of Defence.

Ian Flindall is a surgical registrar in general surgery studying for a PhD in mental fatigue and cognitive performance in the medical profession at Imperial College, London. He achieved his MBBS from King's College, London, in 2001, taking time along the way to study for a BSc (Hons) in experimental pathology. His basic surgical training was obtained in Taunton, Somerset. He passed his MRCS (Eng) in 2006 before moving to Scarborough as a research registrar. There, he completed an MSc in science, research and education at the Hull University. He is continuing higher surgical training in London.

Ivan Keogh is professor and head of the Department of Otorhinolaryngology, National University of Ireland, Galway, and consultant otolaryngologist head and neck surgeon, Galway University Hospitals, Galway. Professor Keogh graduated from the National University of Ireland, Galway, in 1992. His speciality training was under the auspices of the Royal College of Surgeons in Ireland Otorhinolaryngology, Head and Neck Training Programme. In 2000–2001, he undertook a research fellowship at the Department of Genetics, Harvard University, and the Massachusetts Eye and Ear Infirmary in Boston, Massachusetts. A doctorate in medicine was awarded in 2006 for this research. Research interests include molecular genetics of hearing loss, safe surgery, human factors and nano-biophotonics of head and neck cancer. An Intercollegiate Speciality Certificate and Certificates of Specialist Training were awarded in 2006. In 2006–2007, he undertook clinical fellowships in otology and anterior skull base surgery at the Portmann Institute, Bordeaux, France, and the University Hospital Inselspital, Bern, Switzerland. He is a founder member of the Galway-based Irish Centre for Patient Safety. In 2012, he was awarded the Benjamin prize for research by the Collegium Oto-Rhino-Laryngologicum Amicitiae Sacrum.

Manoj Kumar is a consultant general and laparoscopic surgeon at the Aberdeen Royal Infirmary, Scotland. He has a keen interest in human factors and holds an MSc in Patient Safety: A Human Factors Approach from the University of Aberdeen. His thesis investigated adverse outcome reporting in surgery, and he went on to initiate and help develop an integrated reporting system. Manoj is part of the Scottish Mortality and Morbidity Review Project Team working on the development of national processes of reporting and learning. He

has been the recipient of an award by the National Patient Safety Agency for his work on antibiotic prescribing. He is actively involved in human factors training of health care and medical staff.

Nikki Maran is a consultant anaesthetist at the Royal Infirmary of Edinburgh with a particular interest in anaesthesia for emergency surgery. She has been involved in the original research projects identifying the non-technical skills used by anaesthetists (ANTS) and surgeons (NOTSS) and has extensive experience in using these frameworks for feedback in real and simulated clinical environments. She has designed and taught courses to help individuals develop their own non-technical skills and to observe and rate non-technical skills in others. Nikki was one of the two original co-directors of the Scottish Clinical Simulation Centre when it was established in Stirling in 1997 and was centre director until 2012. She is now associate medical director for patient safety in the National Health Service Lothian and a member of the Patient Safety Board of the Royal College of Surgeons of Edinburgh.

Craig McIlhenny is a consultant urologist who works in NHS Forth Valley in Scotland. He has a sub-specialty interest in the endourological management of urinary stone disease and malignant ureteric obstruction. His higher surgical training was in the west of Scotland and the United States. He has a special interest in human factors and patient safety. He sits on the RCSEd Patient Safety Board and is a faculty member of the Non-Technical Skills for Surgeons course. He is a trained Crew Resource Management instructor and has provided human factors and team training for operating surgical teams, intensive care unit teams, 'hospital at night' teams and others both in the United Kingdom and abroad. He also has a major interest in surgical training and is currently surgical director of the Faculty of Surgical Trainers at the Royal College of Surgeons of Edinburgh.

Paul O'Connor is a lecturer in primary care and the associate director of the Whitaker Institute, National University of Ireland, Galway, Ireland. He completed a PhD in psychology at the University of Aberdeen, Scotland, in 2002 and then served as a

Medical Service Corps officer in the US Navy until 2010. His research is concerned with improving human performance and safety in high-risk work environments. He has carried out research in a wide range of industrial and military domains. Since taking up post in Ireland, he has worked on human factors research in surgery and with junior doctors.

Sarah Henrickson Parker is assistant professor, Georgetown University Department of Emergency Medicine, and director of Education and Academic Affairs, National Center for Human Factors in Healthcare. Sarah has a BA in psychology from Wittenberg University in Ohio and an MA in human factors and applied cognition from George Mason University, Fairfax, Virginia. She worked at the Mayo Clinic as a human factors researcher on inpatient quality and safety challenges with the Division of Cardiac Surgery, developing safety interventions designed for the cardiac operating room. She was awarded her PhD from the University of Aberdeen, Scotland, for her research developing the Surgeons' Leadership Inventory, a behavioral marker tool for the intra-operative setting. She was a Ruth L. Kirschstein post-doctoral fellow, funded by the Agency for Healthcare Research and Quality (AHRQ), focusing on team co-ordination during trauma resuscitation. She is working on utilizing innovative measurement techniques in situ and in simulation (Robert Wood Johnson Foundation/AHRQ). Dr Parker's research interests include team performance and communication in high-risk settings, medical education on patient safety and human factors applications within health care.

Simon Paterson-Brown qualified from St Mary's Hospital Medical School, London, United Kingdom, in 1982 before training in surgery around London, the Home Counties, Hong Kong and Edinburgh. He has been a consultant general and upper gastrointestinal surgeon and honorary senior lecturer in the Royal Infirmary of Edinburgh since 1994. His main clinical interests are benign and malignant oesophago-gastric surgery and emergency surgery. He has published works on emergency surgery, laparoscopic surgery, upper gastrointestinal surgery, surgical training

and assessment. He is the co-author of the eight-volume *Companion to Specialist Surgical Practice* series (now in its fifth edition). His current interests include patient safety initiatives in surgery, surgical training and assessment. He was involved in the initial research project that developed the Non-Technical Skills for Surgeons (NOTSS) taxonomy, and with his co-workers he developed NOTSS courses, which have been run through the auspices of the Royal College of Surgeons of Edinburgh in Scotland and overseas since 2006. Other courses that have since been developed include the Safer Operative Surgery course for high-performing teams in the operating theatre. He is currently council member and chairman of the Patient Safety Board of the Royal College of Surgeons of Edinburgh.

Ajit K Sachdeva is the founding director of the Division of Education at the American College of Surgeons. Dr Sachdeva also serves as adjunct professor of surgery at the Feinberg School of Medicine at Northwestern University. Previously, he was the Leon C. Sunstein, Jr, professor of medical and health sciences education; professor and vice chairman for Educational Affairs, Department of Surgery; director, Division of Surgical Education; associate dean for Medical Education; and director of the Academic Center for Educational Excellence at MCP Hahnemann School of Medicine. Dr Sachdeva also served as chief of Surgical Services at the Philadelphia Veterans Affairs Medical Center. He received the Distinguished Educator Award (Lifetime Achievement Award) from the Association for Surgical Education; Margaret Hay Edwards, MD Achievement Medal from the American Association for Cancer Education; Award for Outstanding Contributions to Healthcare Simulation from the Society for Simulation in Healthcare; Frances M. Maitland Award from the Alliance for Continuing Medical Education; Lindback Award for Distinguished Teaching; Blockley-Osler Award for Excellence in Clinical Teaching; and Gold Medal in the Excellence in Government Awards Program. He has served as chairman of the Scientific Review Group Education Subcommittee (Study Section) of the National Cancer Institute and on the boards of the Accreditation Council for Continuing Medical Education and the Accreditation Council for Graduate Medical Education. He has served as president of the Association for Surgical Education, American Association for Cancer Education, Alliance for Clinical Education and Council of Medical Specialty Societies.

Douglas Smink is an associate professor in surgery at Harvard Medical School and a minimally invasive general surgeon at Brigham and Women's Hospital. His clinical practice focuses on abdominal wall hernias and gastroesophageal reflux disease. At Brigham and Women's Hospital, Dr Smink is the vice chair for education in the Department of Surgery, as well as the program director of the general surgery residency and the associate medical director of the Neil and Elise Wallace STRATUS Center for Medical Simulation. In his research, Dr Smink focuses on simulation in surgical education, particularly around team training of nontechnical skills.

Thoralf M Sundt III is the chief of cardiac surgery at Massachusetts General Hospital (MGH) and the Edward D. Churchill professor of surgery at Harvard Medical School. Prior to this, he was a consultant and professor of surgery at the Mayo Clinic. His clinical focus has been on surgery for the correction of acquired cardiovascular conditions in adults, and he is an internationally recognized thought-leader on the management of thoracic aortic diseases and reparative valve surgery. In addition to the more traditional lines of basic and clinical investigation, he has become interested in the science of health care delivery and the disciplines of human factors and systems engineering. On a national level, he was the first chair of the Workforce on Patient Safety for the Society of Thoracic Surgeons and played a central role in establishing a research program in patient safety while at the Mayo Clinic that was productive of original contributions to the surgical literature. At MGH, he is collaborating with investigators from the Harvard Business School and the Harvard School of Public Health studying intra-operative communication and leadership behaviours. He has spoken nationally and internationally on the subject of medical error, decision making and teamwork.

Stephen Tobin is associate professor of surgery and dean of Education at the Royal Australasian College of Surgeons in Melbourne, Australia. Stephen trained at the University of Melbourne and St Vincent's Hospital, Melbourne, graduating MBBS in 1981 and achieving a fellowship of the RACS in general surgery in 1989. He then worked for 2 years in England, specializing in colorectal surgery. He now holds fellowships from RCS England, RCS Ireland and CSSANZ. In 1992, he commenced practice in general and colorectal surgery in Ballarat, Victoria, Australia, founding the Central Highlands Surgeons, now comprising four surgeons. He was the RACS surgical supervisor for 9 years. His post-graduate clinical education studies were done at the University of New South Wales from 2000 to 2003, before a sabbatical period in Portsmouth, United Kingdom. He is a faculty for the Surgical Teachers' Course and has associate professor appointments at the Deakin University and the University of Notre Dame, where he has developed an online curriculum and continues to teach medical students, within the practice. He also holds an honorary clinical associate professor appointment at the University of Melbourne. Stephen commenced as dean of education at the Royal Australasian College of Surgeons in August 2012. Recent initiatives there include Academy of Surgical Educators, Foundation Skills Course for Surgical Educators and the JDoc pre-vocational program. In this role, he contributes to collaborative leadership of RACS surgical education and professional development. He completed a masters in surgical education at the University of Melbourne in 2014 and continues in clinical practice within the Ballarat medical system with the assistance of his surgical colleagues.

Akira Tsuburaya is a gastrointestinal surgeon and associate professor of surgery at Yokohama City University Medical Center in Japan. He is currently a visiting professor at Tokyo Medical University, and from 1994 to 2013 was the chief of gastrointestinal surgery at Kanagawa Cancer Center in Yokohama. Dr Tsuburaya is a national leader on non-technical skills in surgery in Japan. Since 2007, he has organized annual meetings on NOTSS and led the research group that translated the NOTSS behaviour rating tool into Japanese.

He is currently working on e-learning materials for J-NOTSS assessors and designing a trial of NOTSS and error reduction in a sample of Japanese hospitals.

George G Youngson is emeritus professor of paediatric surgery at the Royal Aberdeen Children's Hospital and University of Aberdeen, Scotland. He is a past vice president of the Royal College of Surgeons of Edinburgh and is the founder of its Patient Safety Board. His interests and contributions have included re-configuration of children's surgical services in Scotland, surgical education and clinical human factors as they affect surgical performance. He has been involved in the delivery of the NOTSS masterclass in various continents, including Asia, Europe, China, Africa and the United States.

Steven Yule is an assistant professor of surgery at Harvard Medical School. He is also director of education and research at the Neil and Elise Wallace STRATUS Center for Medical Simulation at Brigham and Women's Hospital in Boston, Massachusetts. He is also on faculty at Ariadne Labs for health systems innovation, the Center for Surgery and Public Health and the Academy at Harvard Medical School in Boston. His training is in organizational psychology and human factors, and he holds faculty positions in psychology (Aberdeen, Scotland) and surgery (Harvard). Dr Yule has been involved in the development of a number of assessment tools including NOTSS, SPLINTS and the Surgical Leadership Inventory. He has led the development of curricula in non-technical skills for surgical trainees and practising surgeons in the United Kingdom and United States, most notably the NOTSS masterclass at the Royal College of Surgeons of Edinburgh since 2006 and the NOTSS workshop at the American College of Surgeons Annual Clinical Congress since 2013. At Harvard, he established the Non-Technical Skills Lab (http://scholar.harvard.edu/ntsl), which brings together social scientists, health services researchers, educators, surgeons and other clinicians with a core mission of enhancing the understanding of the critical role of clinicians' social and cognitive skills in team performance and the quality and safety of patient care. Central to this is the role of simulation and behaviour assessment tools to support professional development in high-, middle- and low-resource environments around the world. He regularly speaks nationally and internationally on non-technical skills, safety and medical simulation.

PART I

Surgical performance: Recognition of the challenge

1

Intraoperative performance, non-technical skills and surgical safety

GEORGE G YOUNGSON

1.1 INTRODUCTION

There are many factors which will influence and determine a surgeon's intraoperative performance, but there is a traditional emphasis placed on the value of comprehensive knowledge, sound surgical technique and good manual dexterity. The importance of these elements of the surgical skill set is recognized by all; but they are, by themselves, insufficient to ensure the best patient outcome. There is another complementary set of skills termed 'non-technical skills' which needs to be integrated into the surgeon's repertoire to optimize surgical performance. This book explores the area of non-technical skills and outlines why these are important in contributing to the understanding of what makes a good surgeon.

1.2 SURGICAL SKILLS

1.2.1 SKILLS AT OUTSET

You may or may not recall the first incision you made, but more than likely it was accompanied by a number of considerations, thoughts and emotions, including a strong sense of responsibility and accountability. Performing that action well so that recovery ensued was, and remains, a central tenet of surgical care. With increasing seniority and increasing responsibility for patient care, the surgeon's actions necessarily become more complex and more demanding. The implications of the intervention made and decisions taken become more significant and potentially more hazardous. Therefore, the risk for the patient must be matched with the requisite level of skill from the surgeon. Acquisition of that skill occurs steadily with time, with repetition and ideally with tuition. This clearly applies to technical skills which are taught through illustration, observation, and learning by attempting to reproduce the actions of an expert. Some of these skills can be practised on simulators with different levels of fidelity, but there is usually a strong wish for those involved in surgical training to have hands-on practice and exposure to the real thing as much as possible.

Acquisition and development of the dexterity and technique needed in operative surgery therefore have primacy of place in the ambitions of every young doctor involved in surgical training. And yet – crucially – processes of thought, judgment, analysis and evaluation of risk and choice of manoeuvre or procedure are all of equal status to the craft aspect in determining the outcome of a surgical procedure. A keen mind and sharp thinking must accompany the precision of sound surgical technique, as does the ability to co-ordinate and collaborate with others and to lead the surgical team. These additional competencies also need to be acquired with time and supervised repetitive practice. In essence, these are the surgeon's non-technical skills that need to be defined and recognized before their use can be taught, developed, evaluated and implemented.

Whereas there is a wealth of published literature dealing with surgical procedures and surgical technique, the same is not true for non-technical skills. This book is one of the few resources detailing and describing surgeons' non-technical skills, and this first chapter outlines the skill set involved and provides examples of the types of challenges that are addressed and resolved by the application of non-technical skills.

The contribution of non-technical skills to surgical excellence is set out, and the factors that impact their development and use are discussed. This book highlights the different aspects of surgical performance and the variables (including those in the theatre environment, as well as the personal attributes of the surgeon) which will determine the acquisition, use and display of surgical skill.

1.2.2 WHAT GOOD SURGEONS DO WELL

Consider those attributes possessed by the surgeon whom you would choose to treat your family members – 'the surgeon's surgeon'. He or she will likely be an expert in many ways. The need for wise patient selection, good preoperative management and vigilant post-operative care are all essential, but the quality of operative skill and standard of performance during the operative procedure is a major determinant of outcome and it is the feature that will likely guide your choice. These attributes will also be accompanied by technical prowess, compassion and diligence, but these features alone will not always secure the best surgical outcome. Skills like composure, precision and attention to detail, high levels of knowledge and experience in treating the condition, knowing what to do and when and ability to get the best out of others as well as himself or herself are all needed. Further, it is during the intraoperative period that non-technical skills make their prime contribution to surgical performance and outcome, and they are therefore outlined here.

A well-exposed and tidy operative field along with gentle tissue handling, smooth and fluid movements, good co-ordination of the surgical team, sustained focus on the procedure with low-volume but relaxed interactions, communications and conversations all describe the surgical environment and practice of the surgeon who is in control of the operation. The tempo and flow of movement is smooth and unhurried, the dialogue is similarly relaxed and yet coherent and pertinent and there is a communal focus on the detail of the operation with attentive responses from all theatre staff involved. Rapid actions, when required, are still controlled and without alarm. This requires composure and competence and represents a situation where the patient is going to do well. It is thus usually quite obvious when a surgeon is in control of the operative procedure. The creation of these conditions is in large measure down to the concerted actions and the confidence of thought, movement and communication instilled by the surgeon in other team members. The good surgeon is thus in charge of self, team, circumstances and conditions within the operating theatre.

The absence of these conditions, by contradistinction, produces a disproportionately disruptive effect on the progress of the operation and creates a potentially hazardous intraoperative environment, which may predispose the patient to a higher risk of complications and adverse events during the surgery as well as in the post-operative period.

The way in which the individual surgeon acts, thinks and behaves therefore constitutes his or her non-technical skills and their deployment promotes high-quality and safe surgery, whereas deficiencies in these areas create problems and form the basis of adverse outcomes in the majority of cases involving surgical error.

1.3 NON-TECHNICAL SKILLS

1.3.1 NOTSS (NON-TECHNICAL SKILLS FOR SURGEONS)

Non-technical skills are defined as the cognitive and social skills that underpin knowledge and expertise in high demand workplaces.[1] They include the thinking skills and personal interactions that are required to accompany the appropriate level of surgical knowledge and technical competence in pursuit of surgical excellence. Non-technical skills can be arranged according to a variety of classifications, but the Non-Technical Skills for Surgeons (NOTSS) taxonomy outlined in detail in this book consists of four major categories of skill that allow the definition and the rating of surgeons' performance at the operating table.[2] These are as follows:

1. Situation awareness
2. Decision making
3. Communication and teamwork
4. Leadership

These four categories all contain elements of performance which can be discretely and explicitly identified, thus allowing an evaluation of surgical performance to emerge which may form the basis of training, debriefing or assessment, particularly if used in a formative fashion.

Non-technical skills in surgery have to date been appreciated for their importance in an intuitive rather than an explicit fashion. Until recently, however, surgeons have lacked the benefit of a specific definition, vocabulary or classification which allows the identification of the elements and categories involved in successful operative surgery. NOTSS fills that gap.

NOTSS has to date been restricted to intra-operative performance and is now being evaluated to identify whether or not it can encompass the surgeon's activities outside the operating room (OR). While cognitive, interpersonal and communication skills are, of course, recognized as essential ingredients of effective clinical practice outside the OR, non-technical skills as used in the context of this book exclusively relate to the performance of the surgeon carrying out an operative procedure. This book, therefore, looks at custom and practice in the OR; it describes and analyses many of the factors that influence the surgeon's performance, ranging from the decisions made through to the management of the entire theatre team. The focus of the book is on the individual surgeon's non-technical skills set; but there is also recognition of the impact of other influences which provoke variation in performance between surgeons, e.g. personality, fatigue, stress, self-confidence, self-efficacy as well as fluctuation within individual performance by virtue of the nature, complexity of the task, ability of the team and effect of the environment. These other factors, although not included as non-technical skills, are referred to throughout the book, when and where they affect performance.

1.3.2 NON-TECHNICAL SKILLS IN ELECTIVE AND EMERGENCY SETTINGS

Just as elective surgery and emergency surgery differ on a variety of counts, non-technical skills are applied and utilized differently by the surgeon under these different circumstances. Apart from obvious differences such as the performance of elective surgery during daytime hours and the often night-time performance of emergencies, the demands placed on the surgeon's abilities may also be quite different, e.g. the surgical team of elective surgery is usually fairly constant and enjoys a certain familiarity and predictability to the operative schedule. The emergency team by contradistinction may not share that same association or familiarity, and the lack of predictability of findings and choice of which procedure is to be performed places different demands on the teamworking and communication skills of the surgeon with other team members during emergency procedures. The use of non-technical skills thus varies and may require different emphasis during different circumstances.

1.3.3 NON-TECHNICAL SKILLS AND THE ELECTIVE CASE

Paradoxically, most errors are perpetrated during routine (as opposed to emergency) surgery, and this may be attributable to the fact that vigilance levels may be allowed to become low, possibly as a consequence of familiarity and certain presumptions being made.[3]

> Errors were most often the result of a lack of diligence and performing ordinary tasks as opposed to a lack of extraordinary skills.
>
> *Rogers et al.*[3]

Familiarity with the planned procedure, the predictable nature of the operative findings and the high level of preparation that accompanies elective surgery may produce a relaxation of focus (particularly during the routine phases of a protracted elective operation) and may promote a certain amount of automaticity of thought and action that makes the surgeon susceptible to error. Conversion from that automatic mode to a purposeful or mindful status requires being alert to the possibility of changes in circumstances and early recognition of cues signifying an alteration in the status of the procedure. Cue recognition is therefore an important feature of surgical performance which depends on experience, awareness

and recognition of patterns (Chapter 4). Being aware, slowing down and anticipating and predicting imminent events all require that a certain level of vigilance is maintained.[4]

1.3.4 NON-TECHNICAL SKILLS AND THE EMERGENCY CASE

By contrast, during emergency surgery the focus of and demands made on the surgeon's concentration and attention may expose other frailties and a predisposition to error caused by a range of different and unwelcome processes, e.g. fixation, inattentional blindness and confirmation bias. These terms are all outlined in subsequent chapters, but they are phenomena exposed by virtue of the finite capacity of the surgeon's functioning mental ability particularly when faced with a crisis situation. Wholesale application of the surgeon's attention and concentration on one specific aspect of the operative procedure may be potentially detrimental to other concurrent aspects of the case. Further, whereas rapid and unpredicted change in circumstances can complicate the routine, as well as the emergency procedure, accepting that concentration levels are also high in complex and challenging elective surgery, the relative unpredictability of the emergency case adds another dimension to the demands placed on the surgeons' attention. Surgeons therefore need to be able to indulge in vigilant and anticipatory behaviour on a constant basis, and this is particularly the case for the surgeon who is undertaking an emergency procedure.

Reactions to emergency situations also clearly affect performance. While retention of composure is an aspiration for all surgeons at all times, the reality can be something different and remaining calm during difficult intraoperative emergencies carries with it the best chance of remaining focused on the task and at the same time retaining enough mental capacity for making the best choices and exhibiting the best judgment and managing others (Chapter 4). This ability and facility is acquired slowly and the characteristics which determine the extent and rate of acquisition are hazy, but repeated exposure and exemplary illustrative behaviour are both valuable and valued.

Emergency surgery also requires the ability to respond and recover after being startled by an unpredicted and unexpected emergency situation; the startle effect and its management are discussed in Chapter 4. Crisis management is therefore increasingly gaining importance in training and in our simulation laboratories[5] and is recognized as utilizing a wide range of non-technical skills (see Chapter 10).

1.4 WHAT NON-TECHNICAL SKILLS ARE NOT

Firstly, it is important to emphasize at the outset that the application of non-technical skills is not discretionary and only for use as befitting certain occasions. These skills permeate every element of any surgical procedure, but it is acknowledged that their use may be intensified in response to complexity and during demanding periods of an operation.

Secondly, attention to non-technical skills is not required only for remediation of poor performance. The evaluation and rating of non-technical skills are not intended as an antidote for a lack of due diligence or vigilance or only to be applied to difficult people or difficult situations. Non-technical skills

are a constant and integral part of the surgical repertoire in all situations and circumstances, and good deployment is required for safe performance.

Thirdly, non-technical skills are about cognitive ability and exhibited interpersonal behaviours rather than a reflection of the surgeon's underlying personality or attitudes. Clearly, the former may be influenced by the latter, but the NOTSS rating system concentrates on those skills that can be observed or inferred while the surgeon is operating rather than being used to evaluate personality traits.

1.5 FACTORS INFLUENCING SURGICAL PERFORMANCE

The performance of a surgeon and the skill level displayed are dependent on and influenced by a wide range of factors. Figure 1.1 outlines a range of factors that individually and collectively impact surgical performance. These include individual attributes such as technical ability, dexterity, knowledge, training and education and experience. Beyond these, however, there are many other concurrent influences which affect how technical skills

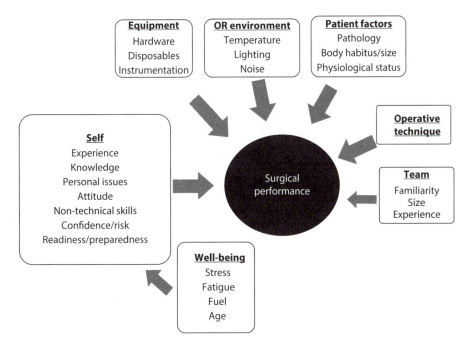

Figure 1.1 Factors influencing surgical performance.

are used. These include factors that are particular to individual patients, such as their pathology and disease process (which affect the quality of tissue and its handling properties), their body size and shape and their physiological status. The composition of the surgical team including the level of familiarity with one another, size of the team and experiences of the individual members will also determine the level of surgical performance, as do the operating conditions of the environment, e.g. temperature, lighting and noise. The available technology and equipment, including the quality and functionality of instrumentation and other adjuncts such as imaging, will all combine to affect the quality of surgery that each patient receives. Some of these factors are outlined in detail in this book, whereas others, including surgical technique, belong to a more traditional library of surgical practice.

Figure 1.1 shows many of the influences and pressures that determine the performance of the individual surgeon and, although this book will not deal with all the detail involved in this list of factors (see the work by Pennathur et al.[6] for relevant literature references), emphasis will be placed on those factors that relate to non-technical skills and those other factors that may influence them.

1.5.1 SURGICAL PERFORMANCE AND EQUIPMENT

The responsibility for familiarity with and safe functioning of surgical equipment resides with the user, i.e. the surgeon, but the variables involved in settings, connections and equipment compatibility standards are such that there is often a heavy dependency of the surgeon on nursing staff (the scrub nurse in particular) to ensure that the equipment is ready for use when needed. There is often an expectation by the surgeon that routinely used equipment such as diathermy will be preset to commonly used settings and that other equipment such as suction tubing/devices are available and working, and it is only when there is malfunction of such equipment that the surgeon's familiarity with this routine technology is tested. This test sometimes exposes the presumptions about that familiarity with usage to be poorly founded.

Anticipating the use of non-routine equipment is aided by some form of preparation and mental rehearsal, and explicit requests of specific items assist forward planning. This availability for use is well served by prior notification of intention to use; but there are circumstances, often during emergency situations, when equipment may need to be requested at short notice and its availability is not assured. Pre-usage identification can be best accommodated by preoperative briefings (which are distinct from the World Health Organization's Safer Surgery Checklists), a manoeuvre/action that also contributes to developing a shared understanding of the objectives of the surgery and one that allows good preparation in good time (see Chapters 6 and 7).

Other factors such as patients' and surgeons' position and posture affect the task. Ergonomics is a science concerned with the 'fit' between people and their work. It puts people first, taking account of their capabilities and limitations. Ergonomics aims to make sure that tasks, equipment, information and environment fit each worker. The ergonomics involved in the OR can have a distinct effect on the performance of the surgeon and predispose to fatigue at best or repetitive strain injury at worst, so posture and factors such as body position are important elements of surgery. This aspect of surgical performance is often not addressed in a conscious fashion, and the impacts of poor posture and subsequent muscle fatigue with the potential for degradation of surgical performance need to be actively considered. This should constitute a part of the surgical team's shared situation awareness. An awareness of the effect of ergonomics on surgical performance and the requirements of an optimal operating position and other physical features of operative surgery (e.g. lighting and visual aids) should therefore be a conscious decision for the surgeon if fatigue is to be avoided in the short term and somatic complaints (e.g. neck and back pain) are to be avoided in the longer term.

1.5.2 SURGICAL PERFORMANCE AND THE TEAM

While there may be a perception that the operating team is the ultimate clinical example of close teamwork, empirical data have been published that suggest that there is an ongoing low level of unease, disagreement and aggression in many ORs,[7] which, if nothing else, is indicative of the complex nature of interpersonal behaviours working together in this environment. Committed individuals working with a common aim but sometimes to differing timescales and agendas, in a closed environment, may have disagreement amplified and exacerbated into aggressive behaviours, particularly if other stressors are inadequately managed. The potential for significant conflict is recognized as a feature of virtually all work environments, but the close proximity of different health care disciplines working intensively together can highlight tensions in interpersonal relationships that potentially prejudice performance if not managed appropriately and can accordingly constitute a threat to patient safety.

The most challenging behaviours and attitudes emanate from those who fail to demonstrate respect for their co-workers, and these range from aggressive and disruptive behaviour expressed verbally through the use of belittlement, humiliation, harassment and intimidation through to actions recognized as passive aggression and being generally obstructive or simply 'difficult'. This creates a hostile and toxic environment and significant amounts of stress and burnout within the team, which can result in high staff turnover rates and failure of continuity and familiarity.[8] These tensions constitute a significant barrier to the delivery of safe care and can permeate through all aspects of thinking and codes of conduct. Such behaviours are not unique to the OR but are often tolerated here to a greater extent than would be the case in other work environments.

Conflict resolution within the team is therefore an important consideration when looking at safety culture, human factors and non-technical skills. Although it is not a component part of the NOTSS taxonomy as such, there are multiple factors that can result in conflict and aggression in the operating theatre and support the need for understanding the consequences of good and poor teamwork, communication and leadership (see Chapters 6 and 7).

Additionally, staffing discontinuity caused by serial changes in members of the team particularly during protracted surgery can result in disruption of continuity to the flow of surgery and a reduction in consistent appreciation of the objectives of the operative procedure by all those team members.

The sequence of tasks and an understanding of the details of the operative challenges may be unappreciated by the replacement members of the scrub team supporting the surgeon. Reiteration of the requisite steps should be used to help maintain and re-establish shared situation awareness.

On most occasions, however, proficiency of team performance is the norm and seems to be almost invisible. Safety can thus be considered to be a 'silent' phenomenon. By contradistinction, disruptive and incompetent teamwork is conspicuous and is usually evident to all. Competence is expected and usually attracts no comment, with excellence often only being identified in exceptional situations where the demands are extraordinarily high. The NOTSS taxonomy helps provide an appreciation of excellence beyond adequacy in those areas that are crucial to good surgery and helps to build on good practice and encourage good codes of behaviour. The surgeon's contribution to teamwork is outlined in detail in this book (see Chapter 6).

The lessons learned from other high-risk industries particularly in relation to teamwork can be applied to surgical performance in the operating theatre (see Chapter 2). This is particularly the case in high-risk and time-limited procedures where team co-ordination is essential (e.g. a ruptured abdominal aortic aneurysm that needs rapid aortic cross-clamping, the urgent arterial haemorrhage that needs control and repair, the complete airway loss that needs an emergency crico-thyroidotomy or tracheostomy, or the cardiac tamponade that needs immediate evacuation). Teamwork, composure, a single leading voice and a clearly articulated plan all make it possible to survive such a catastrophe. Responding to those crises, and more besides, draws on a range of skills and competence that depend on the collective attributes of the team members as much as they depend on the individual clinical skills to execute a manoeuvre, intervention or procedure.

1.5.3 SURGICAL PERFORMANCE AND THE OPERATING THEATRE ENVIRONMENT

The environment of the OR is a unique and complex work setting. It is virtually encapsulated with tightly managed access, initially borne out of a need for bacteriological control and security. Those barriers (both physical and those imposed by protocol), which were established to avoid contamination and the risks of sepsis, as well as designed to provide privacy and protection of patient confidentiality, have also created an environment that is exempt from open and public scrutiny. It is therefore one in which certain individual behaviours and conduct are occasionally seen and tolerated in a way that would not be the case in other social or workplace situations. The role of surgeon confers the privilege of a high level of trust, authority and autonomy; but the relative seclusion of the operating theatre environment can, on occasion, also allow that autonomy and assertiveness to drift beyond discipline and order and into bullying or abusive behaviours, which can have a detrimental impact on patient safety.[9] The actions required of a surgeon are thus on display and clear for all the team to see in every OR, in every continent; but there have been surprisingly few attempts at trying to catalogue them or codify the behaviours – both good and bad behaviours, which lead to accomplished surgery or, alternatively, to disarray – either temporary or more lasting.

The physical environment of the OR, in terms of both size and layout, can influence performance in a number of ways. A contained and restricted space makes the presence and flux of personnel more conspicuous. Excessive flow and passage of staff through the OR with numerous entrances and exits can contribute to the creation of distractions, as well as constituting a hazard through an increased potential for infection. Surplus personnel may also contribute to background noise level, and if accompanied by the practice of playing music (designed to soothe) then the clatter of noise produced by the combined output of conversation (particularly if non-clinical in subject matter), monitor alarms and essential and non-essential conversations can act as potent distracters to the concentration of the surgeon. So, management of team size is a relevant consideration but one that often receives no clear management by any single team member.

The physical layout of the OR and variation in patient positioning can result in different orientation options, which have been associated with surgical error – particularly wrong-side surgery as a consequence of spatial disorientation.[10] This potential for disorientation increases when the surgeon is operating in an unfamiliar OR (as is often the case in emergency surgery) and when there are several patients presenting sequentially with similar/same conditions but on different sides. This is aggravated by last-minute changes in the order of the theatre list. These can all disrupt the surgeons' awareness of polarity and orientation with potential for misidentification of the side of the intended surgery. Situation awareness in the OR needs to extend to the physical aspects and configuration of the OR environment as well as the operative field if surgical performance is to be optimized. Other physical properties of the environment including theatre temperature, lighting control, height of the table, prolonged standing/sitting, use of microscopes, screen placement and angles in minimally invasive surgery and importantly the position of the patient can all affect the surgeon's perception of the field, and the interplays between human performance, ergonomics, the technology in use and the environment and its administration are all key features and components of the scientific study of human factors in surgical practice. Control of these many factors and variables is a task best placed against surgical leadership and one that is best identified and articulated by the surgeon and shared with other members of the operating team.

1.6 SURGICAL ERROR

While hazards in the OR environment have also traditionally been seen as associated with the risks imposed by the physical characteristics of that environment (temperature control, fires, gas explosions, contamination by fluids, sharps, radiation, etc.), errors produced by the individual surgeon, the surgical team, or policies operated by the health organization itself are now appreciated as an equal if not more of a risk in causing harm to patients.[11] While errors in technique are an obvious cause of intraoperative and post-operative complications, deficiencies in other aspects of surgical performance are also hazardous for patients' well-being. It is the errors which are a consequence of deficiency in non-technical skills that are highlighted in this book, as are the advantages and benefits to performance at the individual and team levels that accrue from high-level deployment of non-technical skills.

For example, the surgeon's concentration during the operation can be interrupted by a wide range of distractions, and the awareness, interpretation and appreciation of anatomy, the decisions made and sequence of steps to be carried out in the operation are examples of what may be affected by disturbance to the surgeon's concentration (e.g. by background noises, chatter, pagers, alarms and telephone messages).[12]

Communications between team members may be compromised by poor interpersonal relations. Information can be given in the wrong manner or at the wrong time from the recipient's perspective. Exchange of information may not be confirmed and hence receipt not registered.[13] Unduly assertive behaviour by senior staff particularly during episodes of urgency can intimidate and create hierarchy gradients which may suppress important subsequent communication coming from junior members of the operating team.[14] A balance is needed between the need to protect the surgeon's concentration by filtering unwelcome and unnecessary interruptions and ensuring the maintenance of an open communication channel that allows transfer of crucially important information even at times of heightened tension (see Chapters 6 and 7).

Surgeons themselves, at a personal level, may be subject to suboptimal performance due to a number of pressures and may be affected by virtue of stress in their private lives, by fatigue or variation in their physical well-being (e.g. hypoglycaemia on account of missing meals through pressure of work). They may be ill or affected by prescribed (and unprescribed) medication. By recognizing and characterizing these factors, the surgeon can identify error-prone circumstances and situations and through self-reflection and self-calibration can possibly recognize periods when he or she is vulnerable to committing an error. Identifying this aspect of performance limitation is an important exercise in self-awareness and permits better planning of future actions and activities and may help decide on what tasks and challenge to contend with, when they might happen and what to postpone.

As seen in the following chapters, fatigue, stress and other aspects of personal fitness have not been included as categories within the NOTSS classification and rating process because their scale, extent and measurement in the intraoperative setting are difficult to quantify and evaluate, although coping with pressure is one of the elements in the leadership category. Nonetheless, the relevance of these aspects of human performance limitation to non-technical skills in general is considered and will be outlined.

All these factors – distractions, personal limitations, scheduling delays, staffing changes, etc. – are examples of the kind of pressures that may affect the surgeon with potential detriment to performance; but all can be accommodated and managed, at least in large measure, by applying good non-technical skills.

1.6.1 NEVER (AND OTHER ADVERSE) EVENTS

The catastrophic form of surgical error such as that found in 'never events' (e.g. wrong side/site, wrong patient, wrong prosthesis inserted and retained instrument/swab) is deemed to be rare on an individual surgeon basis, and yet these events are reported as occurring approximately 80 times per week in the United States[15] and 329 times in the 12-month period during 2012–2013 in the United Kingdom.[16] Moreover, wrong-site and wrong-side operations continue unabated despite the implementation of mitigating strategies such as the universal protocol[17] and the WHO surgical checklist.[18,19] Never events take place in full view of other members of the operating team who are usually experienced practitioners in their own fields, either nursing or anaesthetic, posing a number of unanswered questions such as the following: why is a never event allowed to happen by other team members who are involved in the surgery and observing it taking place?[16] Why are no corrective actions implemented to avert the error? Additionally, this type of error is usually performed in a technically adequate fashion, but the procedure is the wrong one and the consequences are devastating.

This type of error is thus attributable more to deficiencies in non-technical skills such as situation awareness, decision making and communication than it is to deficiencies in the craft aspect of surgery. Additionally, decision-based errors such as the wrong choice of procedure (albeit in the correct patient and at the correct time) for any given condition are not usually included in any register of adverse events, have no obligate reporting mechanism and tend to receive less comment or external criticism and recrimination than a never event.

Remedies to protect against error, capture and correct early error or have a damage limitation process have been necessary for some time, and a variety of processes and procedures have been attempted to obviate unintentional harm occurring during surgery. The chief one among these has been the development of checklists and other similar tools (see Chapter 11 for quality improvement driver diagrams) that specifically focus on the awareness of individuals and the theatre team on the correctness of the procedures about to be undertaken. The contribution of non-technical skills to the utility and implementation of the surgical checklist is an important consideration and is discussed later in this book (see Chapters 6, 7 and 11).

1.6.2 ERROR AND CHECKLISTS

In recognition of the risk of error that may accompany surgery, a range of measures have been instituted in ORs across the world. The implementation of surgical briefings, checklists and standards such as the universal protocol[20] and the WHO surgical safety checklist has gone some way in reducing morbidity as a consequence of error and improving outcome following operation;[18,19] however, why these beneficial effects are achieved without any obvious change in the skill set of the surgical team and its constituent individual members remains unclear. The checklist approach could work at least in part, by liberating the surgeons' attention from other uses and responsibilities and allowing it to be deployed in thinking through other aspects of the operation. Further, the checklist is not the only mechanism for protecting against surgical error and awareness must be retained of other contributory factors that may lead to error and are not accommodated by the checklist (e.g. malfunctioning equipment, inappropriate level of staffing and assistance and discontinuity of staff presence throughout the procedure). However, inconsistent and poorly executed checklists by reluctant and recalcitrant users have been shown to not only reduce their effectiveness[21] but

also actually pose a threat to safe practice,[22] posing a question to their value.[23]

The benefits of the surgical checklist also derive from an understanding of what it achieves and why it achieves it rather than merely its application as well as making a contribution to the culture of safety in the OR. In this aspect, blueprinting the WHO checklist components against the NOTSS taxonomy is of considerable interest as it demonstrates the application and implications of non-technical skills in contributing to safe practice (see Chapter 11) and makes the proposal that the benefits and advantages afforded by the WHO checklist are, in part, obtained through individual and team use of non-technical skills.

1.6.3 ANALYSING ERROR

The typical operating theatre is a busy workplace with pressures frequently escalating as the operating schedule progresses during the day. Changes in the order of the list, last-minute amendments to staffing arrangements, communication difficulties, time pressures and interpersonal conflict can all conspire to make a normally complex environment more difficult still. These and similar situations constitute a test of the surgeons' ability to cope and also constitute a potential risk to the patient's safety with a predisposition to error developing as a consequence of these changes.

When a surgical procedure goes wrong in the operating theatre, the term 'accident' is seldom used in relation to the failure. Instead, the term 'surgical error' is in common parlance, but implicit in that term is the attribution of the accident to a poor level of performance by the individual surgeon. Approximately 10% of hospitalized patients are unintentionally injured as a result of mishaps during their treatment. Surgical patients are at highest risk of suffering in this way,[24] and the literature on intraoperative surgical error and complications shows that non-technical aspects of performance such as diagnostic failure or breakdowns in teamwork and information sharing[25] lead to higher risks of major complication or death. An estimated 50% of all surgical errors occur within the operating theatre, and of these 40–50% are deemed entirely preventable[24,26] and perhaps most alarming is the finding that most errors occur during routine surgery rather than in complex and demanding situations.[3] This latter observation suggests that it is reduced vigilance and decreased awareness that poses a threat to the safety of patients rather than deficient operative technique.

Although technical errors can and do contribute to poor surgical outcomes, a lack of application or the use of poor non-technical skills are all the more influential in contributing to surgical error. Any investigation into surgical error and adverse surgical events is therefore required to evaluate the level of surgical skill shown, and this is an intensely personal challenge to the surgeon. It is perhaps because of the directly attributable origins of the mistake to the individual surgeon that there has been some resistance to accepting the scale and ubiquitous nature of surgical error and makes it all the more challenging and sensitive an issue for surgeons to address.

Whereas intraoperative error may be discussed in house at morbidity and mortality meetings and at surgical rounds (and may attract critical comment in these venues), it is rare for non-technical skills to be the focus of any critical analysis at these meetings. Moreover, it is extremely unusual for any regulatory or policy change to accrue from the internal departmental analysis that evaluates morbidity and mortality on a case by case basis. Indeed, any learning tends to be limited to the participants in the individual review meeting, and the extent to which an understanding of the causes of the error are fully scrutinized and evaluated is again often inconsistent, subjective and discretionary. In the absence of any obligate external systematic approach to analyse intraoperative errors as may occur in other industries (e.g. the aviation accident investigation board), the opportunity to systematize causality and to introduce error-trapping techniques that can be learned by all in training and in practice is still a distant goal.

The surgical equivalent of aviation's cockpit voice recorder does not yet exist in ORs in spite of the possibility for substantial adverse intraoperative events (e.g. never events) occurring on a regular basis. However, routine video recording of endoscopic surgery is emerging as a practice in some centres as an attempt to try and identify the quality of surgical technique being employed.[27] Perhaps, this and other forms of routine performance capture methods might allow analysis of the factors that contribute to assessment of good or poor performance and in turn to training in the process of behavioural rating, which is an important element of the NOTSS system. The ultimate goal would be consistent display of high standards of professional codes of conduct and eradication of unacceptable alternatives.

1.6.4 DAY-TO-DAY PERFORMANCE

In the day-to-day performance of surgery, more mundane responsibilities exist for the surgeon and the flow of patients through the OR and completion of the operating list on time is a regular source of challenge. Indeed, the rate of progress of individual operations as well as the whole operating session is a responsibility the surgeon shares with other members of the operating team; but the pace of the operating list often appears to the surgeon to be dictated more by the other team members (and indeed factors outside the operating theatre, e.g. transfer arrangements of patients to and from the theatre and to and from the surgical ward). While the responsibility for generation of the operating list in some organizations resides with the surgeon, the level of control over the factors determining that pace of progress is finite and is, on occasion, challenging to the surgeon's patience and temperament. The accumulation of minor disruptions to the progress of the operating list and the lack of co-ordination of events to which little individual attention is paid and hence no action is taken (as opposed to an obvious single delay, which is often attended to promptly) can be a source of frustration. On those occasions where the list is not flowing properly, cooperation and communication among the staff may often be assumed and taken for granted as opposed to be deserving of specific remedial attention and effort.

> The single biggest problem with communication is the illusion that it has taken place.
>
> *attributed to George Bernard Shaw*

Disruptions to progress during an operating list come from a variety of sources. A complete portfolio of data, information and documentation relating to each patient may not always be present in spite of protocol suggesting that it ought to be so. Omissions, and conflicting information (particularly in relation to the laterality of procedure), especially if they only become apparent at the last minute, are particularly problematic because they place an added pressure on whether to proceed or whether to possibly abandon the case. The implication of case cancellation with all that involves for patient expectation, patient well-being, efficient use of theatre time and the need to reschedule constitutes an inconvenience at best and is a decision that may be often viewed as the last option, a decision often made in frustrating circumstances and yet one potentially with high consequences for the surgical outcome and patient well-being. In some settings, this may also have a financial implication for surgeon and hospital practice. However, such instances can disturb and disrupt composure before starting a case and may produce a legacy of behaviours that are displayed during the intraoperative phase and constitute a challenge to the surgeon's leadership behaviours. How should you lead the rest of the team when faced with uncertainty?

All these factors, which represent the constant list of problems needing to be actively managed in the OR, test the surgeons' non-technical skills, and failure of effective management may predispose to a situation where error becomes a real risk. Appreciation and good execution of non-technical skills is key to mitigating these factors and to making the OR a safer place.

1.7 ABOUT THIS BOOK

This book is about the intraoperative performance of surgeons and the contribution of non-technical skills. It deals with the ordinary workings of everyday OR activity rather than concentrating predominantly on surgical crises, surgical misadventures or surgical catastrophes. Although it clearly has relevance for the entire surgical team, the focus is on the individual surgeon and his or her skill set and how interactions between surgeon and other team members can promote optimal individual, as well as optimal team, performance. It is about the

choices that must be made during surgery and the actions that must be taken. The primary focus of the book is the surgeon's performance during the operation as opposed to different aspects of the care given during the pre- or post-operative phases of surgical care.

The book has been structured into three sections.

The first section 'Surgical Performance: Recognition of the Challenge' outlines those aspects of operative performance that are reliant on and influenced by non-technical skills, as well as the background to NOTSS. Chapter 1 reviews factors that influence surgical performance; risks, challenges and hazards contained in the OR environment; interactions between surgeons and staff, surgeons and instrumentation used; as well as surgical error and its sources. Chapter 2 gives an outline of the evolution of the non-technical skills approach in other industries, most notably aviation, and explains how it was first adopted in clinical specialties, such as anaesthesia. Chapter 3 provides a description of NOTSS, which is a system that allows structured observation, rating and feedback of a surgeon's behaviours in the OR. The chapter describes how this was devised and developed to be applicable in surgical practice.

The second section of the book 'Underpinning Concepts' describes all components of a surgeon's non-technical skills in detail. It outlines and explains the underpinning concepts involved in cognition, the thinking during operative surgery (e.g. decision making) and the social/interpersonal behaviours (e.g. communication and working with other members of the surgical team), as well as referencing the underpinning research contributing to the understanding of non-technical skills. Much of this research comes from domains outside medicine (especially that found in the psychology literature). Further, many applied practices employed in other high-risk industries and professions are relevant to surgical practice and some of these are mentioned. This section highlights the importance and relevance of the four NOTSS categories in different situations, and the potential benefit to patient outcome, as well as highlighting ways for improving the effectiveness and efficiency of the surgical team. The cognitive categories are discussed in Chapters 4 and 5. The next two chapters deal with social skills;

Chapter 6 discusses teamwork and communication skills, whereas Chapter 7 covers intraoperative leadership. In Chapter 8, the strategies required by a surgeon to cope with performance-shaping factors, such as stress and fatigue while operating, are outlined.

The third section 'Implementation and Improvement' outlines the mechanisms by which non-technical skills are acquired and their inclusion and integration into surgical curricula worldwide. Training is reviewed in Chapter 9 in relation to teaching, observing, assessing and coaching non-technical skills. Different methods of providing feedback and showing how this impacts learning and behaviour are presented, as are some of the methods used for creating online teaching tools. Chapter 10 looks at methods of assessing a surgeon's non-technical skills, both in a formative session as well as during summative judgment, e.g. for licensing. The section concludes with Chapter 11, which provides some anticipation of how non-technical skills may become critically important when evaluating surgical performance in the future and when used by those charged with assessing quality and ensuring safe practice in ORs.

As will be seen, non-technical skills permeate every aspect of surgical performance and are essential components of high-quality operative practice. The following chapters expand and amplify all these effects and their relevance to expert delivery of operative care.

1.7.1 USING THE BOOK

The intended audience for this book is primarily surgeons spanning the whole spectrum of seniority and experience, with aspects of learning that should be formative for the surgical novice in his or her early years, and this book also includes content that should stimulate and promote reflection in the experienced and accomplished. Although it may be a 'start-to-finish' read for some, it has been written with the purpose of introducing surgeons to new literature, new aspects to their operative performance and possibly new concepts.

For most surgeons, however, these will not be new skills; but rather, this book provides a fresh look at skills which already exist but may be under- or unappreciated in their importance and, indeed, the book

is intended to promote their further use. It has, therefore, been written with learning and development in mind and, although it may be used for reference purposes, it is mainly presented as a tool and adjunct to develop, improve and enhance clinical practice.

The international authorship and readership present challenges in presentation of the terminology and language used herein to represent different grades of surgeons working in different jurisdictions and different surgical practices (e.g. consultant/attending, resident/trainee/registrar, operating theatre/OR and anaesthetist/anaesthesiologist). It is anticipated, however, that such terms are widely recognizable and that the readers can interpret and apply the terminology as befits their own locality and practice.

REFERENCES

1. Flin R, Martin L. Behavioural marker systems in aviation. *Int J Aviat Psychol.* 2001;11:95–118.
2. Yule S, Flin R, Maran N, Rowley DR, Youngson GG, Paterson-Brown S. Surgeons' non-technical skills in the operating room: Reliability testing of the NOTSS behaviour rating system. *World J Surg.* 2008;32:548–56.
3. Rogers SO, Gawande AA, Kwaan M, Puopolo AL, Yoon C, Brennan TA et al. Analysis of surgical errors in closed malpractice claims at 4 liability insurers. *Surgery.* 2006;140(1):25–33.
4. Moulton CA, Regehr G, Lingard L, Merritt C, McRae H. Slowing down to stay out of trouble in the operating room remaining attentive in automaticity. *Acad Med.* 2010;85:1571–7.
5. Moorthy K, Munz Y, Forrest D, Pandey V, Undre S, Vincent C et al. Surgical crisis management skills training and assessment: A simulation-based approach to enhancing operative room performance. *Ann Surg.* 2006;244:139–47.
6. Pennathur P, Thompson D, Abernathy J, Matinez E, Provonost P, Kim G et al. Technologies in the wild (TiW): Human factors implication for patient safety in the cardiovascular operating room. *Ergonomics.* 2013;56:205–19.

7. Coe R, Gould D. Disagreement and aggression in the operating theatre. *J Adv Nur.* 2008;61:609–18.

8. Leape L, Shore MF, Dienstag JL, Mayer RJ, Edgman-Levitan S, Meyer GS et al. A culture of respect, part 1: The nature and causes of disrespectful behaviour by physicians. *Acad Med.* 2012;87:845–58.

9. Flin R. Rudeness at work. *BMJ.* 2010;340:c2480.

10. Cohen FC, Mendelssohn D, Bernstein M. Wrong sided craniotomy. *J Neurosurg.* 2010;113:461–73.

11. Gawande AA, Thomas EJ, Zinner MJ, Brennan TA. The incidence and nature of surgical adverse events in Colorado and Utah in 1992. *Surgery.* 1999;126:66–75.

12. Healey AM, Sevdalis N, Vincent CA. Measuring intraoperative interference from distraction and interruptions observed in the operating theatre. *Ergonomics.* 2006;49:589–604.

13. Greenberg CL, Regenbogen SE, Studdart DM, Lipsitz SR, Rogers SO, Zinner MJ et al. Patterns of communication breakdowns resulting in injury to surgical patients. *J Am Coll Surg.* 2007;204:533–40.

14. Weldon SM, Korkiakangs T, Bezemer J, Kneebone R. Communication in the operating theatre. *Brit J Surg.* 2013;100:1677–88.

15. Mehtsun WT, Ibrahim AM, Diener-West M, Provonost P, Makary MA. Surgical never events in the United States. *Surgery.* 2013;153:465–71.

16. *Patient Safety Domain. Standardise, Educate, Harmonise. Commissioning the Conditions for Safer Surgery.* NHS England: Never Events Task Force Report. Patient Safety Domain. http://www.england.nhs.uk/wp-content/uploads/2014/02/sur-nev-ev-tf-rep.pdf. Accessed March 22, 2015.

17. Stahel PF, Sabel AL, Victoroff MS, Varnell J, Lembitz A, Boyle DJ et al. Wrong-site and wrong-patient procedures in the Universal Protocol era. An analysis of a prospective database of physician self-reported occurrences wrong-site and wrong-patient procedures. *Arch Surg.* 2010;145:978–84.

18. Haynes AB, Weiser TG, Berry WR, Lipsitz SR, Breizat A-HS, Dellinger EP et al. A surgical safety checklist to reduce morbidity and mortality in a global population. *N Engl J Med.* 2009 Jan 29;360(5):491–9.

19. de Vries EN, Prins HA, Crolla RMPH, Outer den AJ, van Andel G, van Helden SH et al. Effect of a comprehensive surgical safety system on patient outcomes. *N Engl J Med.* 2010 Nov 11;363(20):1928–37.

20. American College of Surgeons, Statement on ensuring correct patient, correct site, and correct procedure surgery. *Bull Am Coll Surg.* 2002;87:26.

21. Pickering SP, Robertson ER, Griffin D, Hadi M, Morgan LJ, Catchpole KC et al. Compliance and use of World Health Organisation checklist in UK operating theatres. *Brit J Surg.* 2013;100:1664–70.

22. Rydenfalt C, Ek A, Larsson PA. Safety checklist compliance in a false sense of safety; new directions for research. *BMJ Qual Saf.* 2014;23:183–6.

23. Urbach DR, Govindarajan A, Saskin R, Wilton AS, Baxter NN. Introduction of surgical safety checklists in Ontario Canada. *N Eng J Med.* 2014;370:1029–38.

24. Anderson O, Davis R, Hanna GB, Vincent CA. Surgical adverse events: A systematic review. *Am J Surg.* 2013;206:253–62.

25. Mazzocco K, Petitti DB, Fong KT, Bonacum D, Brookey J, Graham S et al. Surgical team behaviors and patient outcomes. *Am J Surg.* 2009;197:678–85.

26. Gawande AA, Thomas EJ, Zinner MJ, Brennan TA. The incidence and nature of surgical adverse events in Colorado and Utah in 1992. *Surgery.* 1999;126:66–75.

27. Birkmeyer JD, Finks JF, Reilly AOO, Oerline M, Carlin AM, Nunn AR et al. Surgical skill and complication rates after bariatric surgery. *N Eng J Med.* 2013;369:1434–42.

2

Human factors: The science behind non-technical skills

RHONA FLIN AND MANOJ KUMAR

In this operational environment, there are hierarchical, multidisciplinary teams (often several nationalities and mostly males) working on complex situations that are characterized by high risks and time pressure. There is a 'can-do' work culture.

Analysis of the adverse event which occurred on April 20, 2010 revealed failures in situation awareness (missed warning signals), decision making (confirmation bias), teamwork and leadership.

2.1 INTRODUCTION

The aforementioned description comes not from an operating room but from an industrial environment that also requires non-technical skills for operational crews, namely, an offshore drilling rig.[1] The adverse event mentioned is the blowout on the *Deepwater Horizon* oil rig in the Gulf of Mexico in 2010 that killed 11 men, injured another 50, and caused an enormous oil spill. Investigations revealed causal factors relating not only to technical equipment, such as the blowout preventer, but also to failures in the cognitive and teamwork skills of the crew drilling the high-pressure well.[2] In 1988, the loss of the North Sea oil platform *Piper Alpha*, with 167 deaths, was partly caused by poor communication at shift handover, compounded by leadership failures.[3] Shipping accidents, such as groundings and collisions, are frequently characterized by failures in bridge leadership or crew assertiveness, as well as corporate weaknesses.[4,5] Although human error cannot be eliminated, in high-risk industries there

17

is now an awareness of the organizational and human factors that can help to reduce or mitigate error and are thus protective for safety.

In this chapter, we move out of the operating room to provide a background to the non-technical skills approach. We begin by introducing the field of human factors and then describe how one aspect of it, from psychology (on non-technical skills), relates to developing a better understanding of human thinking and social behaviour in the workplace. Other aspects of human factors science that focus on the organizational setting, work culture, task environment, design and operation of software and technical equipment are not considered here.

2.2 HUMAN FACTORS SCIENCE

The term 'human factors' refers to 'environmental, organisational and job factors, and human and individual characteristics which influence behaviour at work in a way which can affect health, safety and job performance'.[6] Human factors is a multidisciplinary endeavour with scientists being drawn from psychology (the science of mind and behaviour), physiology and engineering, as well as other specialties. Ergonomics, the application of human sciences to the design of objects, systems and environments for human use, is a core component. In a work context, human factors research examines the environmental, organizational, technical and job factors of humans interacting with systems, as well as the physiological and psychological characteristics which influence human behaviour at work. The military and the aviation industry have the longest history of applying human factors principles to enhance the design of equipment, work environments and human performance. Today, many industrial sectors have specialist bodies advising on the application of human factors science to their workplaces.

In the world of health care, there was traditionally a rather limited interest in human factors. But realization of the pervasive rates of iatrogenic injury that motivated the patient safety movement (see Chapter 1) caused attention to be turned to the safety management techniques in industry, especially methods derived from human factors science. Martin Bromiley (an airline pilot whose wife died due

to an anaesthetic accident which had non-technical causes: see Preface) established in the United Kingdom in 2007 the first Clinical Human Factors Group (www.chfg.org). Coming from an industry that incorporated a human factors approach into all aspects of safety management, he was dismayed to find how little awareness there was of the role of human factors in patient safety.[7] His efforts to introduce human factors into clinical training and also into incident investigation have contributed to the recent UK government's initiatives to bring human factors into health care,[8] with similar trends becoming apparent in other countries.[9]

There are a multitude of human and organizational factors that can be related to human error.[10,11] A simplified framework (Figure 2.1) shows the principal themes from human factors science, all of which can be applied to health care.

The patient is portrayed as the central element and the presence of external influences should also be acknowledged, for example, from national culture or government, as safety is influenced by regulatory and commercial pressures, the working environment and management demands. There are many similar frameworks displaying key factors influencing patient safety outcomes: these are often portrayed as systems diagrams. Figure 2.2 is an example, indicating postulated relationships between organizational aspects, human factors, errors and safety outcomes. Non-technical skills along with technical skills, would be located in the box labelled 'Worker behaviours/human error' in Figure 2.2.

Comprehensive texts and reports on human factors for patient safety are available,[9,13] as well as guides on how to implement human factors principles and techniques in health care.[14] There are also accident analysis techniques that examine human factors causes, and these can be applied to adverse events in hospitals.[15,16] One of the dominant models of accident causation is shown in Section 2.2.1.

2.2.1 'SWISS CHEESE' MODEL OF ACCIDENTS

'… It is often the best people who make the worst mistakes – error is not the monopoly of an unfortunate few'.

This statement by the psychologist James Reason[17] captures the importance of human factors

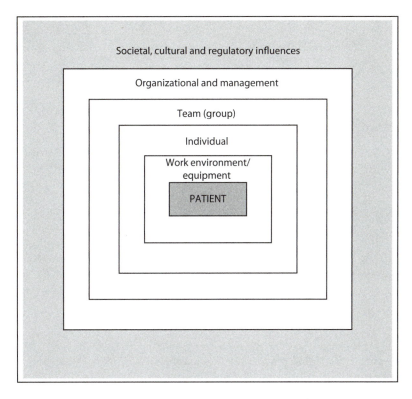

Figure 2.1 Organizational and human factors in health care. (Adapted from Moray N, *Ergonomics*, 43, 868–88, 2000.)

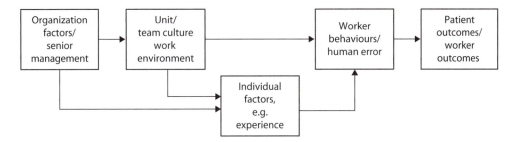

Figure 2.2 Systems diagram of factors influencing patient safety. (From Flin R et al., *Human Factors and Patient Safety. Review of Topics and Tools*, World Health Organization, Geneva, Switzerland, 2009.)

and non-technical skills while acknowledging the fallibility of the interaction of human beings within their environment. Many surgeons will be familiar with his 'Swiss cheese' model[18] (Figure 2.3), which describes the imperfections in the multiple layers of defences (defences in depth) in a complex organizational system to prevent harm. However, like the cheese slices, these defences all have holes in them and accidents are usually caused by the alignment of flaws in an organization's defences.

The defects occur due to two reasons: active failures and latent conditions.

Active failures are described as unsafe acts committed by individuals or teams and can present as slips, lapses, mistakes or procedural violations. These have a short-lived impact on the defences. Latent conditions are issues that are often inherent within an existing system (i.e. resident pathogens). They can result in creating the following: (1) an environment that incites error

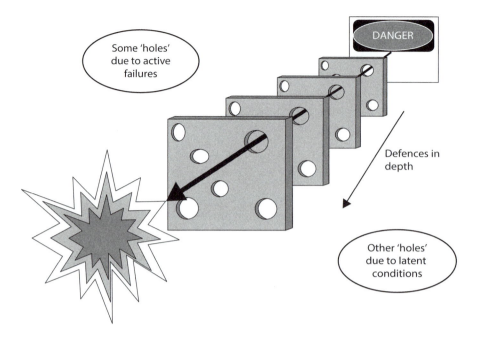

Figure 2.3 An accident trajectory passing through corresponding holes in the layers of organizational defences. (From Reason J, *Managing the Risks of Organizational Accidents*, Aldershot, UK: Ashgate, 1997. With permission.)

such as understaffing, fatigue and inadequate or inappropriate equipment and (2) weaknesses in the defences, such as unattainable or impractical standards, system design or policies. Latent conditions often go unnoticed until they are juxtaposed with active failures, resulting in a negative outcome. Understanding this model and applying it in health care assists in transforming risk management from a reactive system to a proactive system.

The model highlights that the operational personnel (e.g. a surgical team) represents the final line of protection of the organization's defences. They not only are responsible for the active failures that can contribute to losses and injuries but also, more importantly, can detect and correct their own and others' errors. (Pilots make about two errors per flight segment, but most of these are caught and corrected by the aircrew.[19]) Moreover, operating room staff can also recognize and remedy problems, such as equipment malfunctions, and can cope with a wide variety of conditions. Although human error is inevitable and pervasive, as Reason[20] emphasizes, workers can also be heroes by providing the essential resilience and expertise to enable the smooth functioning of imperfect technical systems in safety-critical work environments, such as an OR.

For those wishing to develop their knowledge of human factors, there are training courses ranging from university postgraduate degree programmes to very short courses of 2 or 3 days, and introductory web-based tutorials. Many of the short courses in health care focus on raising awareness of non-technical skills based on the Crew Resource Management (CRM) training given in airlines and other safety-critical industries (see Section 2.4). The World Health Organization's patient safety course for medical students contains one module on human factors, and a number of medical schools are now introducing human factors and patient safety into their undergraduate programmes. It should be noted that an acquisition of human factors expertise will not be achieved by attending a single workshop or seminar. The application of human factors techniques by personnel who lack the appropriate training and experience may also be ineffective or lead to inappropriate interventions.

As indicated earlier, the term human factors refers to a wide-ranging subject applied to human–computer interaction, equipment design, effects of the work environment on human performance and many other topics. The non-technical skills component that focuses on the individual worker, usually in a team context, is only a small part of this field. In the following sections, we describe the following:

1. How non-technical skills were first identified in aviation
2. A behavioural rating system called NOTECHS that was developed to rate these skills from observing pilots at work
3. The migration of this approach into health care

2.3 EVOLUTION OF NON-TECHNICAL SKILLS

Although some surgeons have, quite appropriately, questioned the relevance of pilots' behaviour to operative surgery, it is important to acknowledge that the significance of non-technical skills was first appreciated in aviation. There are also surgeons, anaesthetists and other health care professionals from operating theatres who readily acknowledge the similarities of teamwork and decision-making processes faced in their work environment to those of a flight deck.[21] The time pressures of completing an operating list, status hierarchy within teams and challenges or distractions in communications in an operating theatre are familiar constraints experienced in these two environments. The comparisons made with the aviation industry to facilitate an understanding of the principles of systems safety and error causation have benefitted many clinicians. Although there are human factors lessons to be learnt from other domains, such as the military or nuclear power industry who also utilize this approach, it may be easier for clinicians to derive analogies from the aviation industry due to the degree of familiarity with air flight.[22] It is hence worth emphasizing that the science of human factors is not specialty or profession specific and lessons learned from high-risk industries that adopt this approach may have an educational role in improving surgical outcomes and are thus worthy of consideration.

We now explain how the aviation sector realized that technical skills alone did not guarantee safe flight and what was done to identify pilots' non-technical skills. The term 'non-technical skills' was adopted by the European civil aviation regulator in relation to airline pilots' behaviour on the flight deck. Behavioural rating systems, such as NOTECHS (see Section 2.5), were developed so that pilots' non-technical skills could be assessed for feedback during training or more formally for licensing.

2.4 NON-TECHNICAL SKILLS FOR PILOTS

In the 1970s, a series of major aviation accidents occurred that puzzled investigators: the planes were being flown by experienced crews and there had been no primary technical failures. Accident investigators began to look for other causal factors. In Europe, the seminal event was the Tenerife crash in 1977, in which two Boeing 747 jets collided on the Los Rodeos runway killing all 234 passengers and 14 crew on the KLM plane and 335 of 396 people on the Pan Am plane. Analysis of the accident revealed problems in communication with air traffic control, team co-ordination, decision making, fatigue and leadership behaviours.[23]

Around the same time, United Airlines experienced a sequence of accidents, again without primary technical failures: this pattern of what appeared to be 'pilot error' was now beginning to raise concern. In 1979, a National Aeronautics and Space Administration meeting for aviation psychologists and airline pilots discussed possible causes and solutions. One strong source of evidence came from the cockpit voice recorders which stored an audio recording* from the flight deck. Complementary research findings emerged from flight simulations which recreated accident precursor conditions and observed the pilots' behaviour. The data began to expose the human factors influencing pilots' decisions and actions.[24] These included the effects of a status hierarchy on the flight deck which discouraged co-pilots from speaking up and questioning captains' decisions. When they did make a challenge, they tended to do this with

* Since 2008, 2 hours are usually recorded.

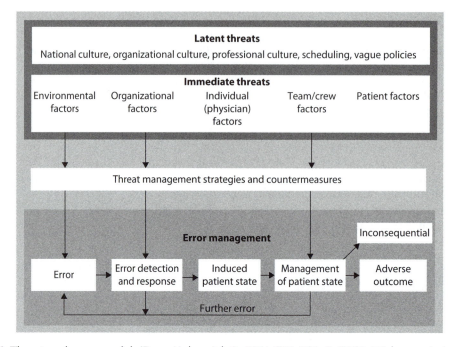

Figure 2.4 Threat and error model. (From Helmreich R, *BMJ*, 320, 781–5, 2000. With permission.)

insufficient assertiveness, using mitigated speech.[25] There were also deficiencies found in decision making and situation awareness. Sometimes, the captain's leadership was inappropriate for the situation or the crew did not co-ordinate their actions or communicate effectively as a team. The inability to adapt behaviour to cope with stress and fatigue was another factor.[26]

It was now clear that technical skills were not sufficient to ensure safe flight and that new training would need to be devised to ensure that pilots understood the importance of their cognitive and teamwork skills, as well as their flying skills. Research programmes were commissioned for aviation psychologists to study flight crews. This was to determine how pilots' behaviours contributed to safe and efficient flight operations or produced performances that were characterized by more errors and poorer decisions. Interviews with pilots and questionnaire surveys examined attitudes to safety, teamwork and personality variables. The analysis of accident investigations began to pay more attention to these human factors. Confidential incident reporting systems* enabled pilots to provide more

information on the precursors to unsafe situations. From these various sources, the pilots' non-technical skills for safe flight could be described. Using this evidence base, airlines designed special training to raise awareness of the importance of these skills, to provide the underpinning scientific knowledge and to give practice for skill development. These courses were initially called Cockpit Resource Management; they were subsequently renamed as Crew Resource Management (CRM) when cabin crews were involved. The UK civil aviation regulator defines CRM as 'a management system which makes optimum use of all available resources – equipment, procedures and people – to promote safety and enhance efficiency of flightdeck operations'.[27]

Although pilots had well-established principles of good airmanship, there was no explicit framework, so the critical behaviour patterns had been transmitted in an informal, inconsistent manner from one generation of pilots to the next. Perhaps not surprisingly, early CRM training courses were not always received well by airline or military pilots, especially if they were not perceived as being sufficiently relevant to flight operations. It quickly became apparent that the material and case examples in CRM training needed to be carefully

* See CORESS for UK surgeons (Confidential Reporting System for Surgery, www.coress.org.uk).

tailored to realistic task situations and challenges. The threat and error model devised by psychologist Bob Helmreich[10] effectively captured the realities of flight conditions and showed how these could lead to pilot error (Figure 2.4 shows this model adapted for health care). Threat and error management became part of many CRM courses and is still used today by a number of airlines.

In the United Kingdom, the Kegworth plane crash in 1989[28] (where British Midland pilots mistakenly shut off the working engine when the other engine was on fire) was such a strong demonstration that human error and teamwork failures could contribute to fatal accidents that the UK's Civil Aviation Authority took the view that CRM had to be introduced even though at the time there were only a few scientific studies on its effectiveness. By the 1990s, CRM training for pilots had been widely introduced in aviation, driven by national regulators and the influence of the International Civil Aviation Organization. Today, CRM training is mandatory in most countries, including the United Kingdom. CRM courses tend to consist of 2 to 3 days of basic CRM training, with some level of refresher training thereafter. There is also simulator training related to CRM where pilots can demonstrate their CRM skills in both routine and non-normal flight scenarios.[27] There are various books providing advice on designing CRM training for pilots[26,29,30]: These may have human factors content of interest to surgeons. Evaluation studies of CRM training[31] tend to show positive effects, although these tend to be for pilots' knowledge, attitudes or behaviours rather than outcome measures such as aircraft accidents, which are very uncommon.

2.5 NOTECHS: NON-TECHNICAL SKILLS FOR PILOTS

In this section, we describe how the airline industry began to develop methods of assessing pilots' non-technical (CRM) skills. Particular attention is given to the European NOTECHS tool, as its development method and design criteria were adapted for the development of the surgical NOTSS tool, as described in Chapter 3.

2.5.1 DESIGNING THE NOTECHS SYSTEM

In the United States, the regulator[32] allowed airlines to develop their own CRM training programmes; but the airlines also had to demonstrate their evaluation, e.g. by assessing crew performance. In Europe, the regulator was concerned as to whether CRM training was transferring onto the flight deck: 'the flight crew must be assessed on their CRM skills [. . .] to: provide feedback to the crew collectively and individually and serve to identify retraining; and be used to improve the CRM training system'.[33] This required a method for evaluating pilots' CRM/non-technical skills that could be applied across European airlines. In response, a research team of airline pilots and psychologists (from Germany, France, the Netherlands and the United Kingdom) was set up in 1996 to work on the NOTECHS (non-technical skills) project. They were asked to identify or develop a feasible, efficient method for assessing an individual pilot's non-technical (CRM) skills (not for assessing the crew as a whole).

A review of available behaviour-rating systems for pilots[34] showed that none was suitable for adoption or adaptation – the systems were too complex to be used across Europe, were too specific to a particular airline or rated crews rather than individual pilots. Therefore, a new one had to be designed. Airline captains with experience in behaviour-rating methods to assess pilots advised on the content and on practical requirements. The resulting NOTECHS system[35,36] had four categories, situation awareness, decision making, cooperation and leadership and managerial skills, each with component elements. Two points should be noted with respect to the system components. The category communication is featured in a number of rating systems but was not shown in NOTECHS as a separate category. This is because communication skills were inherent in all four categories, and almost all the listed behaviours involve communication. A category of 'personal awareness' skills (e.g. coping with stress or fatigue) was considered but rejected due to difficulties in observing, or inferring, except in the most extreme cases. Examples of observable behaviours (behavioural

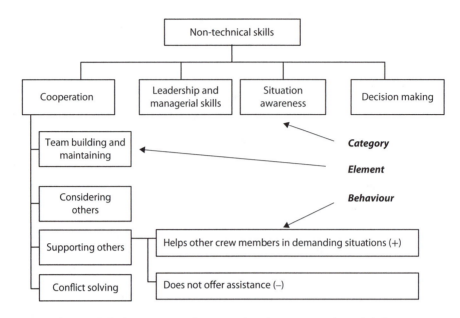

Figure 2.5 Non-Technical Skills for Surgeons framework (pilots' non-technical skills).

markers) illustrated good and poor performance on each element (Figure 2.5).

To ensure fairness and objectivity in NOTECHS ratings, a set of 'operational principles' was established,[36] and these are listed here because they were found to be relevant for the development of the NOTSS system for rating surgeons' non-technical skills (described in Chapter 3):

1. Only observable behaviour is to be assessed. The evaluation must exclude reference to a crew member's personality or emotional attitude and should be based only on observable behaviour. Behavioural markers were designed to support an objective judgement.
2. Need for technical consequence. For a pilot's non-technical skills to be rated as unacceptable, flight safety must be actually (or potentially) compromised. This requires a related objective technical consequence.
3. Acceptable or unacceptable rating required. The JAR-OPS (European aviation operational requirements) requires the airlines to indicate whether the observed non-technical skills are acceptable or unacceptable.
4. Repetition required. Repetition of unacceptable behaviour during the check must be observed to conclude that there is a significant problem. If, according to the JAR-paragraph concerned, the nature of a technical failure allows for a second attempt, this should be granted, regardless of the non-technical rating.
5. Explanation required. For each category rated as unacceptable, the examiner must: a) indicate the element (s) in that category where the unacceptable behaviour was observed; b) explain where the observed non-technical skills (potentially) led to safety consequences; and c) give a free-text explanation on each of the categories rated unacceptable, using standard phraseology.

Advice for users of the NOTECHS system was prepared and is shown in Box 2.1.

BOX 2.1: Advice for users of the NOTECHS system

It was acknowledged that this type of evaluation based on observing and judging a pilot's behaviours during in-flight task performance would, in general, be more subjective than judging technical performance data (e.g. speed or flap settings). The NOTECHS designers tried to produce a rating system that would minimize ambiguities in the evaluation of non-technical skills and emphasized that several considerations should be noted by system users,[35] which are as follows:

1. The first related to the unit of observation and measurement, that is, the NOTECHS system was designed to be used to assess individual pilots rather than a crew composed of a captain and a co-pilot. When rating an entire crew as a unit, it can be difficult to disentangle and rate the individual contributions to overall crew performance. It should be noted that the same issue already exists during operational and licensing checks when considering technical performance of pilots. The NOTECHS system did not solve this problem in some magical fashion; rather, the designers proposed that the system should assist the examiners to objectively point to behaviours that are related more to one crew member than the other, thus allowing them to differentiate their judgements of the two crew members.
2. A second factor related to the possible concern that raters might not be judging the pilots' non-technical skills on an appropriate basis. However, the NOTECHS system requires the instructor/examiner to justify the ratings and any associated criticisms at a professional level, and with a standardized vocabulary. Furthermore, the assessor's judgement of non-technical skills should not be based on a vague global impression or on an isolated behaviour or action. Therefore, it was advised that repetition of the behaviour during the flight is usually required to explicitly identify the nature of the problem reflected in the rating scores.

The NOTECHS method was essentially designed to help the examiner/instructor captains to look beyond technical failure during recurrent checks or training, and to help point out possible underlying deficiencies in non-technical competence. It was recommended that the evaluation of a pilot's non-technical skills using NOTECHS should not provoke a failed (not acceptable) rating without a related technical consequence, leading to compromised flight safety. Some airlines are now changing this so that a failure on non-technical skills alone will be possible. A NOTECHS assessment could provide useful insights into the deficiencies in non-technical skills (e.g. situation awareness) contributing to technical failure (e.g. an 'altitude bust'). Used in this way, the method could provide valuable assistance for debriefing and tailored retraining. The prototype NOTECHS system was designed for the assessment of a pilot's non-technical skills in the flight simulator or during flight operations.

2.5.2 TESTING THE NOTECHS SYSTEM

The testing of the basic usability and psychometric properties of the NOTECHS system was then conducted, along with an examination of the effects of national cultural differences within Europe. An experimental rating task was based on eight video scenarios filmed in a Boeing 757 simulator with airline pilots as the actors. The scenarios simulated flight situations with predefined behaviours (from the NOTECHS elements) exhibited by the pilots at varying standards. The pilots' behaviours were rated using the NOTECHS system by 105 instructors from 14 airlines across 12 European countries. Many of them had experience in using behavioural rating systems for pilot assessment, although they had not used the NOTECHS system. Each experimental session had a morning of briefing and practice on the NOTECHS method. In the afternoon, the instructors were asked to individually rate the captain's and the first officer's behaviours displayed in each scenario, using the NOTECHS score forms. The results indicated that the majority of the instructors were consistent in their ratings, there was an acceptable level of accuracy and they were very satisfied with the NOTECHS rating system.[37] Cultural differences (relating to five European regions) were found to be less significant than other biographical variables, for example, proficiency in English language, experience with non-technical skills evaluation and role perceptions of captain and first officer.[38] An operational trial of NOTECHS was run, with several airlines confirming the applicability and feasibility of the system in real check events for pilots.[39]

These tests showed that NOTECHS was usable by airline instructors and appeared to have acceptable psychometric properties. Users of NOTECHS are expected to be certified flight instructors and authorized examiners. Their recommended training period with NOTECHS is 2 full days or longer (depending on the level of previous experience in rating pilots' non-technical skills). In most countries, there are competence standards for CRM instructors and examiners.[40] Airline pilots already have some knowledge of relevant psychological concepts (e.g. human memory) from their examination on human performance and limitations, which is a licensing requirement.[41] It was recommended that most of the training should be devoted to building an understanding of the NOTECHS method, the specific use of the rating form, the calibration process of judgment, and the debriefing phase. In debriefing, an emphasis is placed on skill components rather than on more 'global' analyses of performance, as the tool was designed for feedback and identification of training needs.

In summary, NOTECHS was primarily designed as a practical tool for instructors and examiners, although it has also been used in research studies.[42-44] It was written in professional aviation language to assist in debriefing and communicating clear advice for improvements. Several European airlines (KLM, Lufthansa and Alitalia) developed their own rating systems, some of which made use of the NOTECHS framework in their design, whereas other airlines initially used NOTECHS, or adapted versions of it as part of proficiency evaluation (Finnair, Eastern Airways, Gulf Air and

Flight AF447 crashed into the Atlantic Ocean in June 2009, killing all 288 passengers. It is now known that it experienced a series of events relating to both technical and non-technical factors.[46,47] As described in the Swiss cheese model, shown in Section 2.2.1, it was not a single error but rather a series of multiple errors that resulted in this catastrophic incident during what is described as the safest period in flying, the cruising phase. The tragic chain of events began with the captain's decision to fly through a storm (when other pilots flying on the same route decided to avoid it). He left the cockpit (2 hours into the flight) to take a nap, leaving the two co-pilots in control. Commercial pilots are not permitted to fly more than 8 or 9 hours, depending on the start time of the pilot's flight duty period.[48] The less experienced co-pilot was told by the captain to fly the aircraft.

The instrument that monitors airspeed then froze due to a combination of weather and technical issues that were waiting to be addressed in the coming days. This resulted in a faulty airspeed gauge causing the autopilot to disengage. The 'startle effect' (physiological and emotional response to a surprising/threatening event) that affected the crew is highlighted in transcripts of the flight recorder. In a clearly stressful period, the wrong manoeuvre was then carried out by one of the co-pilots. The plane started to stall, resulting in alarms being set off. The dynamics and interaction between the crew that ensued pointed to a breakdown in communication, loss of situation awareness and a lack of leadership. These events occurred despite everyone in that cockpit having received CRM training. New research is under way to study startle effects in pilots and how these may be overcome[49] so that this may be incorporated in CRM training.

Iberia). In the United Kingdom, mandatory regulations from the Civil Aviation Authority require a formal incorporation of non-technical (CRM)

skills into all levels of training and checking of flight crew members' performance.

Although the airline industry places considerable reliance on CRM training and for European air operators the regulator is issuing new CRM guidance,[45] there are still occasional accidents in which CRM skills have not been adequately employed. The findings from the investigation into the loss of Air France flight 447 teach us that errors can still occur in ultra-safe industries and that CRM and human factors training is not a finite process but one that has to be continually adapted to meet current challenges.

The CRM approach to identify and train non-technical skills has now been adopted in other industrial sectors, and we give a brief description of this in Section 2.6 before discussing its applications in health care in Section 2.7.

2.6 NON-TECHNICAL SKILLS IN OTHER INDUSTRIES

As the aviation CRM training became established on an international basis, trainers in other high-risk work settings, such as the nuclear power industry, military and merchant navy, began to look at the non-technical skills required in their own operational settings. Accident analyses started to consider the behaviour patterns of frontline operators and how they were being affected by work conditions and organizational culture. By the late 1990s, CRM training was being introduced in other sectors, most notably the nuclear power industry and maritime companies.[26,50] Competence assurance systems for safety-critical personnel, such as nuclear power plant control room operators, began to include, in some countries, evaluation of their non-technical skills as a key component of licensing and revalidation.[51] The energy sector, following recent major accidents such as the *Deepwater Horizon* blowout, has recently issued guidance advising the introduction of CRM training both in general[52] and more specifically for hydrocarbon wells operations.[53] The mining and rail industries use CRM training, as do the emergency services.[54]

2.7 NON-TECHNICAL SKILLS IN HEALTH CARE

In contrast to the focus on non-technical skills in aviation and other industries, as described earlier, very little attention had traditionally been paid in medical or nursing education to human error, human performance limitations or the behavioural components of safe medical practice. It is understandable that a single air disaster will inevitably result in massive media coverage and expected horror from the general public. But, as discussed in Chapter 1, a significant level of morbidity and mortality in health care is deemed preventable but still does not always get the attention it deserves. As we have explained, the increasing awareness of the science of human factors and of non-technical skills within health care has stimulated greater reflection on the methods employed to identify, report, analyse, learn and understand adverse outcome in surgery and medical specialties.[55,56] The traditional view that individual clinicians are solely responsible for adverse outcomes is rightly being challenged. The human, organizational and technical reasons behind health-care professionals becoming involved in adverse outcomes are better identified through human factor analysis. This ensures that appropriate measures are taken to protect patient safety rather than approaching adverse outcomes with a simplistic view of individual failure. This by no means translates to creating an environment without individual accountability or responsibility but rather builds a better understanding of adverse outcomes ensuring that a healthy, responsible relationship exists between the individual, systems and organization as a whole to provide the best outcome for every patient. Non-technical skills can have a direct, indirect or cumulative effect on outcome.

The initial interest in a non-technical skills approach for health care professionals came from the anaesthesiologists when they began to develop clinical simulators for anaesthetic training. Although they knew that non-technical skills such as situation awareness, decision making and teamwork influenced outcomes, they did not have any suitable taxonomies or behavioural rating systems for training and assessing these skills. In Scotland, a team of anaesthetists and psychologists worked together to undertake the necessary task analysis to develop a new framework on anaesthetists' non-technical skills, called Anaesthetists' Non-Technical Skills (ANTS).[57] This tool and its development are described in Appendix 2A, along with information on related non-technical skills tools for scrub practitioners (SPLINTS)[58] and anaesthetic practitioners (ANTS-AP).[59]

Following the release of ANTS, a number of systems have been devised using similar methods of task analysis for other health-care professionals, such as emergency physicians[60] and junior doctors.[61] In the last decade, CRM or non-technical skills training courses have been developed for health care practitioners,[62,63] and these are discussed in relation to surgery in Chapters 6 and 9.

2.8 SUMMARY

Human factors science provides a set of theories, methods and tools for understanding and enhancing human performance in the workplace. Analysis of major accidents in aviation, which included a human factors investigation, revealed the importance of non-technical skills. It was recognized that technical competence alone would not guarantee efficient and safe flight operations, and so pilots' non-technical skills were identified, trained and assessed. This approach has now been adopted in other safety-critical industries and in health care. Chapter 3 describes the development of a non-technical skills framework for surgeons, with particular reference to the NOTSS tool.

APPENDIX 2A NON-TECHNICAL SKILLS FRAMEWORKS FOR ANAESTHETISTS, SCRUB PRACTITIONERS AND ANAESTHETIC ASSISTANTS

2A.1 ANAESTHETISTS' NON-TECHNICAL SKILLS

Anaesthesiologists in the United States became aware of aviation Crew Resource Management (CRM) training and immediately appreciated its significance in their own work; for instance, an anaesthetic crisis resource management course was devised as part of a simulation-centre training programme.[64] With the introduction of higher fidelity simulation facilities for anaesthetists, clinical trainers realized that they needed to have methods for measuring anaesthetists' non-technical skills (e.g. decision making or teamwork), in addition to their technical performance.

In 1998, a team of anaesthetists and psychologists (who had worked on the aviation non-technical skills for pilots [NOTECHS] studies) began a project to design an Anaesthetists' Non-Technical Skills (ANTS) system (Figure 2A.1a). The skill set was derived from data on anaesthetists' behaviour gathered from a literature review, observations, interviews, surveys and incident analysis.[65–67] The ANTS rating tool was formulated

to meet a set of design criteria, similar to those of NOTECHS, such as suitability for practical use in the operating theatre or a simulation setting. (For detailed reports and papers, see http://www.abdn.ac.uk/iprc/ants.)

The resulting ANTS skills framework (Figure 2A.1b) has four categories: situation awareness, decision making, task management and teamworking, with component elements and examples of good and poor behaviours for each element.

Managing stress and coping with fatigue were not included as explicit categories in ANTS due to the difficulty of judging these states, which can be concealed unless extreme; moreover, they influence other behaviours that can be rated. However, it was advised that the skills to cope with fatigue and stress should be covered in a CRM/non-technical skills course for anaesthetists. Leadership was not set as a separate category but incorporated into teamworking, because there are times where the anaesthetist may lead the theatre team. A four-point scale for ANTS was devised for rating observed behaviours with respect to the

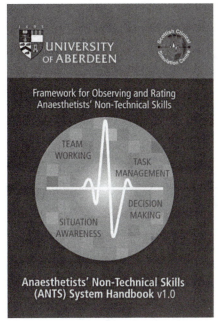

(a)

Categories	Elements
Task management	– Planning and preparing – Prioritizing – Providing and maintaining standards – Identifying and utilising resources
Teamworking	– Co-ordinating activities with team members – Exchanging information – Using authority and assertiveness – Assessing capabilities – Supporting others
Situation awareness	– Gathering information – Recognizing and understanding – Anticipating
Decision making	– Identifying options – Balancing risks and selecting options – Re-evaluating

e.g. behavioural markers for good practice

– Confirms roles and responsibilities of team members

– Discusses case with surgeons or colleagues

– Considers requirements of others before acting

– Cooperates with others to achieve goals

e.g. behavioural markers for poor practice

– Reduces level of monitoring because of distractions

– Responds to individual cues without confirmation

– Does not alter physical layout of workspace to improve data visibility

– Does not ask questions to orient self to situation during hand over

(b)

Figure 2A.1 Anaesthetists' non-technical skills **(a)** handbook and **(b)** framework. (**[a]** Courtesy of the University of Aberdeen.)

elements and categories. The descriptors on the rating scale not only are performance levels but also emphasized their relevance for patient safety. The ANTS ratings can be made where anaesthesia is being delivered, normally in the operating room or anaesthetic room (or in simulator facilities). The tool was designed to be used by experienced anaesthetists to rate the non-technical skills of another anaesthetist who has achieved basic technical competence.

An evaluation of the ANTS behaviour-rating method was undertaken with 50 consultant anaesthetists in Scotland, who were given 4 hours of training on the system and subsequently rated the non-technical skills of consultant anaesthetists in eight videotaped scenarios. Although the amount of training was minimal, the levels of rater accuracy were acceptable and inter-rater reliability approached an acceptable level.[68] The raters had experience in giving feedback on technical skills but had no previous experience of behaviour rating and were given only introductory training in the ANTS system. Therefore, given their limited familiarity and practice with the system, it was concluded that these findings were sufficient to move on to usability trials. The first measures of usability and acceptability from consultants and trainees were promising, and so the system was released in 2004 and made available free of charge via the website to anaesthetists for non-commercial use. See the study by Flin et al.[69] for details on how ANTS has been used in practice in hospital anaesthetic departments, as well as in simulation centres.[70] It has been translated into a number of other languages (see the ANTS website given earlier for details).

2A.2 SCRUB PRACTITIONERS' INTRA-OPERATIVE LIST OF NON-TECHNICAL SKILLS

To develop a non-technical skills rating system for the scrub practitioner, a multidisciplinary team of perioperative practitioners, psychologists, and a consultant surgeon conducted a similar set of task analyses as used for ANTS: reviewing the literature, interviewing scrub practitioners and surgeons and conducting observations in the operating room.[71,72] Panels of experienced scrub practitioners refined the skill list to produce the Scrub Practitioners' List of Intraoperative Non-Technical Skills (SPLINTS) taxonomy.[73] This prototype contained three skill categories, each with three underlying elements, and the panels also provided examples of good and poor behaviours to assist users of the SPLINTS system (see Table 2A.1).

A handbook (Figure 2A.2) was produced to help scrub practitioners use the system in practice and to assess non-technical performance in the operating theatre. The rating scale for the SPLINTS system was the same as that for ANTS: 1 = poor, 2 = marginal, 3 = acceptable, 4 = good and NR = not required (for occasions where that skill was not necessary).

To test the reliability and sensitivity of the SPLINTS system, experienced scrub practitioners ($n = 34$) attended a session consisting of a 4-hour training and testing workshop covering background regarding human factors and non-technical skills, as well as instruction on the SPLINTS rating method. Participants then rated the performance of the scrub practitioner from videotapes of simulated surgical scenarios (e.g. a swab/sponge is missing from a count or organizing equipment when a laparoscopic case has to be converted to an open procedure). The scenarios were designed to show the full range of behaviours that were to be scored using the four-point scale.

Acceptable inter-rater agreement[74] was achieved and, given the short training time, this was encouraging. The practitioners felt the SPLINTS system contained the essential skills and was a potentially usable tool for the operating room. The system has been tried out in a number of hospitals in the United Kingdom and beyond and has been translated into Japanese. Details of SPLINTS and related papers can be found at www.abdn.ac.uk/iprc/splints.

2A.3 ANAESTHETIC PRACTITIONERS' NON-TECHNICAL SKILLS

A new tool, ANTS-AP, has been developed for the assessment of anaesthetic practitioners, such as nurses and operating department

Table 2A.1 SPLINTS skill categories, elements and behavioural examples for good (✓) and poor (×) performance

Category	Element	Behavioural examples
Situation awareness	Gathering information	✓ Watches surgical procedure × Fixates on one task
	Recognizing and understanding information	✓ Reacts to conversational cues exchanged between other team members × Does not change own activity level when appropriate
	Anticipating	✓ Times requests appropriately × Asks for items late
Communication and teamwork	Acting assertively	✓ Gives clear instructions/requests to team members × Fails or is slow to communicate requirements
	Exchanging information	✓ Uses non-verbal signals where appropriate × Fails to articulate problems in a timely manner
	Co-ordinating with others	✓ Deals appropriately with interruptions from others × Ignores requests of others
Task management	Planning and preparing	✓ Organizes equipment × Opens sterile equipment/supplies indiscriminately
	Providing and maintaining standards	✓ Protects sterile field and instrumentation × Fails to check equipment settings/relies on others to do so
	Coping with pressure	✓ Does not rise to others' emotional outbursts × Raises voice unnecessarily

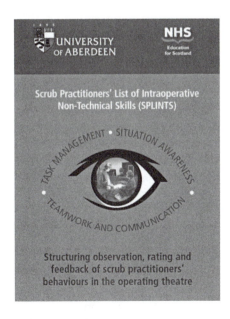

Figure 2A.2 Scrub Practitioners' List of Intraoperative Non-Technical Skills (SPLINTS) handbook. (Courtesy of the University of Aberdeen.)

practitioners, who assist the anaesthetist. This was designed using similar forms of task analysis[75,76] and evaluated[77] using the same methods as ANTS and SPLINTS. Details can be found on the website www.abdn.ac.uk/iprc/ants-ap. A similar system has recently been developed in Denmark for nurse anaesthetists.[78]

HUMAN FACTORS WEBSITES

Clinical Human Factors Group: www.chfg.org.
Eurocontrol (European air traffic control): www.eurocontol.int/humanfactors.
Health and Safety Executive: www.hse.gov.uk/humanfactors.
Human Factors and Ergonomics Society (United States): www.hfes.org.
Institute for Ergonomics and Human Factors (United Kingdom): www.ergonomics.org.uk.

REFERENCES

1. Flin R. Non-technical skills: Enhancing safety in operating theatres (and drilling rigs). *J Perioper Pract.* 2014;24:58–60.
2. Roberts R, Flin R, Cleland J. Staying in the zone. Offshore drillers' situation awareness. *Human Factors.* 2015;57:573–590.
3. Cullen D. *The Public Inquiry into the Piper Alpha Disaster (Cm 1310).* London, United Kingdom: HMSO; 1990.
4. Hetherington C, Flin R, Mearns K. Safety at sea. Human factors in shipping. *J Safety Res.* 2006;37:401–11.
5. Schroder-Hinrichs J, Hollnagel E. From Titanic to Costa Concordia – a century of lessons not learned. *JoMA.* 2012;11:151–67.
6. HSE. *Reducing Error and Influencing Behaviour.* London, United Kingdom: HSE Books; 1999. p. 2.
7. Bromiley M. Have you ever made a mistake? *RCoA Bulletin.* 2008;48:2242–5.
8. NHS England. *Human Factors in Healthcare. A Concordat from the National Quality Board.* 2013. [Accessed September 15, 2014.] Available from: www.england.nhs.uk.
9. Carayon P. (Ed.). *Handbook of Human Factors and Ergonomics in Healthcare and Patient Safety* (2nd ed). New York: CRC Press; 2011.
10. Helmreich R. On error management: Lessons from aviation. *BMJ.* 2000;320:781–5.
11. Reason J. *Human Error.* Cambridge, United Kingdom: Cambridge University Press; 1990.
12. Moray N. Culture, politics and ergonomics. *Ergonomics.* 2000;43:868–88.
13. Flin R, Winter J, Sarac C, Raduma M. *Human Factors and Patient Safety. Review of Topics and Tools.* Report of WHO/IER/PSP/2009.05. Geneva, Switzerland: World Health Organization; 2009. [Accessed April 13, 2015.] Available from: www.abdn.ac.uk/iprc.
14. Carthey J, Clarke J. *Implementing Human Factors in Healthcare. 'How to' Guide.* 2010. [Accessed April 13, 2015.] Available from: www.patientsafetyfirst.nhs.uk.
15. Flin R, Fioratou E, Frerk C, Trotter C, Cook T. Human factors in the development of complications of airway management: Preliminary evaluation of an interview tool. *Anaesthesia.* 2013;68:817–25.
16. Taylor-Adams S, Vincent C, Stanhope N. Applying human factors methods to the investigation and analysis of clinical adverse events. *Safety Sci.* 1999;31:143–59.
17. Reason J. Human error. Models and management. *BMJ.* 2000;320:768–70.
18. Reason J. *Managing the Risks of Organizational Accidents.* Aldershot, United Kingdom: Ashgate; 1997.
19. Helmreich R, Klinect J, Wilhelm J. Managing threat and error: Data from line operations. In G. Edkins, P. Pfister (Eds.). *Innovation and Consolidation in Aviation.* Aldershot, United Kingdom: Ashgate; 2003.
20. Reason J. *The Human Contribution. Unsafe Acts, Accidents and Heroic Recoveries.* Aldershot, United Kingdom: Ashgate; 2008.
21. Hugh T. New strategies to prevent laparoscopic bile duct injury – surgeons can learn from pilots. *Surgery.* 2002;132:826–35.
22. Catchpole K. Spreading human factors expertise in health care: Untangling the knots in people and systems. *BMJ Qual Saf.* 2013;22:793–7.
23. Weick K. The vulnerable system: An analysis of the Tenerife air disaster. In P. Frost, L. Moore, M. Louis, C. Lundberg (Eds.). *Reframing Organizational Culture.* London, United Kingdom: Sage; 1991.
24. Beaty D. *The Naked Pilot: The Human Factor in Aircraft Accidents.* Marlborough, United Kingdom: Airlife; 1995.
25. Fischer U, Orasanu J. 'Say it again, Sam!' Effective communication strategies to mitigate pilot error. In Jensen R, *Proceedings of the 10th International Symposium on Aviation Psychology.* Columbus, Ohio; May 1999.
26. Kanki B, Anca J, Helmreich R. (Eds.). *Crew Resource Management* (2nd ed). San Diego, California: Academic Press; 2010.
27. CAA. *Flight-Crew Human Factors Handbook.* CAP 737. Gatwick, United Kingdom: Civil Aviation Authority; 2014. Available from: www.caa .co.uk. p. 1.
28. AAIB. *Aircraft Accident Report 4/10 Report on the Accident to Boeing 737-400*

G-OBME Near Kegworth, Leicestershire on 8 January 1989. Farnborough, England: Air Accident Investigation Branch; 1989.

29. Jensen R. *Pilot Judgment and Crew Resource Management*. Aldershot, United Kingdom: Ashgate; 1995.

30. Macleod N. *Building Safe Systems in Aviation. A CRM Developers Handbook*. Aldershot, United Kingdom: Ashgate; 2005.

31. Salas E, Wilson K, Burke C, Wightman D, Howse W. Crew resource management training research and practice: A review, lessons learned and needs. In R. Williges (Ed.). *Review of Human Factors and Ergonomics*, Volume 2. Santa Monica, California: Human Factors and Ergonomics Society; 2006.

32. FAA. *Advisory Circular 120-54A. Advanced Qualification Program*. Washington: Federal Aviation Administration; 2006.

33. Joint Aviation Authorities. JAR OPS 1.940, 1.945, 1.955, and 1.965. Hoofdorp, The Netherlands: Joint Aviation Authorities; 2001.

34. Flin R, Martin L. Behavioural markers for Crew Resource Management: A review of current practice. *Int J Aviat Psychol*. 2001;11:95–118.

35. Avermaete J, Kruijsen E (Eds.). *NOTECHS. The Evaluation of Nontechnical Skills of Multi-Pilot Aircrew in Relation to the JAR-FCL Requirements*. Final report NLR-CR-98443. Amsterdam, the Netherlands: National Aerospace Laboratory (NLR); 1998.

36. Flin R, Martin L, Goeters K, Hoermann J, Amalberti R, Valot C et al. Development of the NOTECHS (Non-Technical Skills) system for assessing pilots' CRM skills. *Human Factors and Aerospace Safety*. 2003;3:95–117.

37. O'Connor P, Hormann H-J, Flin R, Lodge M, Goeters K-M, JARTEL group. Developing a method for evaluating crew resource management skills: A European perspective. *Int J Aviat Psychol*. 2002;12:265–88.

38. Hörmann J. Cultural variations of perceptions of crew behaviour in multi-pilot aircraft. *Le Travail Humain* (Human Work). 2001;64:247–68.

39. Andlauer E, JARTEL group. *Joint Aviation Requirements – Translation and Elaboration*. JARTEL Project Report to DG-TREN European Commission. Paris, France: Sofreavia; 2001.

40. CAA. *The Crew Resource Management Instructor (CRMI) and Crew Resource Management Instructor Examiner (CRMIE) Accreditation Framework*. Standards Doc. 29. Version 5. Gatwick, United Kingdom: Civil Aviation Authority; 2013.

41. Campbell R, Bagshaw M. *Human Performance and Limitations in Aviation* (3rd ed). Oxford, United Kingdom: Blackwell; 2002.

42. Goeters K-M. Evaluation of the effects of CRM training by the assessment of non-technical skills under LOFT. *Human Factors and Aerospace Safety*. 2012;2:71–86.

43. Hausler R, Klampfer B, Amacher A, Naef W. Behavioural markers in analysing team performance of cockpit crews. In R. Dietrich, T. Childress (Eds.). *Group Interaction in High Risk Environments*. Aldershot, United Kingdom: Ashgate; 2004.

44. Thomas M. Predictors of threat and error management: Identification of core non-technical skills and implications for training systems design. *Int J Aviat Psychol*. 2004;14:207–31.

45. EASA. *Notice of Proposed Amendment: Crew Resource Management*. NPA 2014–17. Cologne, Germany: European Aviation Safety Agency; 2014. [Accessed April 13, 2015.] Available from: www.easa.europa.eu.

46. BEA. *Final Report. Flight AF 447 on 1st June 2009 A330-203*. Paris, France: Bureau d'enquetes et d'analyses pour la securite d'aviation civile; 2012.

47. Bhangu A, Bhangu S, Stevenson J, Bowley D. Lessons for surgeons in the final moments of Air France flight 447. *World J Surg*. 2013;37:1185–92.

48. Federal Aviation Administration. 14 CFR Parts 117, 119, and 121. Docket No.: FAA-2009-1093; Amdt. Nos. 117-1, 119-16, 121-357. RIN 2120–AJ58. Flight Crew Member Duty and Rest Requirements. 2009.

[Accessed April 13, 2015.] Available from: http://www.faa.gov/regulations.

49. Martin W, Murray P, Bates P. Startle, freeze and denial: An analysis of pathological pilot reactions during unexpected events. In *Proceedings of the 65th International Air Safety Seminar*. Washington: Flight Safety Foundation; 2012.

50. Flin R, O'Connor P, Mearns K. Crew Resource Management: Improving teamwork in high reliability industries. *Team Perform Manag*. 2002;8:68–78.

51. Flin R. *Safe in Their Hands? Licensing and Competence Assurance for Safety-Critical Roles in High Risk Industries*. Report for the Department of Health, London. Aberdeen, United Kingdom: University of Aberdeen; 2008. Available from: www.abdn.ac.uk/iprc.

52. Energy Institute. *Crew Resource Management for the Energy Industries*. London, United Kingdom: Energy Institute; 2014. Available from: www.energyinstitute.org.

53. OGP. *Wells Operations Crew Resource Management. Report 501*. London, United Kingdom: Oil and Gas Producers; 2014. Available from: www.ogp.org.

54. Okray R, Lubnau T. *Crew Resource Management for the Fire Service*. Tulsa, Oklahoma: PennWell; 2004.

55. Szekendi M, Barnard C, Creamer, J, Noskin, G. Using patient safety morbidity and mortality conferences to promote transparency and a culture of safety. *Jt Comm J Qual Patient Saf*. 2010;36:3–9.

56. Russ A, Fairbanks R, Karsh B, Militello L, Saleem J, Wears R. The science of human factors: Separating fact from fiction. *BMJ Qual Saf Health Care*. 2013;22:11 964–966.

57. Fletcher G, Flin R, McGeorge P, Glavin R, Maran N, Patey R. Anaesthetists' Non-Technical Skills (ANTS). Evaluation of a behavioural marker system. *Brit J Anaesth*. 2003;90:580–8.

58. Mitchell L, Flin R, Yule S, Mitchell J, Coutts K, Youngson G. Evaluation of the Scrub Practitioners' List of Intraoperative Non-Technical Skills (SPLINTS) system. *Int J Nurs Stud*. 2012;49:201–11.

59. Rutherford J, Flin R, Mitchell L. Attitudes to teamwork and safety in anaesthetic assistants. *Brit J Anaesth*. 2012;109:21–6.

60. Flowerdew L, Brown R, Vincent C, Woloshynowych M. Development and validation of a tool to assess emergency physicians' nontechnical skills. *Ann Emerg Med*. 2012;59:376–85.

61. Mellanby E, Hume M, Glavin R, Skinner J, Maran N. Non-technical skills for junior doctors in acute care. *Postgrad Med J*. (in press).

62. Musson D, Helmreich R. Team training and resource management in health care: Current issues and future directions. *Harvard Health Policy Rev*. 2004;5:25–35.

63. Van Noord I, Bruijne M, Twisk J, van Dyck C, Wagner C. More explicit communication after classroom-based crew resource management training: Results of a pragmatic trial. *J Eval Clin Pract*. 2015;21:137–144.

64. Gaba D, Howard S, Flanagan B, Smith B, Fish K, Botney R. Assessment of clinical performance during simulated crises using both technical and behavioural ratings. *Anesthesiology*. 1998;89:8–18.

65. Fletcher G, McGeorge P, Flin R, Glavin R, Maran N. The role of non-technical skills in anaesthesia: A review of current literature. *Brit J Anaesth*. 2002;88:418–29.

66. Flin R, Fletcher G, McGeorge P, Sutherland A, Patey R. Anaesthetists' attitudes to teamwork and safety. *Anaesthesia*. 2003;58:233–42.

67. Fletcher G, Flin R, McGeorge P, Glavin R, Maran N, Patey R. Development of a prototype behavioural marker system for anaesthetists' non-technical skills. *Cogn Technol Work*. 2004;6:165–71.

68. Fletcher G, McGeorge P, Flin R, Glavin R, Maran N. Anaesthetists' non-technical skills (ANTS). Evaluation of a behavioural marker system. *Brit J Anaesth*. 2003;90:580–8.

69. Flin R, Glavin R, Patey R, Maran N. Anaesthetists' non-technical skills. *Brit J Anaesth*. 2010;105: 38–44.

70. Graham J, Hocking G, Giles E. Anaesthesia non-technical skills: Can anaesthetists be

trained to reliably use this behavioural marker system in 1 day? *Brit J Anaesth.* 2010;104:440–5.

71. Mitchell L, Flin R. Non-technical skills of the operating theatre scrub nurse: Literature review. *J Adv Nurs.* 2008;63:15–24.

72. Mitchell L, Flin R, Mitchell J, Coutts K, Youngson G. Thinking ahead of the surgeon. An interview study to identify scrub nurses' non-technical skills. *Int J Nurs Stud.* 2011;48:818–28.

73. Mitchell L, Flin R, Yule S, Mitchell J, Coutts K, Youngson G. Developing the Scrub Practitioners' List of Intraoperative Non-Technical Skills (SPLINTS) system. *J Eval Clin Pract.* 2013;19:317–23.

74. Mitchell L, Flin R, Mitchell J, Coutts K, Youngson G. Evaluation of the Scrub Practitioners' List of Intraoperative Non-Technical Skills (SPLINTS) system. *Int J Nurs Stud.* 2012;49:201–11.

75. Rutherford J, Flin R, Mitchell L. Anaesthetic assistants' non-technical skills. A literature review. *Brit J Anaesth.* 2012;109:27–31.

76. Rutherford J, Flin R, Mitchell L. Attitudes to teamwork and safety in anaesthetic assistants. *Brit J Anaesth.* 2012;109:21–6.

77. Rutherford J, Flin R, Irwin A, McFadyen A. 2015 (in press) The evaluation of the ANTS-AP behaviour rating system to assess the non-technical skills used by anaesthetic nurses and ODPs. *Anaesthesia.*

78. Lyk-Jensen H, Jepsen R, Spananger L, Dieckmann P, Ostergaard D. Assessing nurse anaesthetists' non-technical skills in the operating room. *Acta Anaesthesiol Scand.* 2014;58:794–801.

Non-technical skills for surgeons: The NOTSS behaviour marker system

STEVEN YULE AND DOUGLAS S SMINK

3.1 OVERVIEW

This chapter presents the rationale for non-technical skills in surgery and outlines the approach used to design, test and implement the Non-Technical Skills for Surgeons (NOTSS) system. It is also intended as a review of the state of the art of over 10 years of development, research and implementation science around NOTSS. A brief introduction to each of the four categories (situation awareness, decision making, communication and teamwork and leadership) is made along with illustrative observations of behaviour from the operating room. Since the original NOTSS tool was released in May 2006, it has been adopted and adapted by research groups and national associations in several countries around the world.

In this chapter, a broad spectrum of these initiatives is examined, with descriptions of the current state of NOTSS implementation in Europe, North America, Asia, Africa and Australasia.

3.1.1 BACKGROUND

An estimated 10% of hospitalized patients in high-income countries experience an unintended injury or complication not caused by the patient's underlying disease process.[1,2] Surgical patients are at highest risk of suffering in this way,[3] and more than half of these surgical adverse events are preventable.[4] Furthermore, the literature on intraoperative surgical error and complications shows that non-technical aspects of performance, such as diagnostic failure[5] or breakdowns in teamwork and information sharing,[6] lead to a higher risk of major complication or death. These 'non-technical skills'[7] are essential for safe and effective surgery for patients and form the basis of long and successful surgical careers. As we will see throughout this book, deliberate practice either individually or in teams can enhance behaviour. Much of this is simulation based (see Chapter 9). In fact, the American Heart Association recently stated that 'scenario training can successfully assess and train surgical staff in non-technical skills and integration of those skills with already known technical skills'[8] in a paper highlighting strategies to improve patient safety in the cardiac operating room.[9] Several non-technical skills were listed in the 'Top Ten Things to Know', aimed at surgeons, researchers, educators and policy-holders – stakeholders who have influence on the state of safety in the operating room. Although surgical educators have focused on Accreditation Council for Graduate Medical Education (ACGME) core competencies such as professionalism and interpersonal and communication skills for more than a decade, this focus has been largely outside the operating room (see Section IV.A.5 of ACGME 'Program Requirements for Graduate Medical Education in General Surgery'[10]). Despite the importance of non-technical skills in the operating room, most instruction to date has focused on technical skill. Recent interventions to introduce non-technical skills education in surgery, either as stand-alone modules[11] or integrated with technical skills training, have driven a need for valid and reliable tools to assess these skills, identify training needs and evaluate the impact of learning on subsequent behaviour. One leader in implementing non-technical skills is the Royal College of Surgeons in Ireland who has developed and runs a successful human factors and patient safety programme for all surgical trainees in the country.[12] This comprises modules on basic surgical training and non-technical skills.

Other high-risk industries, especially aviation and energy sectors, have responded to similar challenges by developing behaviour assessment tools to integrate assessment of non-technical skills as part of professional culture, requiring trainees to demonstrate competence in these skills before they commence front-line work. There is a growing realization that reducing the burden of operative complications for surgical patients below current levels is multifaceted and will not occur by solely relying on surgeons' technical skill. In fact, many of the influences on surgical outcomes are outside the control of the surgeon in the intraoperative phase and may be referred to as organizational or system factors.[13,14] Although novel surgical techniques or other treatments will continue to evolve as surgeons innovate, the greatest magnitude of impact that is available is in surgeons' non-technical skills: how they gather and use information, leverage the shared experience in the operating room at critical moments, galvanize team members to act and inspire others to question and speak up when they feel something is not right.

One of the challenges is that the underpinning knowledge of non-technical skills was largely absent from the training of the majority of board-certified surgeons operating today. This knowledge is required early in medical and surgical careers, to complement the acquisition of technical skills and medical knowledge. To become a proficient surgeon and ready for graduation from training into independent practice, many surgeons reflect on their management of the operating room and seek out ways to deliberately practice and improve these non-technical skills. Valid and reliable assessment of non-technical skills is required throughout training to facilitate learning. It is against this backdrop that the NOTSS[15] behaviour assessment tool for surgery was proposed in 2002, with development process initially focusing on the approaches and methods used by other high-risk industries that already used such tools to structure learning and evaluation of non-technical skills at work. Behaviour rating systems provide a language and framework for surgeons and surgical teams to reflect on performance in the operating room and support safe practices. Several other surgery-specific behaviour rating systems now exist, such as Observational Teamwork Assessment for Surgery (OTAS)[16] and Oxford-NOTECHS.[17] This chapter focuses on the development, testing, implementation and adaption of the NOTSS system.

3.1.2 APPROACHES IN HIGH-RISK INDUSTRY

As described in Chapter 2, analyses of adverse events and incidents in other high-risk industries, such as civil aviation, offshore oil exploration and nuclear power generation, have resulted in the development of non-technical skills training. This is more commonly called 'Crew Resource Management' training,[18] and behaviour rating systems have been developed specifically for different professional groups to assess these non-technical skills in a formal and explicit manner. These behaviour rating tools can be placed in the basket of 'workplace assessment tools', more commonly used to evaluate performance of professionals on the job, identify learning gaps, focus on training needs and provide feedback for continual improvement. One such example is the NOTECHS (non-technical skills for pilots) system,[19] which is used to observe and rate pilots' behaviour in the cockpit during both simulated flight and real flight. NOTECHS is a hierarchical system, comprising categories and elements of non-technical skills (see Chapter 2), and is one example of a behaviour rating tool to assess non-technical skills of civil aviation pilots in European airlines. This has also been adapted in a 'top down' manner for assessing surgical teams by at least three groups.[20–22] Although there is continuing debate about the relevance of adopting methods of aviation safety to improve health care safety,[23,24] a different approach is to develop specific behaviour rating systems for use in the operating room

('by surgeons for surgeons'). This takes more time to design but allows explicit focus on the skills judged to be relevant for the profession from a 'bottom up' perspective.

These behavioural rating systems are synonymously referred to as 'behaviour marker systems' and 'behaviour assessment tools'; they are methods to observe, categorize and rate identified behaviours that contribute to superior or substandard performance based on a taxonomy of skills. A taxonomy is a form of hierarchical grouping of concepts that identify, name and classify items based on shared characteristics. They are predominantly used in the natural sciences, for example, the classifications of organisms and the periodic table. Skills taxonomies arrange behaviours into ordered groupings, often with higher order categories (e.g. situation awareness and leadership) explained by lower order elements of behaviour (gathering information and understanding information). This is akin to surface and deep features. (See Table 3.1 for the NOTSS behaviour rating system, showing the difference between categories and elements.) The tool can be used to guide observations and classify them into either categories or elements depending on the granularity of analysis required. For workplace assessment, a rating scale is also used in conjunction with the taxonomy to allow observers to rate behaviours in different elements and categories of the taxonomy.

These behaviour marker systems are context specific, and if high levels of validity are desired (see Table 10.1) tools must be developed for the profession in which they are to be used. For example, the NOTECHS system (see Chapter 2) was developed by psychologists and pilots and evaluated with training captains, i.e. subject matter experts (SMEs) from civil aviation.[19] In a similar vein, the NOTSS system was developed by psychologists, surgeons, and other operating room team members and evaluated by panels of consultant surgeons in Scotland.[25] These SMEs are entrenched in the profession that the behaviour rating system is designed to address and provide a rich source of implicit understanding about the required skills for high performance. For effective non-technical skills assessment, the system needs to be explicit, transparent, reliable and valid for the domain in which it is being used. In Section

3.1.3, we describe some of the main behaviour rating tools available for use in surgery.

3.1.3 NON-TECHNICAL SKILLS ASSESSMENT TOOLS IN SURGERY

Non-technical skills are defined as the cognitive and social skills that underpin knowledge and expertise in high-demand workplaces.[7] They enable team members to exchange information about their perceptions on ongoing situations (mental models) to generate a team-level, shared mental model of understanding to support error detection and sharing of critical information.

Methods of improving safety in medicine were originally pioneered in anaesthesia,[26] and some of the first behaviour rating tools were also developed for anaesthetists.[27] More recently, other observational studies have identified the individual, team and organizational factors that appear to underlie surgical performance.[28–34] These observational studies have been used to drive development and adaption of behavioural rating tools in surgery (Table 3.2).

These tools all differ in how they were developed, for whom they were developed and for what purpose they were developed. Observation-based tools to quantify non-technical skills have already begun to be implemented in surgical training

Table 3.1 NOTSS skills taxonomy

Category	Element
Situation awareness	Gathering information
	Understanding information
	Projecting and anticipating future state
Decision making	Considering options
	Selecting and communicating option
	Implementing and reviewing decisions
Communication and teamwork	Exchanging information
	Establishing a shared understanding
	Co-ordinating team activities
Leadership	Setting and maintaining standards
	Supporting others
	Coping with pressure

Table 3.2 Behavioural rating tools in surgery

Behavioural rating tool	Description
NOTSS	*De novo* development with SMEs (surgeons) to observe and rate individual surgeons[15,35]
ANTS	Developed with SMEs (anaesthesiologists) to observe and rate individual anaesthesiologists[27]
SPLINTS	System developed for scrub practitioners focusing on three elements of behaviour in the operating room – situation awareness, decision making and task management[36]
OTAS	Teamwork assessment tool for three operating room sub-teams,[16] developed according to a theory of leadership
Oxford NOTECHS	Amended aviation tool for rating surgical teams[20]
Revised NOTECHS	Amended aviation tool for rating surgical teams[21]
T-NOTECHS	Amended tool for assessing team-level non-technical skills in trauma[37]

programmes, and in simulation education.[38,39] In particular, NOTSS is currently being used by surgeons and researchers in Europe, Australia, Japan and North America. It has been used as the basis for faculty development in train-the-trainer courses offered by the American College of Surgeons,[40] Royal College of Surgeons of Edinburgh,[41] Royal Australasian College of Surgeons[42] and Intercollegiate Surgical Curriculum Project (ISCP) in the United Kingdom.[43] Section 3.2 describes the development of the NOTSS system.

3.2 NOTSS SYSTEM

NOTSS is a behaviour rating system that allows trained assessors to observe, rate and provide feedback on non-technical skills in the operating room. The aim of the NOTSS project was to develop and test an educational system for training and assessing non-technical skills in the intraoperative phase of surgery. NOTSS is based on a skills taxonomy comprising four categories of surgeons' non-technical skills: situation awareness, decision making, communication and teamwork and leadership. This skills taxonomy affords a dual purpose to the system: learning and assessment. For learning, training and education programmes can be based on the skills taxonomy, targeting the categories in isolation or in combination. These are described in more detail in Chapter 9 with advice on developing and implementing training in non-technical skills for surgeons. The other strength of the system is that an assessment of these skills is possible using the rating form, focusing on either

assessing categories, elements or both. In this way, NOTSS can be used for valid and reliable assessment of skill based on observations of real behaviour in the operating room or simulated operating room. Chapter 10 details some of the approaches to assessing the non-technical skills of surgeons in these intraoperative contexts.

NOTSS was released in May 2006 as v1.2,[15,25] a 12-item observational measure with three elements in each of the four categories and example behaviours for each (see Table 3.3). These are the essential non-technical skills surgeons need to perform safely in the operating room. NOTSS allows measurement of several ACGME core competencies, including professionalism, interpersonal and communication skills and systems-based practice (Table 3.4). The skills taxonomy can be used to structure training and assessment in this emerging area of surgical competence. Sections 3.2.1 through 3.2.4 describe the development and testing of the NOTSS system.

3.2.1 DEVELOPMENT OF NOTSS

The system was developed by a multidisciplinary team of psychologists, surgeons and an anaesthetist under funding from the Royal College of Surgeons of Edinburgh and National Health Service Education for Scotland (NES) starting in 2003. Psychologists at the University of Aberdeen, Scotland, led the development. A systematic process was used to develop NOTSS (Figure 3.1), involving SMEs (consultant surgeons) and replicating methods of systems design used for developing methods of assessing behaviour in

Table 3.3 Specific behavioural examples within NOTSS

NOTSS category	Good behaviour	Poor behaviour
Situation awareness	Points out relevant area of anatomy (e.g. bile duct)	Waits for a predicted problem to arise before responding
Decision making	Reaches a decision and clearly communicates it	Selects inappropriate manoeuvre that leads to complication
Communication and teamwork	Listens to concerns of team members	Fails to keep anaesthetist informed about procedure (e.g. to expect bleeding)
Leadership	Delegates tasks to achieve goals	'Freezes' under pressure

Table 3.4 Mapping NOTSS onto ACGME core competencies

ACGME core competency	Related NOTSS category (element)
Professionalism	Situation awareness (projecting and anticipating)
	Leadership (setting and maintaining standards)
Interpersonal and communication skills	Communication and teamwork (exchanging information, establishing a shared understanding, co-ordinating team activities)
Medical knowledge	Decision making (considering and selecting options)
Practice-based learning and improvement	Decision making (implementation and review)
	Leadership (supporting other team members)
Patient care	Situation awareness (gathering and understanding information, predicting future patient state)
	Decision making (selecting and communicating option)
	Leadership (coping with pressure)
Systems-based practice	Communication and teamwork (co-ordinating team activities)

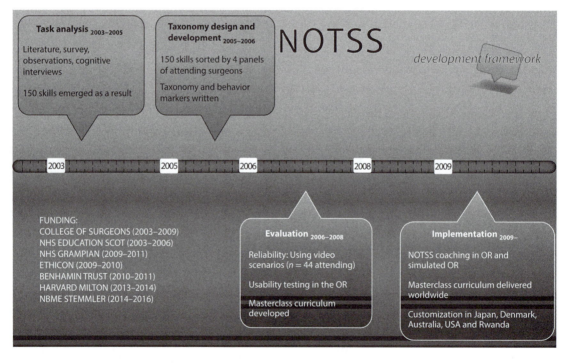

Figure 3.1 Development of the Non-Technical Skills for Surgeons system. (Illustration courtesy of Adrianna Crowell-Kuhnberg.)

other high-demand professions such as civil aviation and nuclear power.[44] An adapted model of systems development[45] was used to guide the iterative evolution of NOTSS through three phases of work, from task analysis[25] through system design to evaluation.[46]

3.2.2 TASK ANALYSIS

Cognitive task analysis has been used in the evolution of a number of behaviour assessment tools. First proposed by Flanagan,[47] the critical incident technique (a type of cognitive interview) is used to elicit tacit knowledge from domain experts. In development of NOTSS, 27 consultant surgeons with expertise in providing surgical care in Scotland were interviewed using this technique to elicit their tacit knowledge of non-technical skills. The interview focused on recalling specific challenging operations elucidating surgeons' use of information, resources, specific strategies and meta-cognition during a specific operative situation. The technique involved discussing a specific operation three times: once by the surgeon, repeated by the interviewer as a method of prompting clarification and additional detail from the surgeon and a third time to examine specific decision points. An interview protocol was designed by the project steering group of psychologists, surgeons and anaesthesiologists with expertise in understanding non-technical skills and the protocol was described by Yule et al.[25] The interviews were recorded digitally, transcribed verbatim and analyzed using the line-by-line coding technique from grounded theory. The outcome was a list of non-technical skills elements used by expert surgeons to manage challenging operative situations and formed the raw data for system design which is described in Section 3.2.3.

3.2.3 ITERATIVE SYSTEM DESIGN

Empirical papers documenting this process are in the surgical, educational and psychology literature. SMEs (consultant surgeons) were involved at all stages of system design, and a steering group chaired by applied psychologists facilitated the process. Different groups of surgeons sorted skills into thematic categories, developed a hierarchical ordering of categories and elements, agreed on surgical language for these concepts and wrote indicative good and poor behaviours for each element. Design criteria ensured that the resulting system was designed by surgeons for surgeons and was written in surgical language, free of technical or psychological jargon. The resulting system is based on a skills taxonomy that makes the required skills explicit (Table 3.1). A set of indicative 'good' and 'poor' behaviours were written for each element, which form the basis of the handbook to guide use of the system,[48] and for training assessors. Example behaviours for each of the four NOTSS categories

are shown in Table 3.2 and highlighted in Chapters 4–7 on the underpinning concepts of NOTSS.

3.2.4 PSYCHOMETRIC TESTING

To assess the system using quantitative methods, a four-point rating scale was selected. Observed skills are rated in NOTSS as follows: 1, poor; 2, marginal; 3, acceptable; and 4, good. Assessments can be made for the categories and/or elements, depending on the purpose of assessment and the degree of granularity required using the NOTSS assessment form (Figure 3.2).

Initial studies have shown promising results regarding the ability of raters to use NOTSS for evaluating both consultant and trainee surgeons' performance in simulated and real operating room settings. In the initial testing of the tool, the inter-rater reliability and sensitivity of the system was examined in a study in which 44 consultant surgeons in Scotland took part. Participants were trained for 3 hours in the conceptual background to the NOTSS tool, underpinning psychology relevant to surgical performance, and principles of behaviour assessment. They then practiced rating behaviour in a series of training video scenarios. These scenarios were filmed in a simulated operating room to show the full range of non-technical skills, both good and poor, for each category and element in the system. In the subsequent experimental phase, participants used NOTSS to assess the behaviour of a target surgeon in seven simulated scenarios filmed in the operating room.[46] The results, analysed using interclass correlation coefficients (ICC) and within-group agreement statistic (r_{WG}), were enlightening. The social skills of communication and teamwork and leadership were rated with an acceptable degree of reliability, but there was more variability between surgeons regarding the cognitive skills of situation awareness and decision making. Given the limited training in a novel area of surgical focus, it was encouraging to see any reliability in ratings at all.

NOTSS was then subject to an independent trial of workplace assessment systems along with Procedure-Based Assessment (PBA) and Objective Structured Assessment of Technical Skill (OSATS) tools to evaluate surgeons' behaviour in real time during operations.[49] This is the biggest trial of NOTSS to date in terms of number of assessments

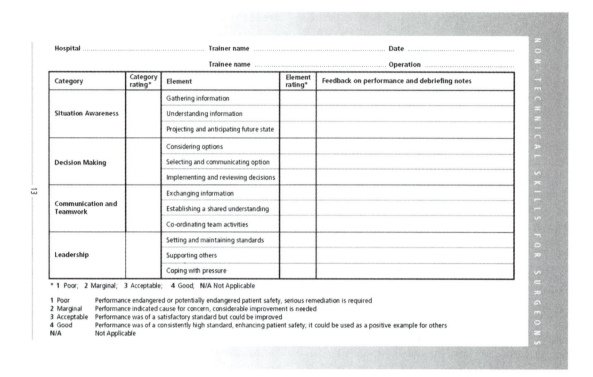

| Hospital .... Trainer name .... Date .... | | | | | |
| Trainee name .... Operation .... | | | | | |

Category	Category rating*	Element	Element rating*	Feedback on performance and debriefing notes
Situation Awareness		Gathering information		
		Understanding information		
		Projecting and anticipating future state		
Decision Making		Considering options		
		Selecting and communicating option		
		Implementing and reviewing decisions		
Communication and Teamwork		Exchanging information		
		Establishing a shared understanding		
		Co-ordinating team activities		
Leadership		Setting and maintaining standards		
		Supporting others		
		Coping with pressure		

* 1 Poor; 2 Marginal; 3 Acceptable; 4 Good; N/A Not Applicable

1 Poor	Performance endangered or potentially endangered patient safety, serious remediation is required
2 Marginal	Performance indicated cause for concern, considerable improvement is needed
3 Acceptable	Performance was of a satisfactory standard but could be improved
4 Good	Performance was of a consistently high standard, enhancing patient safety; it could be used as a positive example for others
N/A	Not Applicable

Figure 3.2 Non-Technical Skills for Surgeons rating form.

made and took place in the United Kingdom, by a research group in Sheffield led by Jonathan Beard. They found that NOTSS was less procedure specific than other assessment tools such as PBA and OSATS. This study also concluded from generalizability analyses that assessments on six occasions were required to make a generalizable assessment of trainees' skill if assessing them on the same operation, whereas eight assessments were required if assessing them during a mix of different operations. Future research is focusing on construct and criterion validity of NOTSS,[50] specifically demonstrating the unique contribution of behaviours measured by using NOTSS in predicting clinically-relevant patient outcomes.

3.3 USING NOTSS

The design criteria used to guide development of NOTSS was selected to ensure that the final system was written in surgical language for suitably trained assessors to observe, rate and provide feedback on non-technical skills in a structured manner. Surgeons have been using NOTSS in the operating room and in simulated settings for assessment,[51] simulation training for individual surgeons[52] and trauma teams,[53] testing generalizability,[54] providing feedback, structuring morbidity and mortality conferences and reflecting on intraoperative incidents.[55] Not all applications require use of the rating scale, for example, in obstetrics a team removed ratings completely to use the structure of NOTSS as a qualitative feedback tool.[56] Other groups have tested NOTSS independently against teamwork assessment tools, finding concurrent validity[57] and comparing self versus assessor ratings.[58]

The design of the assessment form has been locally adapted to fit with other assessment forms (e.g. as part of ISCP implementation), but the principles of NOTSS assessment remain the same across contexts (four-point rating scale to rate four categories and 12 elements of non-technical skills, as originally described). The system is commonly used for providing a single judgement on each category and element for an observation session, be that a complete operation, part operation or a simulated operation. Latterly, some researchers, including those in our own research group, have taken multiple NOTSS assessments in a continuous manner to track changes in behaviour as an operation progresses, but the decision to do this is determined by the particular research or education question being addressed. Other research applications have implemented the NOTSS system for debriefing surgical trainees after real operations and for coaching trainees in non-technical skills after observing them conduct simulated laparoscopic procedures[52,59] in a simulated operating room. See Chapter 10 for a full account of assessing non-technical skills using behaviour observation tools.

The Royal College of Surgeons of Edinburgh has been successfully running a NOTSS masterclass in observing and rating behaviour for attending surgeons since 2006.[41] Faculty development has also occurred for groups in the United States, Japan and Australia. NOTSS has been adopted by the Royal Australasian College of Surgeons as part of their competence assessment[60] and recommended by the ACGME for workplace assessment.[61] A similar system called Anaesthetists Non-Technical Skills (ANTS)[27] was developed previously and Scrub Practitioners, List of Intraoperative Non-Technical Skills (SPLINTS) has subsequently been developed[62] and evaluated[36] for operating room surgical scrub nurses (see Chapter 2).

Since the development of NOTSS and ANTS, there has been a proliferation of behaviour marker tools for many areas of health care. A recent review by Diaz et al. outlines these and present challenges for the wider field, including how to reach consensus on measurement of teamwork, decide standards for reporting psychometric testing and select reliable tools for specific assessment purposes.[63] These challenges are also very relevant for the continual development and refinement of NOTSS to ensure that the tool fits the educational needs of surgeons and surgical trainees. See Chapter 10 for a more in-depth discussion of non-technical skills assessment.

The validity of assessments can be enhanced if the assessment tool relates to underpinning theory. It was Kurt Lewin, widely known as the grandfather of modern social psychology, who said: 'There

is nothing so practical as a good theory'.[64] Although NOTSS is a practical tool, and the assessment categories were developed by surgeons, they relate directly to two of the dominant fields of psychology with unique underpinning theories: cognitive psychology, the study of mental processes (situation awareness and decision making in NOTSS), and social psychology, the study of interpersonal behaviour (communication and teamwork and leadership in NOTSS). The underpinning concepts of the four categories of NOTSS are highlighted in Section 3.4 as a taster of what will be revealed in more depth in the second section of this book, 'Underpinning Concepts' (Chapters 4 through 7).

3.4 UNDERPINNING THEORY OF NON-TECHNICAL SKILLS

Each of the skills in the NOTSS categories (e.g. leadership) has an extensive literature in the psychology, human performance and education realms; however, little of this was derived from studying surgeons. There are now an increasing number of studies on surgeons' cognitive and social skills in the intraoperative phase, and these are described in Chapters 4, 5, 6 and 7 in relation to each NOTSS skill category. In this section, the underpinning psychology of the four main categories of NOTSS behaviour (situation awareness, decision making, communication and teamwork and leadership) is briefly described.

3.4.1 SITUATION AWARENESS

Situation awareness is arguably the most critical non-technical skill, and it is required for accurate decision making, timely communication and appropriate leadership. Situation awareness in NOTSS is defined as 'developing and maintaining a dynamic awareness of the situation in the operating room, based on assembling data from the environment (patient, team, time, displays, equipment); understanding what they mean, and thinking ahead about what may happen next'. According to Endsley's model,[65] situation awareness comprises of three distinct levels (these are called elements in NOTSS, so that is the terminology used here): element 1, gathering information; element 2, interpreting the information (based on experience); and element 3, projecting and anticipating future states based on this interpretation. Chapter 4 outlines the psychological basis of situation awareness and its relevance to intraoperative surgery:

SA1 – Gathering information: Information coming in (to the surgeon) does so from a number of sources including the patient (anatomy), colleagues (verbal and non-verbal cues) and instruments (patient monitors). One of the challenges of surgery in the era of inter-professional teams is for the surgeon to monitor information sources and decide which are important to pay attention to. It is very common for the surgeon to be concentrating so intensely on the current operation that important information is either not seen or heard. This makes successful performance of SA element 2 almost impossible.

SA2 – Understanding information: The surgeon needs not only to receive all the information but also to understand its significance. This will of course require a degree of training and experience, so junior surgeons, not being aware of the significance of certain facts, will respond (or not respond) differently than senior, more experienced surgeons. A common problem in correctly interpreting information is something called 'confirmation bias'. In this instance, information coming in is filtered to allow the surgeon to confirm his or her views, while any information that might suggest another cause is erroneously discarded.

SA3 – Projecting and anticipating future state: Having received and (hopefully) recognized the importance of the information, the surgeon must then anticipate potential future events. Experts spend a lot of time thinking about the future and running mental simulations about what may happen as a result of different courses of future action. This may or may not require a change of plan. Problems with incorrect anticipation may be avoided by discussing options with colleagues and reviewing alternatives. This is all a dynamic situation and will change as the operation progresses.

3.4.2 DECISION MAKING

In NOTSS, decision making is defined as 'skills for diagnosing a situation and reaching a judgement in order to choose an appropriate course of action'.[66] There is now increasing interest in intraoperative judgement.[67] Classical models of decision making propose that this is an *analytical* process: the relative features of options are compared in turn and an optimal course of action is selected. This can be an 'effortful' process and requires both experience and time to come to an acceptable solution.[68] Another common method of decision making applicable to intraoperative surgery is *rule-based* decision making. This method is used by trainee and expert surgeons alike and makes decision making easier as once a situation has been detected a relevant rule can be applied, by following either national guidelines or local protocols. Deciding when to use antibiotic prophylaxis during surgery to reduce the risk of surgical site infection is one example. Experts, however, tend to use a more heuristic-based style called *recognition-primed* decision making (RPD), a type of pattern matching that experts can use to make satisfactory decisions under times of high stress or time pressure.[69] Occasionally, surgeons use *creative* decision making when a totally novel solution is required in the intraoperative environment. For a scientific background on decision making and surgical studies, see Chapter 5. The three decision-making elements of behaviour in NOTSS are described as follows:

DM1 – Considering options: In this element, the skill is generating alternative possibilities or courses of action to solve a problem. Assessing hazards, weighing risks and benefits of potential problems and verbalizing the range of options when there are several viable courses of action form part of the skill set.

DM2 – Selecting and communicating option: This NOTSS element refers to choosing a solution to a problem and telling relevant operating room personnel what the decision is and why it has been chosen. This may involve telling other members of the team what may be obvious to the surgeon, but verbalizing important information is a critical basis on which to establish a shared understanding and in some cases it clarifies ambiguous situations for other team members. The surgeon's role is to make important information clear, concise and explicit for team members to allow them to organize their work as part of a high-performance team.

DM3 – Implementing and reviewing decision: This is the physical act of carrying out the decision that has been made and reviewing the suitability as the operation proceeds. Observable behaviours may include telling people what other alternatives are, how progress can be assessed, and any relevant criteria to refer to when reviewing the efficacy of decisions. Understanding what to do when things are not going according to plan is also an important skill for this element.

3.4.3 COMMUNICATION AND TEAMWORK

Communication and teamwork are the skills required for working in a team context to ensure that everyone has an acceptable shared picture of the situation and can complete tasks effectively. What is essential is that each member of the team has a 'shared mental model' of both what is happening and what is the planned outcome. There are many barriers to communication, which can be both internal and external.

Several studies have clearly shown that a large number of the adverse events that occur in surgery relate to problems with communication,[6,70,71] and a number of general remedies for improving communication within the team have been developed. In Chapter 6, communication and teamwork behaviours for surgeons are examined in detail. The three relevant elements of behavior are described below:

CT1 – Exchanging information: Most surgical procedures typically require teamwork and communication among the members of the surgical team. Exchanging information requires both communication of message and listening. Communication failures at this stage have been shown to result in injury to surgical patients, due to the wrong message being transmitted, the correct message being incorrectly received, the message going to the wrong person (or to no person in particular) or the message being transmitted too early or too late to be effective.[70]

CT2 – Establishing a shared understanding: The goal of exchanging information is to establish a shared understanding. Closed-loop communication, where team members deliberately ensure that there is some read back or acknowledgement of communications can help to ensure this.

CT3 – Co-ordinating team activities: For the team to work as a cohesive unit, their activities must be co-ordinated. Exchanging information and developing a shared understanding enable the team to work together to accomplish common goals. Timing is also important here of efficiency and team synchrony.

3.4.4 LEADERSHIP

In organizations exposed to hazards, there is widespread recognition that leadership is essential for efficient and safe team performance. Leadership has also been shown to be critical for adoption of new technology and learning in the operating room.[72] In the cognitive interviews as part of phase 1 of NOTSS development,[25] surgeons described leadership in the operating room either as entirely their own responsibility or as a shared responsibility between the surgeon, anaesthetist and nursing team leader. During the NOTSS development process, the leadership behaviours were grouped into three elements: setting and maintaining standards, supporting others and coping with pressure. Recent research into surgeons' leadership when operating is presented in Chapter 7. There was a paucity of surgical leadership research when NOTSS was developed, and a recent review of the literature confirms that there is still limited empirical evidence identifying specific leadership skills and associated behaviours enacted by surgeons during operations.[73] There are three leadership elements within NOTSS, described in detail as follows:

L1 – Setting and maintaining standards: A core function of leadership is demonstrating the standards that are expected from other team members. A key failing of leaders is to empha-size the importance of safety but then implic-itly undermine those sentiments by breaking rules and not adhering to high standards of ethical and professional conduct themselves. This sets the tone that those standards are also optional for other team members. For surgeons, examples of this are adhering to guidelines regarding antibiotic use, respect-ing sterility protocols and being transparent regarding errors. Even behaviours such as con-ducting a surgical pause before every operation and providing enough time for others to con-tribute demonstrates the standard that safety and teamwork are high priorities.

L2 – *Supporting others*: Patient safety is the responsibility of every member of the operat-ing room team. Ideally, every team member from the surgeon to the anaesthesiologist to the nurse to the surgical technician, should feel empowered to speak up about potential safety concerns.[74] The surgeon, as a high-status mem-ber of the team, is instrumental in supporting fellow team members to speak up to ensure safety.[75] This could include encouraging others at the beginning of the procedure to speak up if they see something unsafe or by thanking others after they have done so. This helps pro-mote a safe environment both for the current procedure and for future procedures as well. Treating people with respect when they speak up is also essential. However, this element is not solely about speaking up, other relevant 'supporting others' skills include appropri-ate delegation, giving credit for tasks accom-plished, providing constructive criticism, and adjusting ones behaviour to the needs of others.

L3 – *Coping with pressure*: Most surgical pro-cedures progress routinely with only rare instances of anxiety and heightened pressure. Pressure is a part of surgery, however, and cer-tain procedures or events can be very intense. The operating surgeon plays an important role in leading the team through such situations. The surgeon needs to not only make it clear to the team members when there is more pres-sure in a situation but also help the team cope with that pressure. The surgeon can do this by

clearly stating that this is an important phase of the procedure. He or she can also lead by example, keeping composure even in the most difficult of times. In general, the team will appreciate knowing the intensity of the situa-tion and will respond to the surgeon's compo-sure by maintaining their own. (See Chapter 8 for a broader discussion on stress and coping.)

3.5 NON-TECHNICAL SKILLS AT WORK IN THE OPERATING ROOM

3.5.1 SITUATION AWARENESS: LAP CHOLE WITH CHOLANGIOGRAM

A surgeon is performing a laparoscopic cholecys-tectomy for acute cholecystitis. With significant inflammation of the gallbladder, the anatomy of the cystic artery, cystic duct, and common bile duct can be in question. It is the surgeon's responsibility to safely *gather information* about those anatomic structures with techniques like the critical view of safety, an intraoperative cholangiogram, or con-verting to an open cholecystectomy. If an intraop-erative cholangiogram is chosen, the surgeon must *understand the information*, properly interpreting the information provided by the cholangiogram. During the procedure, the surgeon should *project and anticipate future state*, including notifying the team about a decision to perform a cholangiogram or convert to open cholecystectomy, so that the team can obtain the necessary equipment.

3.5.2 DECISION MAKING: EMERGENT INCARCERATED VENTRAL HERNIA REPAIR

Imagine a scenario where the surgeon operates emergently on a patient with an incarcerated ven-tral hernia and concern for ischemic bowel. During the operation, the surgeon reduces the hernia and identifies a 25 cm segment of ischemic small intes-tine. The surgeon must *consider options* 'on the fly': (1) resect the bowel, (2) allow the intestine time to regain circulation, or (3) do a diagnostic test such as giving fluorescein dye to assess perfusion. Assume a bowel resection is performed, the surgeon must then consider options for hernia repair, which again require intraoperative judgment. Options may include placement of prosthetic mesh, placement of biological mesh, or suture repair of the hernia and are, in part, based on the level of ischemia and bowel contamination. At this point, the surgeon must both *select and communicate the option* to the team, so they understand the procedure and obtain the necessary equipment. Finally, the surgeon should *implement and review her decision.* In so doing, the surgeon proceeds with bowel resection and hernia repair but must also constantly assess and review their decision. For instance, if suture repair is selected but the fascia is not able to come together, the surgeon may need to change path and place mesh.

3.5.3 COMMUNICATION AND TEAMWORK: OPEN RUPTURED ABDOMINAL AORTIC ANEURYSM REPAIR

A ruptured abdominal aortic aneurysm is a life-threatening event. Surgical mortality, for patients who actually survive to reach the hospital, is quite high. Communication and teamwork in the operating room are important to operative success. Upon entering the operating room, the surgeon should *exchange information* with the anesthesiologist, even prior to making incision. Decisions should be made about target blood pressure, as well as when to make incision, as patients are at risk for dramatic drop in blood pressure after induction of anesthesia. The surgeon needs to be prepared to operate immediately, and most recommend that the patient be prepped and draped prior to intubation so as to allow quick entry into the abdomen. The surgeon should also *establish a shared understanding* with the entire surgical team. All members must know the gravity and urgency of the procedure and be prepared for the critical events. Part of the surgeon's role is to *coordinate team activities*, which includes confirming that the team is ready to begin, making certain that all necessary retractors, sutures, and vascular grafts are available, and notifying the team when medications such as intravenous heparin (if needed) should be administered.

3.5.4 LEADERSHIP: TOTAL KNEE REPLACEMENT

When performing a total knee replacement, it is essential that the proper sidedness of the procedure be identified. This happens during the surgical safety pause, and it is the responsibility of the surgeon to ensure that a proper timeout is performed. If a team member is distracted during the safety pause, good leadership behavior by the surgeon is to *set and maintain standards* by pausing and asking the team member to re-focus on the safety pause. During the safety pause and throughout the case, all members of the team should feel empowered to speak up with any knowledge that may impact the procedure or patient safety. For instance, a nurse who sees a break in sterile technique should be comfortable speaking up and notifying the team, so that postoperative infection is avoided. One of the surgeon's jobs is to *support others*, creating the environment that fosters the sharing of critical information. Another important role of the surgeon is *coping with pressure.* Although rare, the popliteal artery can be injured during a total knee replacement. If this happens, the surgeon must remain calm, notify the team of the injury and its urgency, and delegate tasks so that the team can address the situation.

3.6 NEW DEVELOPMENTS WITH NOTSS SINCE THE TAXONOMY WAS PUBLISHED

Since the NOTSS tool was released in 2006, an increasing number of researchers, surgeons, societies and organizations all over the world have grown curious about its application. In each country where NOTSS has been implemented, it has been adapted to the local context. This is commonly in the form of translating the skills taxonomy and training materials into the local language; however, in some cases the underpinning taxonomy has been subject to more rigorous examination and customization. Short case studies from countries in five continents where NOTSS has been implemented are described in this section. Examples are drawn from Asia, Europe, North America, Australasia and Africa (Figure 3.3).

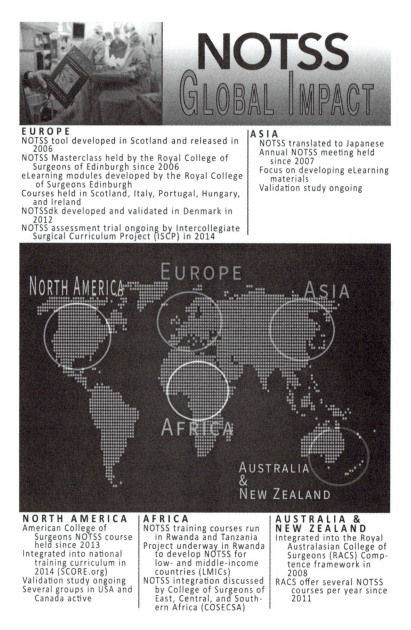

NOTSS GLOBAL IMPACT

EUROPE
NOTSS tool developed in Scotland and released in 2006
NOTSS Masterclass held by the Royal College of Surgeons of Edinburgh since 2006
eLearning modules developed by the Royal College of Surgeons Edinburgh
Courses held in Scotland, Italy, Portugal, Hungary, and Ireland
NOTSSdk developed and validated in Denmark in 2012
NOTSS assessment trial ongoing by Intercollegiate Surgical Curriculum Project (ISCP) in 2014

ASIA
NOTSS translated to Japanese
Annual NOTSS meeting held since 2007
Focus on developing eLearning materials
Validation study ongoing

NORTH AMERICA
American College of Surgeons NOTSS course held since 2013
Integrated into national training curriculum in 2014 (SCORE.org)
Validation study ongoing
Several groups in USA and Canada active

AFRICA
NOTSS training courses run in Rwanda and Tanzania
Project underway in Rwanda to develop NOTSS for low- and middle-income countries (LMICs)
NOTSS integration discussed by College of Surgeons of East, Central, and Southern Africa (COSECSA)

AUSTRALIA & NEW ZEALAND
Integrated into the Royal Australasian College of Surgeons (RACS) Competence framework in 2008
RACS offer several NOTSS courses per year since 2011

Figure 3.3 Non-Technical Skills for Surgeons global impact. (Illustration courtesy of Adrianna Crowell-Kuhnberg.)

3.6.1 ASIA

Perhaps the most widely adopted example of NOTSS comes from Japan.[76] The group is headed by Dr Akira Tsuburaya (Surgeon and Associate Professor, Yokohama City University Medical Center) and colleagues Dr Takahiro Souma (Tokyo) and Dr Yoishi (Nara). In 2008, they translated the NOTSS taxonomy and behaviour markers into Japanese (Figure 3.4); they have also held NOTSS workshops annually since 2007, allied to the Japanese Surgical Society annual conference. The approach has been to build a broad base of support within Japan to run a clinical trial testing the impact of NOTSS implementation on intra-operative adverse event rates. Notably, Japanese

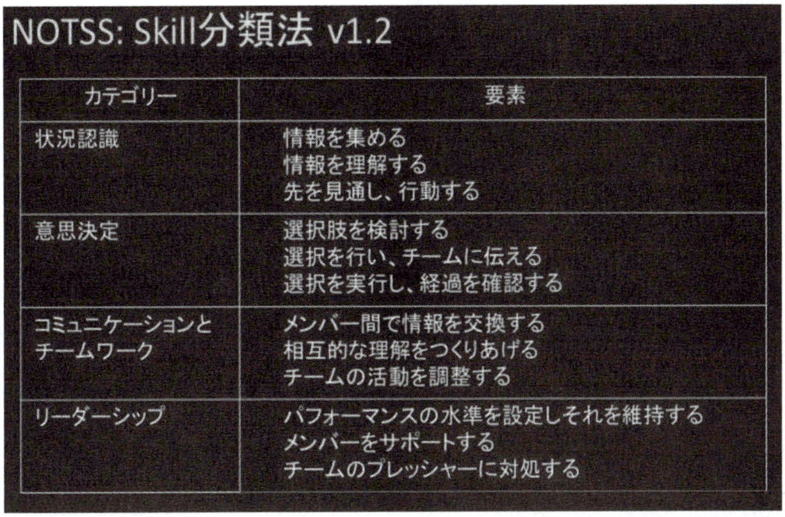

NOTSS: Skill分類法 v1.2

カテゴリー	要素
状況認識	情報を集める 情報を理解する 先を見通し、行動する
意思決定	選択肢を検討する 選択を行い、チームに伝える 選択を実行し、経過を確認する
コミュニケーションと チームワーク	メンバー間で情報を交換する 相互的な理解をつくりあげる チームの活動を調整する
リーダーシップ	パフォーマンスの水準を設定しそれを維持する メンバーをサポートする チームのプレッシャーに対処する

Figure 3.4 Non-Technical Skills for Surgeons taxonomy in Japanese. (Courtesy of Akira Tsuburaya.)

anaesthetists and scrub practitioners[77] have also translated non-technical skill materials, and there has been notable support for non-technical skills relating to patient safety.[78] A recent focus has been on developing eLearning materials.

3.6.2 EUROPE

In the United Kingdom, the Intercollegiate Surgical Curriculum Project (ISCP) is currently implementing NOTSS as a formative assessment tool to help surgeons develop their non-technical skills, aiming to enhance the available suite of assessments for learning. Before participating in the program and completing an assessment, all raters, assigned educational supervisors and clinical supervisors, need to be trained to use the system. The Royal College of Surgeons of Edinburgh has developed e-learning modules for surgical trainees[79] and a train-the-trainers online training programme called 'NOTSS in a box',[80] which is being used for this purpose. For practising surgeons, the Royal College of Surgeons of Edinburgh also provides an annual NOTSS masterclass. This is a 2-day curriculum aimed at developing skills to identify, categorize and assess non-technical skills (see Chapter 9 for more details). These activities are likely to create a desire for more widespread adoption of training and assessment in this area. To scale up the application of NOTSS,

faculty development and training is required. This prompted an expert group to determine consensus guidelines for faculty training in non-technical skills.[81]

NOTSS has also been translated into Italian, and plans are in place for German and French versions. Training courses have been run in Italy, Portugal, Hungary and Ireland. The European Society for Urology has recently run a study using NOTSS, and it is part of their fellowship training. This group has also written about the incorporation of non-technical skills in robotic surgery training.[82] However, the most complete body of work in any European country other than the United Kingdom has been in Denmark. A group from the Danish Institute for Medical Simulation headed by a surgeon, Lene Spanager, has taken the NOTSS tool and replicated portions of the underpinning task analysis in Danish operating theatres to determine the non-technical skills used by surgeons in that context. By conducting cognitive interviews with subject matter experts in Denmark, they identified one additional element of behaviour, 'monitoring own behaviour', and added it to the category situation awareness[83] in a tool referred to as 'NOTSS-dk'. All other categories and elements remained intact in this independent validation of the NOTSS skills taxonomy. In fact, this study is the only one to date that has amended the skills taxonomy. No other studies have changed the underpinning model of four categories and 12 elements. The Danish group tested the validity of NOTSS-dk in a series of (simulated) observations using a five-point rating scale and found that inter-rater reliability was high for both pre-training ratings (Cronbach's alpha = .97) and post-training ratings (Cronbach's alpha = .98). Generalizability analysis showed that two untrained raters or one trained rater were needed to obtain generalizability coefficients greater than .80.[84]

3.6.3 NORTH AMERICA

The first NOTSS workshop was held in May 2011 at the annual meeting of the American Association of Thoracic Surgeons by invitation of Dr Thor Sundt III, Chief of Cardiothoracic surgery at Massachusetts General Hospital. Over 100 cardiothoracic surgeons attended this 3-hour programme, including some from the Northern New England Cardiovascular Disease Group, a consortium of eight hospitals in New Hampshire, Vermont and Maine, who pioneered data and practice sharing to enhance surgical performance and improve safety. This group has engaged NOTSS as part of operating room audits and also studies of non-technical skills in mitral valve replacement and low output failure.[85]

In 2013, NOTSS was incorporated to the *ACS Surgery Weekly Curriculum*[86] and in 2014 it became part of the Surgical Council On Resident Education (SCORE) national curriculum for surgical training. For practising surgeons 1-day NOTSS workshops were held at the American College of Surgeons Annual Clinical Congress in 2013 and 2014, and for programme directors a workshop was held on leadership in NOTSS in 2014 at the Association of Program Directors in Surgery (APDS) annual meeting. To support these sessions, the NOTSS video series was created (www.vimeo.com/notss). To customize the NOTSS skills taxonomy and assessment tool to the context of US surgery, the National Board of Medical Examiners Stemmler medical education fund is sponsoring a 2-year project at Brigham & Women's Hospital, Boston, Massachusetts, led by Harvard Medical School faculty. The research team will develop contextually valid behaviour markers, run a generalizability study using simulation scenarios filmed at the Neil and Elise Wallace STRATUS Center

for Medical Simulation, Boston, and then validate NOTSS in the US in a series of operating room observations.[87] In addition, one group in Canada has been very active in NOTSS research. Grantcharov and Dedy have completed a systematic review[88] and simulation training courses in Toronto.[51]

3.6.4 AFRICA

As surgical workforce training and surgical capacity continue to increase in low- and middle-income countries (LMICs), new strategies for improving surgical care and reducing adverse events are increasingly becoming important worldwide. This view is strongly supported by the World Health Organization's Patient Safety Curriculum Guidelines, which repeatedly recognizes the importance of teaching non-technical skills for team development and performance, individual task proficiency, and teamwork among mixed groups of health care providers in resource poor settings.[89]

NOTSS has already experienced worldwide application as detailed earlier but this is only in high-income countries such as Scotland, England, Canada, the United States, Australia and Japan. Perhaps, a different blend of non-technical skills is required to provide safe and effective surgical care in an LMIC setting that lacks high-tech gadgets, abundant resources and integrated health care delivery systems.

There is evidence of increasing interest in incorporating non-technical skills into surgical training among LMICs such as Rwanda, as evidenced by a recent educational programme focused on teaching non-technical skills to anaesthesiologists.[90] Non-technical skills for surgeons are increasing in importance in other countries in East Africa and have been discussed at annual meetings of the College of Surgeons of East, Central, and Southern Africa (COSECSA).[91] NOTSS workshops have also been delivered in Uganda, Malawi, Zambia and Mozambique. Despite this growing interest, however, there is a lack of culturally appropriate models for teaching non-technical skills in resource-constrained settings common to many LMICs. For any educational tool to function well, it must be designed to function within the three contextual elements of environmental factors, provider factors and patient factors that vary across different settings. There are numerous examples in the literature of health care provider education programmes that highlight lack of contextual fit as a barrier to successful implementation.[92,93] With these differences in mind, a collaboration of surgeons from the Center for Surgery and Public Health, Brigham & Women's Hospital, Harvard Medical School and from University Central Hospital of Kigali (Rwanda) have set out to create a behavioural marker tool to observe, rate, provide feedback on and teach non-technical skills for surgeons operating in Rwanda. This work is being led by John Scott, Robert Riviello and Georges Ntakiyiruta.

The approach is closely following the original method used to create the first version of NOTSS: observations in the operating theatre, cognitive interviews with SMEs and a panel of SMEs to develop a tool that reflects the non-technical skills necessary for expert performance in the Rwandan surgical environment. Finally, this tool will be tested for ease of use, reliability and accuracy using a combination of live and simulated cases in both operating theatres and simulation centres. The final output will be a context-appropriate behavioural marker tool that is built by and for Rwandan surgeons operating in their own clinical settings. A non-technical skills curriculum for East African surgery will follow.

3.6.5 AUSTRALASIA

NOTSS was incorporated by the Royal Australasian College of Surgeons into their professional competence framework in 2008 and revised in 2012.[94] This group have developed a faculty of surgical trainers to run courses in Australia and run approximately one per month[95] based on a video series.[42] A surgical research group in Adelaide is running simulation trials involving NOTSS.

3.7 IMPORTANCE OF NOTSS FOR SURGEONS AND PATIENTS

Non-technical skills are the cognitive and social skills that underpin knowledge and expertise in high-demand workplaces. In the operating room,

surgeons with good non-technical skills can effectively share information about their perceptions of ongoing situations with other team members, elicit critical information from others regarding the task and patient safety and allow the formation of better shared mental representations about the operation in real time. In rare situations when crises occur in the operating room, surgeons use their non-technical skills to delegate tasks and effectively manage challenging operations under time pressure. It stands to reason that demonstrating good non-technical skills during routine operations means that the entire operating room team is more in tune with the surgeons' thought processes and better able to adapt quickly to deal with unexpected events when they occur.

There are several methods of assessing non-technical skills, and in this chapter we have focused on the underpinning theory of the NOTSS system. As described in this chapter, NOTSS makes explicit the main non-technical skills required for safe surgical practice. The system is not intended to provide a comprehensive list of all possible behaviours; it is more of a guide to those that are most likely to have the biggest impact. Other tools have been developed for those wishing to dive deeper into specific categories of behaviour to develop nuanced pictures of surgeons' behaviour in the operating room. For example, the Surgical Leadership Inventory allows assessment of eight leadership behaviours,[73,96,97] and the recently developed Teamwork Monitoring and Management rating scale allows assessment of self and team monitoring behaviours along with communication and leadership related to teamwork and task work.[57] However, as Dietz et al. point out,[63] selection of assessment tools should be driven by the specific purpose for which they are intended, and these two tools are aimed more at generating research data to study non-technical skills rather than at providing usable assessments of behaviour, or of learning for feedback, debriefing, coaching and formative or summative assessment.

The challenge for surgical trainees is that the importance of these skills to clinical performance and patient outcomes has only been realized widely in the past decade, so formal training in these skills with particular emphasis on the operating room is not widespread. A recent review on non-technical skills training for surgical residents found a number of instructional strategies had been trialed, but evidence of their effectiveness is moderate at best.[88] This will improve as the new wave in non-technical skills education and assessment gains support. See Chapter 9 for more discussions on training curricula and learning modalities to enhance non-technical skills.

In times of reduced operating hours and less time to gain practical skills in the operating room during surgical training, the importance of non-technical skills as a framework on which to make the most of medical knowledge and clinical expertise rises. Other high-risk industries responded to similar challenges by integrating simulation training and coaching on non-technical skills for trainees. It may be possible to enhance performance by coaching non-technical skills, and early studies have shown this to be beneficial and welcomed by surgical residents. As with acquisition of any skill, deliberate practice coupled with objective feedback from a trained observer may be able to shorten learning curves. Coaching is in its infancy in health care,[98] with focus on technical skill,[99] but could be a powerful method of improving capacity for non-technical skills in the operating room (see Chapters 9 and 11).

3.8 CONCLUSION

The research to develop and test NOTSS has resulted in a framework for professional training and assessment in an important but underappreciated area of surgical performance. By its uptake across the globe, it seems that NOTSS has universal application across most if not all health jurisdictions. It is thus a major contribution to clinical education and practice globally. However, local customization is important to ensure that the skills taxonomy fits the local work culture and that norms of behaviour are reflected in the behaviour markers. The rating scale may also change to fit local assessment practice, as observed in Denmark with NOTSS-dk.[84] The non-technical skills frameworks and resulting tools developed for training and assessment are being adopted by a number of bodies worldwide both for medical and nursing

trainee education and for continuing professional development. Consultant surgeons and anaesthetists now use these tools in their own training and research. The contribution to patient safety has translated into its integration into undergraduate curricula of a variety of medical schools in the United Kingdom, as well as the General Medical Council-approved curriculum of surgical specialties (www.iscp.ac.uk). The task analysis for developing NOTSS was derived with some refinements from the methods used to devise earlier systems such as ANTS and NOTECHS. This systematic approach has now been adopted by other research teams who have used it to develop similar tools for other medical professions such as emergency medicine[100] and scrub technicians.[36]

To conclude, non-technical skills contribute to nearly half of all surgical errors, and in some cases unnecessary harm and suffering for patients can be avoided not by increasing precision, skill or enhanced therapy but by better (1) situation awareness, (2) intraoperative decision making, (3) teamwork and communication and (4) leadership. It is now possible to assess and quantify these skills in the operating room using NOTSS. Part II of this book provides more detail regarding the underpinning theories and supporting research evidence regarding these four categories of non-technical skills.

REFERENCES

1. Vincent C, Neale G, Woloshynowych M. Adverse events in British hospitals: Preliminary retrospective record review. *BMJ.* 2001;322:517–9.
2. de Vries E, Ramrattan M, Smorenburg S, Gouma D, Boermeester M. The incidence and nature of in-hospital adverse events: A systematic review. *Qual Safe Health Care.* 2008;17(3):216–23.
3. Anderson O, Davis R, Hanna GB, Vincent CA. Surgical adverse events: A systematic review. *Am J Surg.* 2013;206(2):253–62.
4. Gawande A, Zinner M, Studdert D, Brennan T. Analysis of errors reported by surgeons at three teaching hospitals. *Surgery.* 2003;133(6):614–21.

5. Way LW, Stewart L, Gantert W, Liu K, Lee CM, Whang K et al. Causes and prevention of laparoscopic bile duct injuries: Analysis of 252 cases from a human factors and cognitive psychology perspective. *Ann Surg.* 2003 Apr;237(4):460–9.

6. Mazzocco K, Petitti DB, Fong KT, Bonacum D, Brookey J, Graham S et al. Surgical team behaviors and patient outcomes. *Am J Surg.* 2009 May;197(5):678–85.

7. Yule S, Flin R, Paterson-Brown S, Maran N. Non-technical skills for surgeons: A review of the literature. *Surgery.* 2006;139:140–9.

8. AHA. Top ten things to know. Patient safety in the cardiac OR: Human factors and teamwork: American Heart Association. 2013. [Accessed April 17, 2015.] Available from: https://my.americanheart.org/idc/groups/ahamah-public/@wcm/@sop/@smd/documents/downloadable/ucm_454536.pdf.

9. Wahr JA, Prager RL, Abernathy JH, Martinez EA, Salas E, Seifert PC et al. Patient safety in the cardiac operating room: Human factors and teamwork. A scientific statement from the American Heart Association. *Circulation.* 2013; Sep 3;128(10):1139–69.

10. Accreditation Council for Graduate Medical Education. ACGME Program Requirements for Graduate Medical Education in General Surgery. 2011. [Accessed April 17, 2015.] Available from: http://www.acgme.org/acgmeweb/portals/0/pfassets/programrequirements/440_general_surgery_07012014.pdf.

11. Flin R, Yule S, Paterson-Brown S, Maran N, Rowley D, Youngson G. Teaching surgeons about non-technical skills. *The Surgeon.* 2007;5:86–9.

12. Doherty E, O'Keeffe D, Traynor O. Developing a human factors and patient safety programme at the Royal College of Surgeons in Ireland. *The Surgeon.* 2011;9:S38–9.

13. Dekker S, Leveson N. The systems approach to medicine: Controversy and misconceptions. *BMJ Qual Saf.* 2015; Jan;24(1):7–9.

14. Catchpole K, Giddings A, de Leval M, Peek G, Godden P, Utley M et al. Identification of systems failures in successful paediatric cardiac surgery. *Ergonomics.* 2006;49:567–88.

15. Yule S, Flin R, Maran N, Rowley DR, Youngson GG, Paterson-Brown S. Surgeons' non-technical skills in the operating room: Reliability testing of the NOTSS behaviour rating system. *World J Surg.* 2008;32:548–56.

16. Russ S, Hull L, Rout S, Vincent C, Darzi A, Sevdalis N. Observational teamwork assessment for surgery: Feasibility of clinical and nonclinical assessor calibration with short-term training. *Ann Surg.* 2012 Apr;255(4):804–9.

17. Robertson E, Hadi M, Morgan J, Pickering S, Collins G, New S et al. Oxford NOTECHS II: A modified theatre team non-technical skills scoring system. *PLOS One.* 2014;9(3):1–8.

18. Musson D, Helmreich R. Team training and resource management in health care: Current issues and future directions. *Harvard Health Policy Rev.* 2004;5(1):25–35.

19. Flin R, Martin L, Goeters K, Hormann H, Amalberti R, Valot C et al. Development of the NOTECHS (non-technical skills) system for assessing pilots' CRM skills. *Hum Factors Aero Saf.* 2003;3(2):95–117.

20. Mishra A, Catchpole K, McCulloch P. The Oxford NOTECHS system: Reliability and validity of a tool for measuring teamwork behaviour in the operating theatre. *Qual Safe Health Care.* 2009;18:104–8.

21. Sevdalis N, Davis R, Koutantji M, Undre S, Darzi A, Vincent C. Reliability of a revised NOTECHS scale for use in surgical teams. *Am J Surg.* 2008;196:184–90.

22. Steinemann S, Berg B, DiTullio A, Skinner A, Terada K, Anzelon K et al. Assessing teamwork in the trauma bay: Introduction of a modified 'NOTECHS' scale for trauma. *Am J Surg.* 2012;203:69–75.

23. Gaba D. Have we gone too far in translating ideas from aviation to patient safety? No. *BMJ.* 2011;342:c7310.

24. Rogers J. Have we gone too far in translating ideas from aviation to patient safety? Yes. *BMJ*. 2011;342:c7309.

25. Yule S, Flin R, Paterson-Brown S, Maran N, Rowley D. Development of a rating system for surgeons' non-technical skills. *Med Educ*. 2006 Nov;40(11):1098–104.

26. Gaba D, Howard S, Flanagan B, Smith B, Fish K, Botney R. Assessment of clinical performance during simulated crises using both technical and behavioural ratings. *Anesthesiology*. 1998;89:8–18.

27. Fletcher G, Flin R, McGeorge P, Glavin R, Maran N, Patey R. Anaesthetists' non-technical skills (ANTS): Evaluation of a behavioural marker system. *Brit J Anaesth*. 2003;90:580–8.

28. Helmreich R, Davies J. Human factors in the operating room: Interpersonal determinants of safety, efficiency and morale. *Baillieres Clin Anaesthesiol*. 1996;10:277–95.

29. de Leval M, Carthey J, Wright D. Human factors and cardiac surgery: A multi-centre study. *J Thorac Cardiovasc Surg*. 2000;119(4):661–72.

30. Carthey J, de Leval M, Reason J. The human factor in cardiac surgery: Errors and near misses in a high technology medical domain. *Ann Thorac Surg*. 2001;72:300–5.

31. Flin R, O'Connor P, Crichton M. *Safety at the Sharp End*. Aldershot, United Kingdom: Ashgate; 2008.

32. Catchpole K, Giddings A, Wilkinson M. Improving patient safety by identifying latent failures in successful operations. *Surgery*. 2007;142:102–10.

33. Christian CK, Gustafson ML, Roth EM, Sheridan TB, Gandhi TK, Dwyer K et al. A prospective study of patient safety in the operating room. *Surgery*. 2006 Feb;139(2):159–73.

34. Roth E, Christian C, Gustafson M, Sheridan T, Dwyer K, Gandhi T et al. Using field observations as a tool for discovery: Analysing cognitive and collaborative demands in the operating room. *Cogn Technol Work*. 2004;6:148–57.

35. Yule S, Paterson-Brown S. Surgeons' non-technical skills. *Surg Clin North Am*. 2012 Feb;92(1):37–50.

36. Mitchell L, Flin R, Yule S, Mitchell J, Coutts K, Youngson G. Evaluation of the Scrub Practitioners' List of Intraoperative Non-Technical Skills (SPLINTS) system. *Int J Nurs Stud*. 2012;49:201–11.

37. Steinemann S, Berg B, DiTullio A, Skinner A, Terada K, Anzelon K et al. Assessing teamwork in the trauma bay: Introduction of a modified 'NOTECHS' scale for trauma. *Am J Surg*. 2012 Jan;203(1):69–75.

38. Hull L, Arora S, Symons NR, Jalil R, Darzi A, Vincent C et al. Training faculty in nontechnical skill assessment: National guidelines on program requirements. *Ann Surg*. 2013 Aug;258(2):370–5.

39. Scott DJ, Dunnington GL. The new ACS/APDS Skills curriculum: Moving the learning curve out of the operating room. *J Gastrointest Surg*. 2008 Feb;12(2):213–21.

40. American College of Surgeons. Non Technical skills for Surgeons (NOTSS) in the operating room: Behaviors in high performing teams. 2013. Available from: http://web2.facs.org/cc_program_planner/Detail_Session_2013.cfm?CCYEAR=2013&SESSION=PG27&GROUP=PG&KEYWORD=Non-technicalSkillsfor-Surgeons(NOTSS)intheOperatingRoom%3ABehaviorsinHigh-performingTeams.

41. Royal College of Surgeons of Edinburgh. Non-Technical Skills for Surgoens (NOTSS). 2013. Available from: http://www.rcsed.ac.uk/education/educational-resources/non-technical-skills-for-surgeons-(notss).aspx.

42. Royal Australasian College of Surgeons. Non-Technical Skills for Surgeons (NOTSS). 2013. Available from: http://www.surgeons.org/for-health-professionals/register-courses-events/professional-development/non-technical-skills-for-surgeons/.

43. ISCP. Intercollegiate Surgical Curriculum Project. 2014 [Accessed September 30, 2014.] Available from: www.iscp.ac.uk/NewsItem.aspx?enc=ebUWfHYX2WIZtx94qKr4TR999rSVpGR+xzhQpUvFtdk=).

44. Yim H, Kim A, Seong P. Development of a quantitative evaluation method for non-technical skills preparedness of operation teams in nuclear power plants to deal with emergency conditions. *Nucl Eng Des.* 2013;255:212–25.

45. Gordon S. *Systematic Training Programme Design: Maximising Effectiveness and Minimizing Liability.* Englewood Cliffs, New Jersey: Prentice Hall; 1993.

46. Yule S, Flin R, Maran N, Rowley D, Youngson G, Paterson-Brown S. Surgeons' non-technical skills in the operating room: Reliability testing of the NOTSS behavior rating system. *World J Surg.* 2008 Apr;32(4):548–56.

47. Flanagan J. The critical incident technique. *Psychological Bulletin.* 1954;51(4):327–58.

48. Flin R, Yule S, Rowley D, Maran N, Paterson-Brown S. The non-technical skills for surgeons (NOTSS) system handbook v1.2: Structuring observation, rating and feedback of surgeons' behaviours in the operating theatre. Aberdeen, Scotland: University of Aberdeen; 2006.

49. Crossley J, Marriott J, Purdie H, Beard JD. Prospective observational study to evaluate NOTSS (Non-Technical Skills for Surgeons) for assessing trainees' non-technical performance in the operating theatre. *Brit J Surg.* 2011 Jul;98(7):1010–20.

50. Sharma B, Mishra A, Aggarwal R, Grantcharov TP. Non-technical skills assessment in surgery. *Surg Oncol.* 2011 Sep;20(3):169–77.

51. Dedy N, Zevin B, Bonrath E, Grantcharov T (Eds.). *Non-Technical Skills of Surgery Residents: Does Experiential Learning Lead to Competence?* Washington, DC: American College of Surgeons Clinical Congress; 2013.

52. Yule S (Ed.). *Non-Technical Skills Coaching Improves Surgical Residents' Operative Performance: Results from a Randomized Trial in a Simulated Operating Room.* Orlando, Florida: International Meeting on Medical Simulation; 2013.

53. Briggs A, Raja A, Joyce M, Yule S, Jiang W, Lipsitz S et al. (Eds.). *The Impact of Trauma Team Training on Team Leaders' Non-Technical Skills during Simulated Trauma Scenarios.* San Diego, California: Association for Academic Surgery; 2014.

54. Crossley J, Marriott J, Purdie H, Beard JD. Prospective observational study to evaluate NOTSS (Non-Technical Skills for Surgeons) for assessing trainees' non-technical performance in the operating theatre. *Brit J Surg.* 2011;98:1010–20.

55. Siu J, Maran N, Paterson-Brown S. Observation of behavioural markers of non-technical skills in the operating room and their relationship to intra-operative incidents. *Surgeon.* 2014 Jul 9. pii: S1479-666X(14)00075-4. doi: 10.1016/j.surge.2014.06.005. [Epub ahead of print]

56. Jackson S, Brackley K, Landau A, Hayes K. Assessing non-technical skills on the delivery suite: A pilot study. *Clin Teach.* 2014;11:375–80.

57. Pugh C, Cohen E, Kwan C, Cannon-Bowers J. A comparative assessment and gap analysis of commonly used team rating scales. *J Surg Res.* 2014;190:445–50.

58. Arora S, Miskovic D, Hull L, Moorthy K, Aggarwal R, Johannsson H et al. Self vs. expert assessment of technical and non-technical skills in high fidelity simulation. *Am J Surg.* 2011;202:500–6.

59. Kissane-Lee N, Fiedler A, Mazer L, Pozner C, Smink D, Yule S. *Coaching Surgical Residents on Leadership in a Simulated Operating Room: Randomized Controlled Trial.* American College of Surgeons Annual Clinical Congress, Washington, DC; 2013.

60. Dickinson I, Watters D, Graham I, Montgomery P, Collins J. Guide to the assessment of competence and performance in practicing surgeons. *ANZ J Surg.* 2009;79:198–204.

61. Swing S, Clyman S, Holmboe E. Advancing resident assessment in graduate medical education. *J Grad Med Educ.* 2009;1(2):278–86.

62. Mitchell L, Flin R, Yule S, Mitchell J, Coutts K, Youngson G. Thinking ahead of the surgeon. An interview study to identify scrub nurses' non-technical skills. *Int J Nurs Stud.* 2011 Jul;48(7):818–28.

63. Dietz A, Pronovost P, Benson K, Mendez-Tellez P, Dwyer C, Wyskiel R et al. A systematic review of behavioural marker systems in healthcare: What do we know about their attributes, validity and application? *BMJ Qual Saf.* 2014 (online first). doi:10.1136/bmjqs-2013-002457

64. Lewin K. *Field Theory in Social Science: Selected Theoretical Papers.* New York: Harper & Brothers Publishers; 1951. p. 169.

65. Endsley M. Toward a theory of situation awareness in dynamic systems. *Hum Factors.* 1995;37(1):32–64.

66. Flin R, Youngson G, Yule S. How do surgeons make intraoperative decisions? *Qual Saf Health Care.* 2007 Jun;16(3):235–9.

67. Jacklin R, Sevdalis N, Harries C. Judgment analysis: A method for quantitative evaluation of trainee surgeons' judgments of surgical risk. *Am J Surg.* 2008;195:183–8.

68. Pauley K, Flin R, Yule S, Youngson G. Surgeons' intraoperative decision making and risk management. *Am J Surg.* 2011 Oct;202(4):375–81.

69. Klein G. A recognition-primed decision (RPD) model of rapid decision making. In G. Klein, J. Orasanu, R. Calderwood (Eds.). *Decision Making in Action.* New York: Ablex; 1993. pp. 138–47.

70. Greenberg CC, Regenbogen SE, Studdert DM, Lipsitz SR, Rogers SO, Zinner MJ et al. Patterns of communication breakdowns resulting in injury to surgical patients. *J Am Coll Surg.* 2007 Apr;204(4):533–40.

71. Lingard L, Espin S, Whyte S, Regehr G, Baker G, Reznick R. Communication failures in the operating room: An observational classification of recurrent types and effects. *Qual Safe Health Care.* 2004;13:330–4.

72. Edmondson A. Speaking up in the operating room: How team leaders promote learning in interdisciplinary action teams. *J Manage Stud.* 2003;40:1419–52.

73. Henrickson Parker S, Yule S, Flin R, McKinley A. Towards a model of surgeons' leadership in the operating room. *BMJ Qual Saf.* 2011 Jul;20(7):570–9.

74. Yule S. Invited commentary: Speaking up in the OR. *J Am Coll Surg.* 2014;219(5):1007–9.

75. Barzallo Salazar M, Minkoff H, Bayya J, Gillett B, Onoriode H, Weedon J et al. Influence of surgeon behavior on trainee willingness to speak up: A randomized controlled trial. *J Am Coll Surg.* 2014;219(5):1001–7

76. Tsuburaya A. Non-technical skills for surgeons: Desired actions and skills for patient safety (Japanese). *Shukan Igakukai Shinbun* (Weekly Newspaper for Medicine). 2012 Aug 8 http://www.igaku-shoin.co.jp/paperDetail.do?id=PA02989_02.

77. Mitchell L, Flin R. Japanese translation of 'Scrub practitioners: List of intra-operative non-technical skills'. 2011. [Accessed April 19, 2015.] Available from: http://www.abdn.ac.uk/iprc/uploads/files/JapaneseSPLINTSHandbook.pdf.

78. Takahashi R. Introduction to non-technical skills training (Japanese). In K. Nakajima, Y. Kodama (Eds.). *Introduction to Patient Safety.* Tokyo, Japan: Igakushoin; 2010. pp. 35–53.

79. Youngson G. Teaching and assessing non-technical skill. *Surgeon.* 2011;9:S35–7.

80. Royal College of Surgeons of Edinburgh NOTSS Training Website. 2014. [Accessed September 30, 2014.] Available from: http://www.rcsed.ac.uk/NOTSS.

81. Hull L, Arora S, Symons NR, Jalil R, Darzi A, Vincent C et al. Training faculty in nontechnical skill assessment: National guidelines on program requirements. *Ann Surg.* 2013;Aug;258(2):370–5.

82. Brunckhorst O, Khan M, Dasgupta P, Ahmed K. Effective non-technical skills are imperative to robot-assisted surgery. *Br J Urol.* 2014 in press 10.1111/bju.12934

83. Spanager L, Lyk-Jensen H, Dieckmann P, Wettergren A, Rosenberg J, Østergaard D. Customization of a tool to assess Danish surgeons' non-technical skills in the operating room. *Danish Med J.* 2012;59(11):1–6.

84. Spanager L, Beier-Holgersen R, Dieckmann P, Konge L, Rosenberg J, Oestergaard D. Reliable assessment of general surgeons' non-technical skills based on video-recordings of patient simulated scenarios. *Am J Surg*. 2013;206:810–7.

85. Yule S, McRitchie A, DeBord-Smith A, Ross C, Charlesworth D, Malenka D et al. Situation Awareness in Low Cardiac Output Failure. Northern New England Cardiovascular Disease Group Spring meeting 2014, Portsmouth, NH.

86. Yule S, Smink D. Competency-based surgical care: Nontechnical skills in surgery. In Ashley S, ed., *ACS Surgery: Principles and Practice*. 2013. Hamilton, ON: Dekker Publishing.

87. National Board of Medical Examiners Stemmler Fund for Medical Education. 2014. [Accessed September 30, 2014.] Available from: http://www.nbme.org /research/grantsawarded.html.

88. Dedy N, Bonrath E, Zevin B, Grantcharov T. Teaching nontechnical skills in surgical residency: A systematic review of current approaches and outcomes. *Surgery*. 2013; Nov;154(5):1000–8

89. WHO. WHO patient safety curriculum guide: Multi-professional edition. 2014. [Accessed June 13, 2014.] Available from: http://whqlibdoc.who.int/publications /2011/9789241501958_eng.pdf?ua=1.

90. Livingston P, Bailey J, Ntakiyiruta G, Mukwesi C, Whynot S, Brindley P. Development of a simulation and skills centre in East Africa: A Rwandan-Canadian partnership. *Pan Afr Med J*. 2014;17:315.

91. Lane R. Surgical education & training in the COSECSA region. *East Central Afr J Surg*. 2009;14(1):1–12.

92. Choy I, Kitto S, Adu-Aryee N, Okrainec A. Barriers to the uptake of laparoscopic surgery in a lower-middle-income country. *Surg Endosc*. 2013; 27(11):4009–15.

93. Frehywot S, Vovides Y, Talib Z. E-learning in medical education in resource constrained low-and middle-income countries. *Hum Resour Health*. 2013;11(1):1.

94. RACS. *Surgical Competence and Performance: A Guide by the Royal Australasian College of Surgeons*. Department of Professional Standards. Melbourne, Australia: Royal Australasian College of Surgeons (RACS); 2008, 2012.

95. RACS. Royal Australaisian College of Surgeons: Non-Technical Skills for Surgeons (NOTSS). 2014. [Accessed September 30, 2014.] Available from: http://www.surgeons. org/for-health-professionals/register-courses-events/professional-development/ non-technical-skills-for-surgeons/.

96. Henrickson Parker S, Flin R, McKinley A, Yule S. The Surgeons' Leadership Inventory (SLI): A taxonomy and rating system for surgeons' intraoperative leadership skills. *Am J Surg*. 2013 Jun;205(6):745–51.

97. Henrickson Parker S, Flin R, McKinley A, Yule S. Factors influencing surgeons' intraoperative leadership: Analysis of unanticipated events in the operating room. *World J Surg*. 2014;38(1):4–10.

98. Gawande A. Personal best: Top athletes and singers have coaches. Should you? *The New Yorker*. October 3, 2011.

99. Hu YY, Peyre SE, Arriaga AF, Osteen RT, Corso KA, Weiser TG et al. Postgame analysis: Using video-based coaching for continuous professional development. *J Am Coll Surg*. 2012 Jan;214(1):115–24.

100. Flowerdew L, Gaunt A, Spedding J, Bhargava A, Briwn R, Vincent C et al. A multicenter observational study to evaluate a new tool to assess emergency physicians' non-technical skills. *Emerg Med J*. 2013;30:437–43.

PART II

Underpinning concepts

Situation awareness

RHONA FLIN AND SIMON PATERSON-BROWN

The neck of the gallbladder led straight into the tube we were eyeing. So it had to be the right duct. We had exposed a good length of it without a sign of the main bile duct. Everything looked perfect, we agreed. 'Go for it', the attending [surgeon] said.

I slipped in the clip applier … I got the jaws around the duct and was about to fire when my eye caught on the screen, a little globule of fat lying on the top of the duct. That wasn't necessarily anything unusual, but somehow it didn't look right. With the top of the clip applier, I tried to flick it aside, but instead of a little globule, a whole layer of thin unseen tissue came up, and, underneath, we saw that the duct had a fork in it. My heart dropped. If not for that extra fastidiousness, I would have clipped off the main bile duct.

General surgeon[1]

4.1 INTRODUCTION

Situation awareness for a surgeon can be simply explained as 'knowing where you are and what is going on around you'. The aforementioned example illustrates what a critical skill this is for surgeons while operating – to be continuously gathering correct information, making sense of it and anticipating what could go wrong.

The definition of situation awareness for surgeons in the Non-Technical Skills for Surgeons (NOTSS) handbook is: 'Developing and maintaining a dynamic awareness of the situation in the operating room based on assembling data from the environment (patient, team, time, displays, equipment); understanding what they mean, and thinking ahead about what may happen next'. In Chapter 5 on decision making, we also use the closely related term 'situation assessment' to refer

Table 4.1 NOTSS elements of situation awareness

Category	Elements
Situation awareness	Gathering information
	Understanding information
	Projecting and anticipating future state

to the focused evaluation signalled by a change of state in a task that is normally the first part of the decision-making process.

The term situation awareness was first used in military operations, 'gaining an awareness of the enemy before the enemy gained a similar awareness',[2] and it was applied in commercial aviation before being adopted in anaesthesia[3] and in surgery.[4] Situation awareness encompasses the cognitive skills of perception and attention: a continuous monitoring of the task environment, noticing what is going on, detecting any significant changes and anticipating how the situation might develop. This book concentrates on an individual surgeon's skills when operating; therefore, this chapter refers only to cognition during a procedure and does not consider the earlier stage of clinical assessment. Of course, any knowledge gained in the preoperative stage will affect the surgeon's thinking once an invasive procedure has begun.

The component elements in NOTSS for a surgeon's situation awareness are shown in Table 4.1, and these will be discussed in turn.

Section 4.1.1 describes how surgeons have begun to apply this term in their work; then, we examine how the brain processes information, which is followed by a model of situation awareness in a surgical context. After that, we consider the factors that influence a surgeon's intraoperative situation awareness and show how it can be enhanced or diminished.

4.1.1 IDENTIFYING SITUATION AWARENESS IN SURGERY

It goes without saying that surgeons carrying out any operation require a high level of attentional skill, perhaps more so in highly complex procedures than in simpler, routine ones. However, erroneous situation awareness can occur during any operation and perhaps might be more likely in the more routine ones. In a study of 252 laparoscopic bile duct injuries examined for causes relating to 'visual perception, judgement and human error', Way et al.[4] found that the errors stemmed almost entirely (97%) from surgeons' misperception (i.e. incorrect situation awareness) rather than problems related to technical skill or judgement. Furthermore, in 22% of cases the operation was documented as 'routine' and in 75% the surgeons completed the operation without being aware that the common bile duct had been injured. A later study of 42 cases of duct misidentification found that underestimation of risk, cue ambiguity and visual perception ('seeing what you believe') were important factors in misidentification.[5] It is only recently that surgeons

I forced myself to return to the operating theatre and looked into the bloody wound, cautiously exploring it, dreading what I might find. It became apparent that my registrar had completely misunderstood the anatomy and opened the spine at the outer rather than the inner edge of the spinal canal and hence had immediately encountered a nerve root, which, even more incomprehensibly he had then severed. It was an utterly bizarre thing to have done, especially as he had seen dozens of these operations done before, and done many unsupervised on his own. 'I think you've cut straight through the nerve – a complete neurotmesis', I said sadly to my dumb-struck assistant.

Neurosurgeon[10]

When the call came, the doc said, 'You're not going to believe this: now he has a pneumo on the other side'. Looking at the new pictures, it was obvious what I and everyone else had missed earlier: the original x-ray had been put up backwards. The kid's weakened muscles caused his back to curve, skewing his chest and displacing his heart to the right, and the air under pressure in the left chest had made the distortion even worse. Lots of people take a casual look at a chest x-ray and put it on the viewer making sure the heart is on the left, where it belongs; in this case, that casual move caused the x-ray to be flipped. Now, knowing what side the tube was on, it was apparent that the picture had been put up correctly. So there it was: the air pocket on the left, where it had been all the time.

General surgeon[11]

have begun to use the label 'situation awareness' to describe these cognitive processes for the individual surgeon[6] or for the whole surgical team[7–9] (see Chapter 6). Although surgeons may not know this term, most should be able to recall what inaccurate situation awareness feels like, as well as appreciating the consequences.

Retrospective accounts by surgeons when problems related to erroneous situation awareness have occurred might include comments such as the following:

- 'I didn't realise that she had been losing so much blood ... '
- 'We were very surprised when we noticed bile leaking from the area ... '
- 'I didn't notice that we had dissected so close to the ... '
- 'I was so busy attending to the message from the ward that I ... '

- 'I wasn't aware that the retractor had caught the hilum of the spleen ... '
- 'We were convinced that the structure we had isolated was the cystic duct ... '

As can be seen from the elements in Table 4.1, situation awareness is about the surgeon gathering and processing information from the operative site and the theatre environment and using stored memories to make sense of it. A basic model of the human brain's information-processing system is presented in Section 4.2. The cognitive architecture helps to explain both the strengths and the limitations of situation awareness.

4.2 HUMAN MEMORY SYSTEM

The human brain functions as a sophisticated information-processing machine. Although often likened to a computer, there are some tasks that a computer can do much more efficiently, e.g. rapid calculations, and others where the brain is the superior processor, e.g. learning from experience. As there is too much information available in the environment at any one time for the brain to process, humans attend selectively to some things rather than others. The selection is driven partly by the environment, e.g. a sudden noise or change in light attracts attention, but we are also guided by past experience. That is, information stored in memory directs attention to certain cues in the environment, thought to be meaningful or important. This selective attention process essentially forms the basis of situation awareness.

The memory system has been systematically studied since psychology began over 100 years ago. Research into memory capacity and function has resulted in an accepted model of cognitive architecture – the structure of the brain's storage and information-processing system. In essence, there are three linked systems: sensory memory, short-term or working memory, and long-term memory.

4.2.1 SENSORY MEMORY

The sensory memory holds incoming information for very brief periods of time: the iconic memory retains a visual image for about half a second, and for acoustic signals the echoic store lasts for about 2 seconds.[12] We are rarely aware of these transient stores, but when an image persists briefly after the visual stimulus has been removed this is sensory memory. We appear to have little conscious control of these stores; however, the persistence effect provides extra time to process incoming information.

4.2.2 WORKING MEMORY

Of more significance to situation awareness and decision making is the second memory store, which was earlier labelled short-term memory but is now called working memory (Figure 4.1). Working memory essentially contains conscious awareness – it is a limited capacity store (akin to the desktop or working space on a computer). Psychologists used to teach that short-term memory held around seven pieces of information.[13] This was based on memorizing lists of random numbers, but these actually contain minimal information per bit and longer lists could be recalled if the digits were chunked into meaningful units (e.g. familiar dates or dialling codes). More recently, neuroscience has confirmed that the average capacity of working memory is closer to three to five meaningful items.[14]

Maintaining information in working memory is particularly important when engaged in safety-critical tasks. However, working memory not only has a limited storage capacity but is also fragile. Repetition, mental rehearsal or some other kind of intense concentration is required to hold information in working memory (e.g. remembering a number list); otherwise, the memory trace will rapidly decay and the content will be forgotten.

Each person has a certain cognitive capacity for picking up new information and maintaining mental awareness of it (the amount can change depending on conditions). The working memory store may

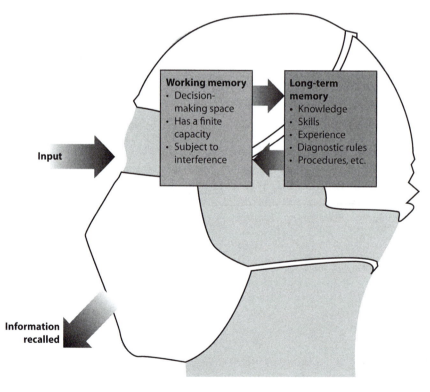

Figure 4.1 Memory stores.

be likened to the capacity of a vessel, such as a beaker. The present information load is represented by the liquid: when the beaker is not full, the person can still manage to attend to incoming information (more liquid). The type of image shown in Figure 4.2 is sometimes used in situation awareness training to represent this metaphor. But when the container is full, no new material can be added unless some of the existing content is removed or displaced. The ideal mental state for surgeons is to have some spare capacity in their working memory in case the information load they have to cope with suddenly rises.

When working memory is about to reach capacity, 'task shedding' may have to take place so that concentration is prioritized and maintained on the most important information. Flitter,[15] a

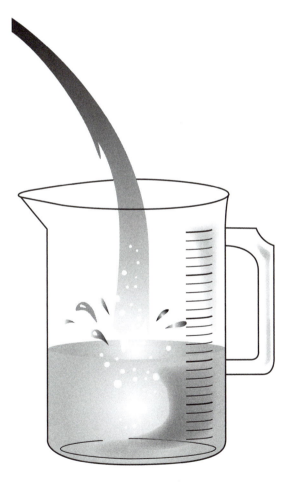

Figure 4.2 Jug represents total situation awareness capacity; liquid represents information and current mental load.

neurosurgeon, describes this level of attention: 'Each individual blood vessel, each single fiber of tissue became the object of attention, determining sequential efforts. Distance was traversed in millimeters rather than inches. Even the sounds in the operating theatre were muted by that view, as if hearing were partly visual.' This surgeon is reducing his attention to the background noise as he focuses his thinking onto the visual image of the operative site. A surgeon asking for quiet, or for music to be turned off, may be trying to protect working memory capacity by minimizing extraneous auditory information – that is, reducing processing capacity.

Again, due to cognitive overload, surgeons may experience nominal aphasia when concentrating on a procedure.

> ... if I'm really concentrating hard on a task, I'll forget the names of instruments I use every day.
>
> *Surgeon*
>
> ... when they [surgeons] ask for something and you give them what you think it is that they need and it's not the thing they said but you know it is what they actually want.
>
> *Scrub nurse*
>
> The surgeon said "give me the buzzy thing" ....
>
> *Scrub nurse[16]*

If a surgeon (or indeed any other member of the operating team) is working through a series of steps in a procedure, then they are using their working memory store to hold the information. Mental arithmetic, such as that required by scrub practitioners to count surgical instruments, makes heavy use of working memory. When an individual engaged in this type of cognitive activity is distracted or interrupted, he or she may forget which steps have been completed. In effect, the new information contained in the distraction erases the material that the working memory store was holding. Knowing when and how to preserve information in working memory is a key aspect of maintaining situation awareness. Distraction is discussed in Section 4.4.

Sometimes, it is necessary to use working memory to hold information about future actions. This is known as prospective memory (e.g. to perform an incidental appendicectomy after an exploratory operation for a different problem or remembering to remove the gall bladder for gallstones in a patient undergoing a radical gastrectomy for cancer, which is in itself a procedure that takes several hours and requires intense concentration and at the end will undoubtedly be associated with some mental fatigue on all sides). In a simulator study with medical students, 26% (73) of intentions to do something at a later time were missed.[17]

With expertise, surgical tasks (e.g. performing an anastomosis) become more automatic – the procedures and actions are well known and easily retrieved from long-term memory. Therefore, this frees up working memory to attend to other tasks, such as instructing a trainee or talking to the anaesthetist, as there is less need for conscious processing to attend to the well-practised tasks. However, such automatic behaviour can cause other problems relating to assumptions and expectations, as in Section 4.3.2.

4.2.3 LONG-TERM MEMORY

The main memory store is called long-term memory. This is a huge repository for all kinds of information the surgeon has acquired and stored over the years (akin to a computer hard drive). It retains personal memories of events (episodic memory), as well as declarative (facts) and procedural knowledge. Semantic memory holds personal likes and dislikes, language and how to perform tasks such as driving or operating – in fact, everything the individual knows. At any moment in time, only a small fraction of this memory store is accessed. For situation awareness, information is being retrieved from the long-term memory store as its relevance to incoming information is recognized, some of which will be transferred into working memory. Certain types of information are easier to recall from long-term memory, e.g. if it is familiar; was recently accessed; or is unusual, salient or of particular personal interest.

4.3 MODEL OF SITUATION AWARENESS

The diagram in Figure 4.3 represents a widely accepted model of situation awareness.[18] The component levels correspond to the three elements shown in Table 4.1.

The three stages (levels) of situation awareness are shown in a linear fashion but in reality will operate in repeating cycles. These are illustrated

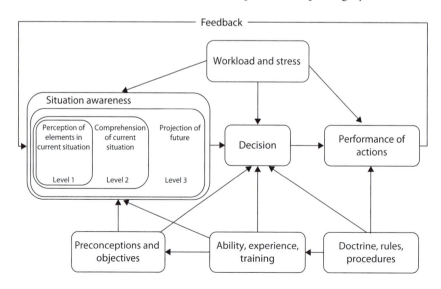

Figure 4.3 Model of situation awareness. (From Endsley M, *Hum Factors*, 37, 32–64, 1995. With permission.)

Table 4.2 Examples of surgeons' situation awareness

Level of situation awareness	Consultant surgeons' statements
Gathering information/perception	'The bone was extremely soft'. 'The spinal fluid was still leaking out'. 'We took the swabs off to find that it was pouring blood'.
Understanding information/ comprehension	'I thought that the most likely thing was that the patient was becoming coagulopathic'. 'It is two hours into the operation and what we do is review the x-rays and stop the operation'. 'Having thought about the situation, we decided …'.
Projection and anticipation	'What we're trying to avoid is …'. 'We decided that it would be technically very difficult to repair the hole in the lining of the spinal canal'.

Source: Flin R et al., Qual Saf Health Care, 16:235–239, 2007.

in Table 4.2 with quotations from interviews with general and orthopaedic surgeons describing challenging cases.[19]

The aforementioned model also indicates factors that can influence situation awareness, such as preconceptions and expectations, experience and task workload. As mentioned earlier, the resulting assessment of the situation usually precedes decision making, which is also influenced by organizational rules and cultural factors. Each of the three elements (levels) of situation awareness (essentially what, so what and now what) are discussed in the following three sections with reference to intraoperative surgery.

4.3.1 GATHERING INFORMATION

The first element of the situation awareness category in NOTSS is gathering information. At the preoperative stage in the operating room, use of the checklist and pre-task briefing help to ensure that basic information (e.g. patient identity, site marking and procedure) is located and shared. Once the procedure has started, this skill element requires attending to visual information, such as the operative field, to understand the anatomy; noticing the position of instruments; monitoring screens, level of blood loss and assistants'/nurses' behaviour; as well as listening to auditory information from alarms, conversation between anaesthetists and sounds of equipment. There will also be attention to tactile information, checking the strength of tissue, level of pulsation or tension of sutures. Kinaesthetic and olfactory information may also provide clues: a sudden smell of faeces suggests an inadvertent bowel injury. Essentially, the surgeon has the opportunity to continuously collect information from the operative field and the theatre environment to monitor the status of the patient, procedure and team's performance. Whether the surgeon picks up all this information will depend on his or her alertness, background noise (distractions) and relationship and understanding with the other members of the operating team. Depending on the task, the surgeon may often need to communicate with other team members to gain the required information. For instance, in cardiac surgery involving cardio pulmonary bypass, the perfusionist (P) will hold key information that the surgeon (S) requires, as the following dialogue recorded by Hazlehurst et al.[8] illustrates:

0:00 s S: Give cardioplegia. Green off.
    P: Green is off.
0:12 s S: Empty the heart.
    S: The heart's full for some reason.
    P: I think that's the way you've got it cranked [kinked].
    S: Not now. I've got a straight shot. Still full.
    P: Emptying out?
    S: It is now.
    P: OK.
    S: Are you holding volume?
    P: No.

The essential role of communication for gathering information and sharing it to achieve a common understanding within a team is discussed in Chapter 6.

In summary, the surgeon has to use many sources to acquire the necessary information before building an interpretation of the situation as illustrated in the next section later.

In the NOTSS system, sample behaviours are given for each element of situation awareness, and Table 4.3 gives examples of behaviours that indicate good or poor situation awareness at the information-gathering stage.

Surgical information gathering: mid-case

When I am trying to cross-clamp the aorta during an operation for a leaking aortic aneurysm, I am **feeling** for the neck with my fingers, pushing the left renal vein away and assessing whether I will need to clamp above the renal arteries. I am **listening** to the anaesthetist's update on the patient's condition and continually **watching** the blood pressure on the monitor, **observing** the response to cross-clamping. In some long, difficult and protracted cases I might even begin to **smell** the early scent of ischaemic bowel.

Vascular surgeon

Attention to small cues (weak signals) and recognizing anomalies are a very important part of the information-gathering phase, even in a routine case that appears to be going to plan, as the quote at the opening of this chapter illustrates. There are many reasons why a surgeon could fail to perceive all the information needed during an operation,[18] such as the following:

- The information was not available.
- The significant cues were difficult to detect.
- There was a failure to notice information that was present.
- Misperception of data.

There are many examples of problems that can occur at the information-gathering stage, for example, narrowing of attention (sometimes called tunnel vision, perceptual set or a fixation error). This happens when attention is so focused on one aspect of the situation that there is a failure to notice other cues, even if they are salient or important. In one anaesthetic fatality, the doctors were so focused on trying to intubate the patient that they failed to notice that a critical amount of time had passed and that she had become dangerously hypoxic.[20] Similarly, surgeons may spend a lot more time than they realize trying to stop bleeding, resulting in significant blood loss, when packing and reassessing the situation would be more appropriate. Attention can easily be distracted

Table 4.3 Behavioural markers for gathering information element (from NOTSS)

Good behaviours	Poor behaviours
Carries out pre-operative checks of patient notes, including investigations and consent	Arrives in theatre late or has to be repeatedly called
Ensures that all relevant/investigations (e.g. imaging) have been reviewed and are available	Does not ask for results until the last minute or not at all
Liaises with anaesthetist regarding anaesthetic plan for patient	Does not consider the views of operating room staff
Optimises operating conditions before starting, e.g. moves table, lights, AV equipment	Fails to listen to anaesthetist
Identifies anatomy/pathology clearly	Fails to review information collected by team
Monitors ongoing blood loss	Asks for information to be read from patient notes during procedure because it has not been read before operation started
Asks anaesthetist for update	

Note: Gathering information refers to seeking information in the operating theatre from operative findings, theatre environment, equipment and people.
AV: audiovisual.

Fixation in surgery

A surgeon is dissecting lymph nodes from the region of the common hepatic artery during a radical gastrectomy. He encounters some minor but persistent bleeding from some lymphatic tissue, which he tries to control. The patient has a large liver, which continually falls down and obscures the view. He asks the assistant to retract (the liver) harder but fails to notice that in so doing the assistant is tearing the liver capsule until suddenly a split in the liver occurs and profuse bleeding ensues. The surgeon had become so fixated on trying to deal with some minor bleeding from lymphatic tissue (which could easily have been controlled with a swab/sponge and dealt with later) that he failed to notice how hard the assistant was pulling on the liver.

from monitoring essential cues because the surgeon is cognitively busy thinking about another aspect of the task to the point of becoming fixated.

It is surprisingly easy to demonstrate the fallibility of human perceptual and memory systems. One type of attentional failure, particularly relevant to dynamic environments, is 'change blindness', where observers fail to notice that key elements have been altered between presentations of the same image. Psychologist Daniel Simons has demonstrated this in a range of intriguing studies.[21] In one of his experiments,[22] a pedestrian was stopped in the street by a stranger who asked for directions. While the directions were being given, some workmen walked between the two people with a huge board so that the stranger could not be seen for a brief period. Astonishingly, half of those giving directions failed to notice that the stranger had been switched for a different person, after the board had been removed. The same effect applies to auditory stimuli, which is called inattentional deafness.[23] For those surgeons who like some low-level background music in their operating theatre, it often comes as quite a surprise when they relax from some task that has required intense concentration to find that they never heard any of the

music despite the fact that it was clearly audible to everyone else in the theatre. This is the task shedding mentioned in Section 4.2.2, but sometimes it can be critical information that is missed or de-prioritized.

We normally engage in some degree of self-monitoring of our current state of awareness or at least notice when we have stopped gathering information relevant to the task in hand. If you have been reading this book and suddenly realized that you have not taken in any of the last three paragraphs, this reveals not only mind wandering but also activation of this monitoring function. Mind wandering or 'zoning out'[24] is when one mentally drifts away from the task in hand 'towards unrelated inner thoughts, fantasies, feelings and other musings'.[24] This 'daydreaming' is a very common experience. It is a form of distraction, but attention shifts to inner thoughts rather than to a different external stimulus. To date, mind wandering has been mainly studied in the laboratory; but for jobs that can involve periods of vigilant monitoring, such as that of anaesthetists, there are clear safety implications. Although zoning out is unlikely to occur for the operating surgeon, surgical assistants may fall into such a state, particularly in long and tedious (for them) operations.

4.3.2 UNDERSTANDING INFORMATION

At the second stage, 'comprehension of the current situation', the surgeon has to process the incoming information to understand what is going on and to appreciate the significance of the cues that have been gathered. If you are operating and suddenly notice intense activity at the end of the table, with the anaesthetist asking for drugs/blood, the circulating nurse being called to help and a new tone from the anaesthetic monitors, these cues together will probably lead you to conclude that an anaesthetic problem is occurring. However, experience might also lead you to reassess where you are in the operation and what might have happened surgically to produce the flurry of activity around the anaesthetist, such as occult, or unnoticed, blood loss or a pneumothorax. The interpretation of the combination of cues is based on knowledge stored in long-term memory as to what patterns of information mean and signify in terms of response. Humans are skilled at pattern matching. So, for an expert this process happens very quickly and with little conscious processing (i.e. limited use of working memory); thus, it feels automatic. But our interpretation of information can also be easily distorted by prior information, context and other factors.

In the operating room, experienced surgeons quickly learn to recognize and comprehend streams of information from the surgical site, monitoring equipment, behaviour of anaesthetists and so on. 'I heard the anaesthetist asking quietly for atropine, and therefore immediately realised that the patient must have developed a bradycardia which might be related to excessive intra-abdominal pressure' (during the early part of a laparoscopic procedure). This process of categorization and comprehension is facilitated by 'mental models', that is, knowledge structures ('schemas') stored in memory that represent particular combinations of cues and their meaning. This could be the anatomy of the lungs, a mental map of the operating suite, the structure of a device (e.g. diathermy), a sequence of task activities or a set of behavioural responses. These schemas are generalized prototypes of classes of things or events rather than specific and detailed representations of every single previous encounter. The following example shows how various cues in combination are used by a surgeon and an anaesthetist to recognize a problem, i.e. make a diagnosis.

Table 4.4 lists on the left side a selection of behaviours that indicate that the surgeon has a good comprehension of what is happening from the available information. On the right side, surgeon's actions that would suggest there is an inadequate understanding of the current situation are listed.

The surgeon's mental model produces expectations about the characteristics of a given situation. With a store of mental models for familiar tasks, a situation does not need to be an exact match to a previous event to be recognized, but it needs to present enough features for a categorization into type. Novices (e.g. junior trainee surgeons) have fewer and less rich mental models. They have to spend more time and mental energy trying to comprehend patterns of cues by a conscious process of systematic analysis and comparison with possible interpretations. Experienced practitioners faced with novel situations also have to

---

Pattern recognition of a problem

When coming off cardio-pulmonary bypass the patient is given protamine to reverse the anticoagulant effects of heparin. If the patient rapidly develops hypotension and tachycardia, the experienced surgeon and anaesthetist will immediately recognise an adverse/allergic reaction to the protamine has occurred and take appropriate steps. Delay in responding is associated with a high mortality and early recognition and treatment essential for a good outcome.

Cardiac surgeon

Table 4.4 Behavioural markers for understanding information element (from NOTSS)

Good behaviours	Poor behaviours
Acts according to information gathered from previous investigation and operative findings	Overlooks or ignores important results
Looks at CT scan and points out relevant area	Misses clear sign (e.g. on CT scan)
Reflects and discusses significance of information	Asks questions which demonstrate lack of understanding
	Discards results that don't 'fit the picture'

Note: Understanding information refers to interpreting the information gathered from the environment and comparing it with existing knowledge to identify the match or mismatch between the situation and the expected state and update one's mental model.

CT: computed tomography.

interpret situations by using significant mental effort (a process that places a high load on working memory).

> ... One of the things he felt he was good at was spotting potential disaster long before anyone else could see it coming – recognizing those minor glitches and anticipating how they would inevitably slide into major ones if they weren't corrected at once. He seemed to have the whole operation mapped out in his mind, and if it began to diverge from the imagined version in his head – a picture of what he'd envisaged happening held over what was actually happening – he could compensate or jig it back onto its track before proceeding.
>
> *Journalist describing a paediatric cardiac surgeon[25]*

As illustrated earlier, the mental model enables the surgeon to (1) direct attention to critical cues, (2) form anticipations regarding future states (including what to expect, as well as what not to expect) based on the projection mechanisms of the model and (3) rapidly make links between recognized types of situations and typical actions.[18]

Military friendly fire (blue on blue) accidents powerfully illustrate the effects of expectations on perception.[26] In northern Iraq in 1994, two American fighter planes erroneously shot down two of their own Black Hawk helicopters carrying 26 peacekeepers. They believed that only enemy aircraft would be present in the sector they were patrolling. 'There is little doubt that what the F-15 pilots expected to see during their visual pass [i.e. enemy Hind aircraft] influenced what they actually saw'. One pilot said, 'I had no doubt when I looked at him that he was a Hind. The Black Hawk did not even cross my mind when I made that visual identification'.[26] An obvious surgical example relates to inadvertently dividing a structure that you do not expect to encounter because of where you think you are: the recurrent laryngeal nerve in thyroid surgery, common bile duct during gall bladder surgery or ureter during a hemi-colectomy.

The mental model for a given task or situation is formed from not only experience but also prior information (e.g. scans, case notes and briefing). The surgical checklist is a type of pre-job briefing designed to ensure that those involved not only check patient identity against the planned procedure but also have an idea of what is to be done, what the risks are, how the risks might be minimized and any specific equipment that might be required. Of course, if the briefing is not accurate, then the wrong mental model may be activated or created, as some surgical never events have unfortunately demonstrated.

Another risk is building a mental model and then failing to review or alter it in the face of incoming information that disagrees with it. In such situations, there is a danger of 'confirmation bias' by accepting only new information that agrees with the active mental model and discarding that which disagrees with it. When the model is in fact wrong for the present situation but incoming information is interpreted as being compatible, 'bending the facts to fit' occurs. It is therefore essential to review the current mental model regularly in the light of any new incoming information to update it and, where necessary, revise the model.

Confirmation bias may have occurred in the hours before the catastrophic blowout on the *Deepwater Horizon* drilling rig in the Gulf of Mexico in 2010, which killed 11 workers and caused an enormous oil spill. The drill crew was running negative pressure tests to confirm that the well was secure, but they became puzzled by a set of anomalous readings. One of the drillers said that these could be explained by a 'bladder effect'.[27] The accident investigation revealed that experienced drilling engineers had never heard of this effect, yet the explanation appeared to provide a plausible mental model for the drill crew who were trying to comprehend why the new readings were still suggesting that the well was not entirely protected.

Confirmation bias may be more likely when one interpretation of the situation spells undesired consequences and/or a significant amount of additional work. For example, a surgeon assessing the anastomosis after a bowel resection may ignore incoming information such as tension and dusky colour, both of which, taken to their logical conclusion, might suggest that the whole anastomosis should be taken down and redone. This is not an easy decision to make at the end of a long and arduous operation. With experience, surgeons gain more and richer mental models of situations and tasks that they acquire over years of work. They also learn the consequences of failing to pay heed to subtle indications during a procedure that their mental model might have to be revised.

When failure to comprehend the situation occurs, there could be multiple reasons, such as[18]

- Lack of/inadequate mental model
- Selecting the wrong mental model
- Over-reliance on default values in the model
- Memory failure when attempting to develop a new model

A key component of understanding an operational situation is the estimation of inherent risk and, not surprisingly, this is influenced by experience, as has been shown for both airline[28] and military[29] pilots. A recent study of surgeons[30] describes sources of information that may signal intraoperative risks or 'threats'—these were related to the patient (unusual anatomy, lack of [or excess] adiposity, adhesions from prior surgery, uncertainty about patient's condition and unexpected findings) and to the task (inaccurate test results, time pressure, visiting surgeons watching the operation and visibility problems associated with laparoscopic surgery or unexpected blood loss). Surgeons also described facing risks from the operating environment (inappropriate patient position and unavailable or broken equipment), from the team (communication problems and undue deference) and from individual staff members (inexperienced assistants and bravado). Trainee surgeons need to learn which cues will be most informative when building their mental models, thus enabling them to make more rapid and more accurate intraoperative risk assessments.

4.3.3 PROJECTING AND ANTICIPATING FUTURE STATE

The third element of situation awareness is projection and anticipation of what might happen next. An understanding of the present status coupled with stored knowledge of previous operations enables the surgeon to think ahead about how the situation is likely to develop in the immediate future. This could be preoperatively recognizing that a big hernia will need a very large mesh, a gastroscope might be used to identify the site of a lesion in the stomach or a colostomy may be required in large bowel surgery.

This anticipatory stage of situation awareness has been described as 'mental simulation of future system state and behaviour to eliminate surprises. On the one hand, the resulting expectancies may facilitate perception because they can make it easier to remain vigilant and to adequately allocate attention. On the other hand, they involve the potential for ignoring or misinterpreting the unexpected'.[31] While operating, this could be understanding that if a certain anatomy is associated with invasion of other structures that are nearby and if dissection continues then major bleeding or injury may occur. For safe execution of a surgical procedure, a surgeon must always be able to think ahead of the current state and anticipate what might happen later in the operation if certain decisions are made.

> A good surgeon [...] can think three dimensionally, knowing how everything is gonna fit together, thinking about all these factors while he's doing each step, thinking three steps ahead about how one thing will affect another, concentrating not just on the thing he's doing but on the things he's gonna be doing.
>
> *Physician's assistant describing a paediatric cardiac surgeon[25]*
>
> If dissection continues and bleeding occurs, vascular clamps may be required, so I ask for them to be got ready in anticipation. Or if I continue here, I might damage the common bile duct, so instead I will change direction and do a sub-total cholecystectomy.
>
> *General surgeon*

Table 4.5 gives sample behaviours from NOTSS indicating that the surgeon is thinking ahead

Table 4.5 Behavioural markers for projecting and anticipating future state element

Good behaviours	Poor behaviours
Plans operating list, taking into account potential delays due to surgical or anaesthetic challenges	Overconfident manoeuvres with no regard for what may go wrong
Verbalises what equipment may be required later in operation	Does not discuss potential problems
Shows evidence of having a contingency plan ('plan B') (e.g. by asking scrub nurse for potentially required equipment to be available in theatre)	Gets into predictable blood loss, then tells anaesthetist
	Waits for a predicted problem to arise before responding
Cites contemporary literature on anticipated clinical event	Operates beyond level of experience

Note: Projecting and anticipating future states refers to predicting what may happen in the near future as a result of possible actions, interventions or nonintervention.

and anticipating or samples of 'Poor behaviours', where the surgeon is apparently not doing this adequately.

Trainee surgeons have to learn that they must be able to predict the effects of their actions considering the consequences and risks of each step of a procedure and always having a backup plan in place. Failures in situation awareness for trainees can be due to the lack of or an inadequate mental model or simply not thinking far enough ahead of the present situation. Common 'warning signals' derived from other professions (aviation[32] and firefighting[33]) that can indicate that you, your trainee or even the whole team could be 'losing' the correct situation awareness would also apply to surgeons. A list of these follows:

Ambiguity: information from two or more sources does not agree (e.g. it looks like the ureter but it does not seem to vermiculate).
Fixation: focusing on one thing (e.g. adjusting a tool) to the exclusion of everything else.
Lack of required information (e.g. when locating a structure).
Failure to maintain critical tasks (e.g. regular review to assess blood loss).
Failure to reach an expected point in a procedure at the anticipated time.
Failure to resolve discrepancies: contradictory data and disagreements.
Confusion: uncertainty about a situation (accompanied by a sense of unease).
A gut feeling that things are not quite right.

4.4 INFLUENCING FACTORS

Cognitive processes, such as situation awareness, are influenced by a number of what can be called 'performance-shaping' factors. Some of these are shown in Figure 4.3.

Two prime factors are fatigue and stress, both of which can reduce the quality of situation awareness. When fatigued, speed and capacity for acquiring and processing new information can be reduced. Less information can be held in working memory (conscious awareness), and it may be more difficult to retain. In medicine, it has been shown that reducing hours of work (and therefore fatigue) was associated with reduced errors.[34] Stress has a similar detrimental effect, partly because preoccupation with personal problems takes up attentional resources. Fatigue and stress are discussed in Chapter 8.

Environmental factors can also affect the surgeon's situation awareness. Operating rooms can be noisy places and this can have an impact on surgeons' ability to hear what is being said, especially when music is being played.[35] Distractions and interruptions (such as phones ringing and doors opening with people coming in and going out) occur surprisingly frequently.[36,37] These have also been documented during resuscitations.[38] One recent study in urology demonstrated that on average one distraction occurred every 10 minutes and an associated reduction in compliance with intraoperative safety checks.[39] When distraction has occurred during a sequence of actions, it is suggested to 'back up' a few steps to ensure the task sequence has been maintained.

Protecting situation awareness for oneself and for other team members may require the surgeon to control some of these environmental or social factors. For instance, not distracting or interrupting co-workers who are trying to retain information in working memory (e.g. scrub nurses counting instruments and an anaesthetist drawing up drugs) is an important part of teamworking. Ward nurses wearing tabards printed with 'DISPENSING DRUGS. DO NOT INTERRUPT' is an attempt to protect their situation awareness during a safety-critical task. In the aviation sector, where distraction has been recognized as a significant hazard, there is advice on how to manage this.[40] Trainee surgeons are even more likely to have their situation awareness disrupted by distraction than experienced seniors. However, higher expertise does not guarantee immunity from distraction and it can be compounded by an emotional response, such as annoyance, that diminishes the surgeon's concentration, as the following example illustrates:

'Save this bone', was what I typically announced to the scrub nurse when beginning the decompression stage of a posterior lateral autologous instrumented lumbar fusion. The procedure involves harvesting small fragments of posterior spinous process and lamina in order to remove pressure from the underlying nerves within the lumbar spinal canal. This portion of the operation may take up to an hour or more, requires continual attention under the operating microscope to prevent damaging the nerves as the bone is removed. Slowly the container in which the nurse was storing the bone fragments filled up with the irreplaceable biological matrix which form the basis for a successful fusion. Having successfully completed the decompression, I asked for the morsels of bone to be returned to me for return to the patient in the fusion bed. As if in slow motion, the container seemed to depart from the hands of the scrub nurse onto the floor as if that had been the plan all along. I could not overcome my distress at what had occurred, my disappointment with the scrub nurse, and the limitations I was now facing in securing the adequate bony fusion that was required to lessen the risk of the screws and rods construct requiring further surgery. This repetitive litany of disappointment and anger, frustration and uncertainty was sufficient to distract me from adequately tightening the locking caps that hold the rods to the pedicle screws in a secure fashion. Neither my surgical assistant nor the scrub nurse pointed out that we had failed to torque these locking caps to their appropriate tension. The surgery was completed after I had harvested a smaller amount of bone for the fusion and the patient was taken into the recovery room. His hospital course appeared uneventful, his wound healed and several weeks later I saw him in the office in a follow-up appointment. 'I hear a click', was how he greeted me in the examining room. Sure enough, I could hear it as well when he repositioned himself on the table.

Neurosurgeon

4.5 TRAINING SITUATION AWARENESS

It is debatable whether basic cognitive capacity and processing speed can be altered by training. However, one study with airline pilots indicated that suitable instructional materials could enhance their situation awareness skills.[41] This kind of training usually focuses on learning the most informative cues, pattern recognition to build richer mental models and practising techniques for effectively gathering information (e.g. scanning instruments) or multitasking or protecting situation awareness. The use of check-lists, briefings or other cognitive aids can also be included as part of the instruction. Guidelines for training situation awareness are available, mostly developed for aviation[32,42] or anaesthesia,[3] although see Graafland et al.[43] for a recent surgical review.

Surgeons are now receiving training on situation awareness, usually as part of non-technical skills (or Crew Resource Management) courses (see Chapter 9). The module on situation awareness is typically designed to achieve an increased level of knowledge and self-awareness by teaching the kind of cognitive material contained in this chapter. Where operating room simulation facilities or task trainers are available, these can be used to practise the development and maintenance of situation awareness when operating. Specific cues and events can be manipulated in simulations, along with levels of workload and distracting conditions. A 'freeze' technique can be used when the scenario is paused and participants are asked to provide their current understanding of the situation as well as their anticipation of how it could unfold.[44] Computer games are now being employed to improve surgeons' situation awareness in laparoscopic procedures,[6] and eye-tracking studies are showing trainee surgeons how their scanning and fixation patterns differ from those of more experienced surgeons.[45]

Recommendations from other professions for maintaining good situation awareness[46] can be included in training courses for surgeons:

1. *Good briefing:* This is so that the surgeon and the rest of the team understand the nature and risks of a case before the operation begins. At the preoperative stage, specific actions can be taken to gather and share information across the team. Use of the pre-task briefing session at the beginning of an operating list allows the whole team to be introduced to each other (so that skill mix, experience, etc., can be understood), specific equipment required to be discussed and potential difficulties to be identified. The World Health Organization checklist before each procedure then focuses on each patient's comorbidity, correct site and procedure; the need (again) for any specific

equipment; the anticipated length of the procedure; any prophylactic measures to be undertaken; and possible problems that could occur.

2. *Planning and preparation:* Time spent preoperatively on thinking about the case can have significant benefits on perception and anticipation once the surgeon starts to operate. Arora et al.[47] demonstrated the benefits of mental rehearsal for novice surgeons' technical skills.

3. *Physical and mental fitness for work:* Surgeons whose physical or mental fitness for duty is diminished (fatigue, infection, stress, physical limitations [e.g. back pain and impaired vision/hearing] and alcohol or drug dependence) are likely to have poorer situation awareness skills. In extreme cases, this would require the surgeon to withdraw from the task due to the potential level of impairment. For more minor conditions, remedial measures can be applied, including informing co-workers of the problem.

4. *Minimizing distraction and interruption:* This is especially during critical phases of a procedure. The concept of the 'sterile cockpit' devised in the aviation industry[48] is now applied by some surgeons to the operating room. The sterile cockpit rule for pilots prohibits crew members from performing non-essential duties or other activities while the aircraft is at a critical stage of the flight (taxiing, taking off, initial climb, final approach and landing). Any crew conversation during these stages must only be about the flight operation.

5. *Self-monitoring:* Noticing that you are working on the wrong mental model is hard to self-detect. Regularly updating one's mental model, i.e. comparing the mental model of the situation with real-world cues, and the interpretations of others may be helpful. Sensitivity to cues that distraction or zoning out is occurring or at least having an awareness of the conditions when this is likely to happen is also important.

6. *Encouraging speaking up:* Asking all staff in the operating room to speak up when they are not sure of what they should do or when they notice something of concern. It is not enough to rely on the operating surgeon's situation

awareness – key information may be located beyond the operative field, which only other team members can see.

> … His eyes were always darting around, as if he were about to say something. His gaze moved from chest to monitor, chest to monitor, chest to anaesthesiologist, chest to monitor, chest to Deb [team member], chest to the opening OR door, chest to monitor.
>
> 'I'm watching' he'll tell me, 'because I want to know right away if there's a problem so Roger can stop doing that or we can adjust. I've got to watch because he can't, and if there's something not right, well then, you don't have very long before you have to react to it – otherwise you've caused a little problem. One little problem leads to another. Little problems turn into bigger problems, so the better you keep these little problems down, the better the picture.'
>
> *Physician's assistant describing working with a paediatric cardiac surgeon[25]*

7. *Time management:* Avoiding the 'hurry-up syndrome' by early planning, preparation and resisting imposed time pressure. A study of 31 aviation accidents[49] found that in 55% of them the pilots were behind schedule. Rushing to complete tasks in a tight time frame is not conducive to good situation awareness and is something very familiar to most surgeons.

4.6 ASSESSING SITUATION AWARENESS

There are a number of techniques for assessing situation awareness, and some of these can be adapted for surgeons. The best developed method is by conducting observations while a surgeon is operating in theatre or in a simulator, typically with the use of behavioural rating scales, such as NOTSS, and this is covered in Chapter 10. There are also generic rating tools, such as the Situation Awareness Rating Scales used by a trained observer watching someone performing a task.[50] In these methods, the observer has to infer the level of the operator's situation awareness from particular behaviours or communications that indicate information gathering, formulation of a mental model or anticipation. Using a rating scale for the surgical team, an observational study of 26 laparoscopic cholecystectomies showed that a higher level of situation awareness was associated with a better technical outcome.[51]

The Situation Awareness Global Assessment Technique (SAGAT)[52] employs the task-freeze technique mentioned earlier, and it has been used in simulation studies with trauma surgeons[53] and ENT (ear, nose and throat) surgeons.[54] The task is stopped and the operator is asked questions to determine his or her current knowledge of the task and related circumstances. For safety-critical occupations, this often has to be conducted in a simulator. Surgical trainers may already use this kind of approach when working with trainees, pausing during the procedure to question the trainee about their understanding of the procedure, current risks and next steps.

Self-rating measures of situation awareness are also available: the Situation Awareness Rating Technique[55] requires the operator to complete a rating scale during a task to determine current level of attentional capacity and understanding of the task status. Other questionnaires have been designed to assess general levels of situation awareness, i.e. as an individual trait rather than as a transient state.[56,57] There is also a mental task load index that has been adapted for surgeons.[58]

Finally, there has been a rapid development of portable electronic devices that can record the surgeon's eye-gaze patterns[45] or film the scene of view (e.g. Google Glass). These techniques have produced a proliferation of studies to determine where surgeons direct their attention when operating[59,60] and may also be used to inform assessments of situation awareness.

4.7 SUMMARY

A surgeon's intraoperative situation awareness involves gathering information and developing an understanding of it to build a mental model of the current situation that can help in the anticipation of future state. The information comes from the operative site, from the operating room environment and from other members of the team. It is important that operating room teams have some degree of shared situation awareness and shared mental models for the task. Team mental models and communication are discussed in Chapter 6.

REFERENCES

1. Gawande A. *Complications: A Surgeon's Notes on an Imperfect Science*. London: Profile Books; 2002. p. 72.
2. Gilson R. Situation awareness. *Hum Factors*. 1995;37:3–4.
3. Gaba D, Howard S, Small S. Situation awareness in anesthesiology. *Hum Factors*. 1995;37:20–31.
4. Way L, Stewart L, Gantert W, Kingsway L, Lee C, Whang K et al. Causes and prevention of laparoscopic bile duct injuries. *Ann Surg*. 2003;237:460–9.
5. Dekker S, Hugh T. Laparoscopic bile duct injury: Understanding the psychology and heuristics of error. *ANZ J Surg*. 2008;78:1109–4.
6. Graafland M, Schijven M. A serious game to improve situation awareness in laparoscopic surgery. In Schouten B et al. (Eds.). *Games for Health*. Wiesbaden, Germany: Springer; 2013.
7. Bleakley A, Allard J, Hobbs A. 'Achieving ensemble': Communication in orthopaedic surgical teams and the development of situation awareness—an observational study using live videotaped examples. *Adv Health Edu*. 2013;18:33–56.
8. Hazlehurst B, McMullen C, Gorman P. Distributed cognition in the heart room: How situation awareness arises from co-ordinated communications during cardiac surgery. *J Biomed Inform*. 2007;40:539–51.
9. Parush A, Kramer C, Foster-Hunt T, Momtahan K, Hunter A, Sohmer B. Communication and team situation awareness in the OR: Implications for augmentative information display. *J Biomed Inform*. 2011;44:477–85.
10. Marsh H. *Do no harm. Stories of Life, Death and Brain Surgery*. London: Weidenfeld & Nicholson; 2014. p. 171.
11. Schwab S. *Cutting remarks. Insights and Recollections of a Surgeon*. Berkeley, California: Frog; 2006. p. 75.
12. Eysenck M, Keane M. *Cognitive Psychology: A Student's Handbook*, 5th ed. Hove: Psychology Press; 2005.
13. Miller G. The magical number seven, plus or minus two: Some limits on our capacity for processing information. *Psychol Rev*. 1956;63:81–97.
14. Cowan N. The Magical Mystery Four. How is working memory capacity limited, and why? *Curr Dir Psychol Sci*. 2010;19:51–7.
15. Flitter M. *Judith's Pavilion. The Haunting Memories of a Neurosurgeon*. South Royalton, Vermont: Steerforth Press; 1997. p. 21.
16. Mitchell L, Flin R, Yule S, Mitchell J, Coutts K, Youngson G. Thinking ahead of the surgeon. An interview study to identify scrub nurses' non-technical skills. *Int J Nurs Stud*. 2011;48:818–28.
17. Dieckmann P, Reddersen S, Wehner T, Rall M. Prospective memory failures as an unexplored threat to patient safety. *Ergonomics*. 2006;49:526–43.
18. Endsley M. Toward a theory of situation awareness in dynamic systems. *Hum Factors*. 1995;37:32–64.
19. Flin R, Youngson G, Yule S. How do surgeons make intraoperative decisions? *Qual Saf Health Care*. 2007;16:235–9.
20. Bromiley M. Have you ever made a mistake? *Bulletin of the Royal College of Anaesthetists*. 2008;48:2242–5.
21. Simons D, Chabris C. Gorillas in our midst. Sustained inattentional blindness for dynamic events. *Perception*. 1999;28:1059–74.
22. Simons D, Levin C. Failure to detect changes to people during a real-world interaction. *Psychon Bull Rev*. 1998;5:644–9.

23. Dalton P, Fraenkel N. Gorillas we have missed. Sustained inattentional deafness for dynamic events. *Cognition.* 2012;124:367–72.

24. Smallwood J, Schooler J. The restless mind. *Psychol Bull.* 2006;132:946–58.

25. Ruhlman M. *Walk on Water. Inside an Elite Paediatric Surgical Unit.* New York: Viking; 2003. pp. 225–226, 236.

26. Snook S. *Friendly Fire: The Accidental Shootdown of US Black Hawks over Northern Iraq.* Princeton, New Jersey: Princeton University Press; 2000. p. 80.

27. Roberts R, Flin R., Cleland J. Staying in the zone. Offshore drillers' situation awareness. *Human Factors.* 2015;57:573–590.

28. Orasanu J, Fischer U. Finding decisions in natural environments: The view from the cockpit. In C. Zsambok, G. Klein (Eds.). *Naturalistic Decision Making.* Mahwah, New Jersey: LEA; 1997.

29. Thomson M, Onkal D, Avcioglu A, Goodwin P. Aviation risk perception: A comparison between experts and novices. *Risk Analysis.* 2004;24:1585–95.

30. Pauley K, Flin R, Yule S, Youngson G. Surgeons' intraoperative decision making and risk assessment. *Am J Surg.* 2011;202:375–81.

31. Sarter N, Woods D. Situation awareness: A critical but ill-defined phenomenon. *Int J Aviat Psychol.* 1991;1:45–57.

32. CAA. Appendix 6. Situation awareness. Appendix 4. Information Processing. *Crew Resource Management (CRM) Training. CAP 737,* 2nd ed. Gatwick, United Kingdom: Civil Aviation Authority; 2006. www.caa.org.

33. Okray R, Lubnau T. *Crew Resource Management for the Fire Service.* Tulsa, Oklahoma: PennWell; 2004.

34. Lockley S, Cronin J, Evans E, Cade B, Lee C, Landrigan C et al. Effect of reducing interns' weekly work hours on sleep and attentional failures. *N Engl J Med.* 2004;351:18, 1829–37.

35. Way J, Long A, Weihing J, Ritchie R, Jones R, Bush M, Shinn JB. Effect of noise on auditory processing in the operating room. *J Am Coll Surg.* 2013;216:933–8.

36. Healey A, Sevdalis N, Vincent C. Measuring intraoperative interference from distraction and interruption observed in the operating theatre. *Ergonomics.* 2006;49:589–604.

37. Sevdalis N, Forrest D, Undre S, Darzi A, Vincent C. Annoyances, disruptions, and interruptions in surgery: The Disruptions in Surgery Index (DiSI). *World J Surg.* 2008;32:1643–50.

38. Marsch S, Tschan F, Semmer N, Spychiger M, Breuer M, Hunziker P. Unnecessary interruptions of cardiac massage during simulated cardiac arrests. *Eur J Anaesthesiol.* 2005;22:831–3.

39. Sevdalis N, Undre S, McDermott J, Giddie J, Diner L, Smith G. Impact of distractions on patient safety: A prospective study using validated instruments. *World J Surg.* 2014;38:751–8.

40. Dismukes K, Young G, Sumwalt R. Cockpit interruptions and distractions. *ASRS Frontline.* 1998;10:1–8. www.asrs.src.nasa. gov/directline.

41. Banbury S, Dudfield H, Hormann J, Soll H. Development and validation of a novel measure to assess the effectiveness of commercial airline pilot situation awareness training. *Int J Aviat Psychol.* 2007;17:131–52.

42. Endsley M, Robertson M. Training for situation awareness in individuals and teams. In M. Endsley, D. Garland (Eds.). *Situation Awareness. Analysis and Measurement.* Mahwah, New Jersey: LEA; 2000.

43. Graafland M, Schraagen JMC, Boermeester MA, Bemelman WA, Schijven MP. Training situational awareness to reduce surgical errors in the operating room. *British Journal of Surgery.* 2015;102(1):16–23.

44. Saus E, Johnson B, Eid J, Riisem P, Andersen R, Thayer J. The effect of brief situational awareness training in a police shooting simulator: An experimental study. *Mil Psychol.* 2006;18:S3–21.

45. Hermens F, Flin R, Ahmed I. Surgeons' eye movements. A literature review. *J Eye Mov Res.* 2013;6:1–11.

46. Flin R, O'Connor P, Crichton M. *Safety at the Sharp End. A Guide to Non-Technical Skills.* Aldershot, United Kingdom: Ashgate; 2008.

47. Arora S, Aggarwal R, Pramudith S, Moran A, Grantcharov T, Kneebone R et al. Mental

practice enhances surgical technical skills: A randomized controlled study. *Ann Surg.* 2011;253:265–70.

48. Walters J. *Crew Resource Management is No Accident.* Wallingford, United Kingdom: Aries; 2002.
49. McElhatton J, Drew C. Time pressure as a causal factor in aviation accidents. In R. Jensen (Ed.). *Proceedings of the Seventh International Symposium on Aviation Psychology.* Columbus, Ohio: Ohio State University Press; 1993.
50. Bell H, Lyon D. Using observer ratings to assess situation awareness. In M. Endsley, D. Garland (Eds.). *Situation Awareness. Analysis and Measurement.* Mahwah, New Jersey: LEA; 2000.
51. Mishra A, Catchpole K, Dale T, McCulloch P. The influence of non-technical performance on technical outcomes in laparoscopic cholecystectomies. *Surgical Endoscopy.* 2008;22:68–73.
52. Endsley M. Design and evaluation for situation awareness enhancement. In *Proceedings of the Human Factors and Ergonomics Society 32nd Annual Meeting,* vol. 1, pp. 97–101. Santa Monica, California: HFES; 1988.
53. Hogan M, Pace D, Hapgood J, Boone D, Taylor R. Use of human patient simulation and the Situation Awareness Global Assessment Technique in practical trauma skills assessment. *Journal of Trauma Injury-Infection and Critical Care.* 2006;5:1047–52.
54. Luz M, Manzey D, Modemann S, Straus G. Less is sometimes more: A comparison of distance-control and navigated-control concepts of image-guided navigation support for surgeons. *Ergonomics.* 2015; 58:383–393.
55. Taylor R. Situation awareness rating technique (SART): The development of a tool for aircrew systems design. In *Situational Awareness in Aerospace Operations.* Neuilly sur Seine, France: NATO-AGARD; 1990.
56. Sneddon A, Mearns K, Flin R. Stress, fatigue, situation awareness and safety in offshore drilling crews. *Safety Sci.* 2013;56:80–8.
57. Wallace J, Chen G. Development and validation of a work-specific measure of cognitive failure: Implications for occupational safety. *J Occup Organ Psychol.* 2005;78:615–32.
58. Wilson M, Poolton J, Malhotra N, Ngo K, Nast R. Development and validation of a surgical workload measure: The Surgery Task Load Index (SURG-TLX). *World J Surg.* 2011;35:1961–9.
59. Tien G, Pucher P, Sodergren M, Yang G, Darzi A. Differences in gaze behaviour of expert and junior surgeons performing open inguinal hernia repair. *Surgical Endoscopy.* 2015;29:405–413.
60. Lutch M, Kohli A, Cates D, Lue A. Google Glass in head and neck surgery. *Otolaryngol Head Neck Surg.* 2014;151(suppl 1):40–1.

5

Decision making

RHONA FLIN AND DOUGLAS S SMINK

I opened the child's abdomen and the entire mid-gut was twisted and very ischaemic. There were multiple areas of frank necrosis and the rest was of dubious viability. He was very septic and haemodynamically quite unstable. I had to decide whether to rapidly carry out an en-bloc resection in order to stabilize the situation, get him off the table and into ITU and think about future prospects in the cold light of day, or whether simply to make a proximal stoma and perform a second look laparotomy the next day.

Pediatric surgeon

5.1 INTRODUCTION

Intra-operative decision making is one of the most important non-technical skills for a surgeon. While diagnosis, decision to operate, choice of procedure and operative plan are normally worked out in advance, surgeons also have to be able to make decisions while operating. This chapter focuses on intra-operative decision making, which can be described as dynamic decision making: having to decide on a course of action while an event is unfolding, sometimes under time pressure. In some cases, there may be minimal opportunity for information gathering or for quiet contemplation of options.

There are many books and articles on surgeons' decision making; however, these mainly consider preoperative diagnosis and judgements on whether to operate and choice of procedure, although *Surgical Intuition*[1] is a notable exception. Surgical manuals delineate the steps to follow in an operation; but these are very technical, specifying anatomical markers, instruments and sequences of actions.[2] Whereas anaesthetists' thought processes have been studied in relation to decision errors[3] and difficult cases,[4] surprisingly few studies have been undertaken on how surgeons make decisions while operating.[5] A recent paper comments, 'Despite its importance, intra-operative decision making is not a focus in surgical education and remains part of the hidden curriculum in surgery'.[6]

While most surgical decision making takes place preoperatively, there are many occasions when decisions are required after the procedure has started. These may be at pre-planned points when due to the patient's condition or the particular procedure a decision point is reached where a choice has to be made. There are also unplanned and unexpected moments in an elective case where a decision may be required. For instance, the anatomy may not be as anticipated, the patient's condition may worsen, an error may occur, equipment can fail or the selected technique may not produce the intended result. Sudden bleeding can require a fast, almost reflex action.

This time I easily open the clip and slip the blades over the aneurysm. I open my hand and the blades close, neatly clipping the aneurysm. The aneurysm, defeated, shrivels since it is no longer filling with high pressure arterial blood. I sigh deeply – I always do when the aneurysm is finally dealt with. But to my horror I find that this second applicator has an even more deadly fault than the first: having closed the clip over the aneurysm, the applicator refuses to release the clip. I cannot move my hand for fear of tearing the minute, fragile aneurysm off the middle cerebral artery and causing a catastrophic haemorrhage. I sit there motionless with my hand frozen in space.

Neurosurgeon[7]

As this example illustrates, the best planned elective operations may still contain a few surprises, necessitating decision making. In emergency cases, there is usually much less time to collect full diagnostic information or to determine exactly which procedure will be appropriate and so more on-task decision making will be required.[8] In the United Kingdom, emergency general surgery is now the largest group of all surgical admissions.[9]

Erroneous or suboptimal decisions during surgery are not uncommon[10-12]; however, many of them will be detected and can be corrected as the procedure progresses. Recognizing errors while operating is a marker of surgical expertise. Other errors (e.g. persisting laparoscopically rather than converting to an open procedure, incorrectly judging tissue to be viable and underestimating tumour margins) may not manifest until after the operation is completed and the patient is recovering – or not. As explained in Chapter 1, the likelihood of surgical errors or a poor decision is influenced by technical, system and safety culture factors, and we also have to consider how the decision was made. The chosen course of action would have made sense to the surgeon at the critical moment. To understand how a high-quality or a suboptimal decision is made, we have to deconstruct the cognitive processes underlying this important non-technical skill.

So, how do surgeons make decisions when operating?

Decision making is defined in the Non-Technical Skills for Surgeons (NOTSS) system as 'skills for diagnosing the situation and reaching a judgement in order to choose an appropriate course of action'. While operating, the surgeon engages in a continuous cycle of monitoring and re-evaluating the progress of the procedure and, when necessary, may decide to alter the plan to meet the demands of the situation. Different decision-making techniques are used depending on circumstances, such as time pressure; task demands; feasibility of options; and what level of constraint, support and resource exists. The elements of intra-operative decision making in NOTSS are shown in Table 5.1.

These NOTSS elements of decision making encompass the skill set for deciding what to do in a given situation. In this chapter, we will also discuss the preceding step of evaluating the present state

Table 5.1 Elements of intra-operative decision making (from NOTSS)

Category	Elements
Decision making	Considering options
	Selecting and communicating option
	Implementing and reviewing decisions

of events (in the NOTSS rating tool, this is encompassed in situation awareness). The term 'situation assessment' is used in this chapter to refer to the moment when the surgeon's ongoing situation awareness indicates that there is a change in the task environment that needs to be consciously considered and that a decision may now be required.

To explain the underlying cognitive processes, this chapter draws on the limited literature on intra-operative decisions (mainly from interview studies) and in places we refer to studies of decision making in other hazardous work settings (naturalistic decision making [NDM]). The aim of NDM researchers is to understand how experienced practitioners make decisions under conditions of high uncertainty, inadequate information, shifting goals and high time pressure and risk, usually working with a team and subject to organizational constraints.[13,14] The NDM approach has been applied in studies of surgeons' decisions while operating,[5,6,15] and so it is adopted as the theoretical background. We introduce a basic model of intra-operative decision making, describe several different methods that surgeons use to make these decisions, discuss influencing factors and offer suggestions for training and assessment of these decision-making skills.

5.2 MODEL OF INTRA-OPERATIVE DECISION MAKING

While a surgeon is operating, a continuous cognitive cycle of situation awareness and decision making is interwoven during task execution. This process consists of monitoring, noticing and evaluating cues to assess the situation; judging progress against the current plan; and then, if necessary, making a decision, implementing it and considering whether the course of action is appropriate. Based on available evidence,[15-21] a model of intra-operative surgical decision making is proposed (Figure 5.1). It shows a three-stage process that is enacted once a decision point is reached or a change occurs in the task environment (e.g. unexpected bleeding). At that moment, an operating surgeon should normally slow down (mentally pause) to do the following:

1. Assess the situation: what is the status or problem? How does this affect my plan? What is the level of risk? How much time do I have?
2. Use a decision method for determining a course of action: what shall I do now?
3. Check the result: is this course of action working?

For very familiar decision points, or microdecisions (e.g. cutting pressure and stitch tension), an expert surgeon will probably experience this as a smooth, continuous mental process, without conscious points of hesitation even though decisions are being made, that would not be obvious to the novice. This is in essence the automatic mode of thinking where decisions are being made intuitively by a practised professional.[2] At other times, even an intuitive decision will be preceded by a momentary pause[18] to think what to do, even though the answer is rapidly accessed from memory and applied.

This framework was informed by a model of in-flight decision making,[22,23] which emphasized the importance of the situation assessment stage. The pilot's estimation of available time and level of risk during situation assessment is critical as this determines the type of decision method employed. When there is little time and high risk, pilots use faster decision strategies, such as applying a known rule or intuition. When there is more time (even with variable risk), they may opt for a slower but more rigorous choice method to systematically

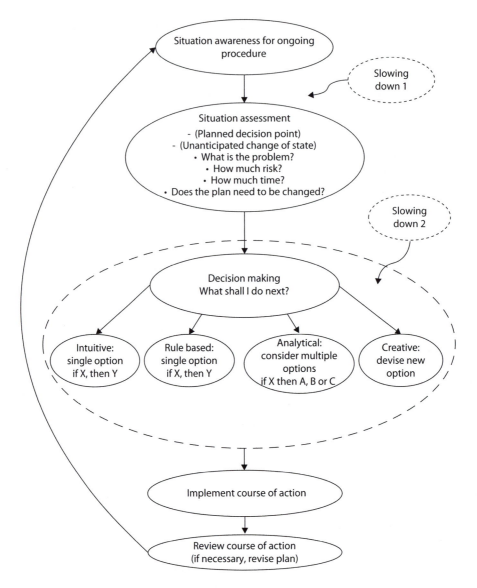

Figure 5.1 Model of surgeons' intra-operative decision making

compare and evaluate alternative courses of action (e.g. the FOR-DEC method [see Section 5.5]).

Essentially, the decision-making method (faster or slower) is selected to meet the demands of the situation. If there is sufficient time, a systematic comparison of options can be considered; but if the event is time critical, such as a sudden high-volume bleeding, then a rapid response must be executed (to at least control the event and if necessary 'buy time' to think). The feedback loop emphasizes the cyclical nature of this process:

surgeons need to maintain situation awareness throughout a procedure, and when any critical change is detected they must take time to re-evaluate the situation and, if necessary, switch from one decision-making mode to another.

Hence, the stages of a surgeon's intra-operative decision making are as follows:

1. What is the problem?
2. What shall I do?
3. Is this working?

5.2.1 SITUATION ASSESSMENT: WHAT IS THE PROBLEM?

As Figure 5.1 illustrates, the first step of the decision-making process is the surgeon's situational diagnosis, collecting clues to build a mental model of what is happening. This situation assessment step is the mental process to systematically survey the task environment: it can be a more conscious state of evaluation than the ongoing situation awareness. It is an attempt to make sense of the current status, usually when there is recognition of a new problem or change of state requiring a decision. Or, it could be triggered by a realization that the preoperative plan is not working. The operating surgeon should be mentally 'in the loop' of the procedure when this happens, so he or she can evaluate the new situation and may even be aware of how it has occurred.

In contrast, a surgeon called in to help with a colleague's problem has to make a rapid assessment from the situation report being given (sometimes in a less than clear fashion); this is akin to the 'size-up' process conducted by a fire ground commander arriving on the scene of an emergency and having to gain an impression of what exactly is happening. This is cognitively demanding and requires a certain level of expertise, but a 'fresh pair of eyes' can be invaluable for the situation assessment phase when the operating team is becoming overwhelmed by a problem or getting trapped into a single interpretation.

In both events (on-task or called in), the situation assessment stage is critical for the surgeon's decision making. Conscious mental effort is directed at identifying and understanding a specific juncture or an emerging problem. It may be that the operative plan has pre-specified decision points where there will be a pause and an assessment of the best course of action. As explained in Chapter 4, as surgeons become more experienced at operating they build a memory bank of typical procedures, anatomical ambiguities, techniques proved to be effective, unusual events and their trajectories. As expertise develops, these become stored as 'schemas' or 'mental models', which allow rapid pattern matching from memory to facilitate the situation assessment process.

Sometimes, a full assessment is impossible or no matching pattern can be found but the surgeon still has to make a decision on the basis of the available information and the estimated risk. It could be that the situation is undiagnosable but the warning signs are clear, so the decision is made to curtail or abandon the procedure. This would equate to helicopter pilots having no idea why their aircraft was violently vibrating but knowing that it was such a dangerous signal that time could be very limited and the risk could be high and that the correct response was to land or ditch into the sea without delay.

If the situation assessment is incorrect, then it is likely that the resulting decision and course of action that is taken in response will be suboptimal or unsuitable. For example, after performing a femoral artery embolectomy for acute limb ischaemia, the surgeon must decide whether or not to proceed with lower extremity fasciotomies to avoid the development of compartment syndrome. This is based on both the time of ischaemia and the appearance of the tissues at operation. Misinterpreting the situation and not doing fasciotomies could result in compartment syndrome, further ischaemic damage and need for return to the operating room. For pilots, more decision errors occur because they misunderstand the situation than when they make a correct assessment followed by the wrong response.[24] This finding may be applicable to experienced surgeons. As explained in Chapter 4, inaccurate situation assessment can arise from a number of factors: cues may be missed, misinterpreted, misdiagnosed or deliberately ignored, resulting in the wrong picture being formed of the problem. In addition, the level of risk or available time may be misjudged.

5.2.2 JUDGING TIME AND RISK

Experienced surgeons are likely to be more accurate at estimating available time to make a decision than their junior colleagues who will tend to underestimate this, especially as anxiety can increase the sense of urgency to act. Advice from one consultant surgeon to his trainees is as follows: 'Don't just do something, stand there'. This signals that there is often time to think before an action is required. Of course, expert surgeons know more strategies ('get out of jail' cards) that they can use to buy time in a problematic situation.

Surgeons' intra-operative risk assessment has been investigated in several studies. Dominguez et al.[25] were interested in decisions to convert during laparoscopic surgery. They interviewed 20 general surgeons (10 senior residents and 10 staff level) who were asked to watch two videotapes of challenging laparoscopic cholecystectomy cases and to think aloud, providing a continuous commentary on the procedure (as if they were doing the case or had been called to help). At three points, the tape was stopped and the surgeons were asked about the procedure, e.g. should it be converted to open surgery? They also rated their 'comfort level' with the operation at each point. The results (as illustrated in the following quotation) showed the importance of situation assessment in surgeons' decision making – judging comfort level, assessing risks, predicting outcomes and also the role of self-monitoring (e.g. 'I'll need to be careful here').

> Judging what was safe was an ongoing activity. Beginning with the initial 'I would just look and see', an incremental, one-step-at-a-time approach was often described by surgeons interviewed. Confidence in identification and potential for injury were judged at each step. This type of ongoing, dynamic decision making, reflecting a complex mingling of facts and risk assessment, is not typically studied in medical decision literature, which tends to focus on diagnosis as an event. Sunk cost reasoning, such as 'I've gotten this far, I might as well continue', was evident in some justifications for continuing laparoscopically. Comfort was a well-established part of their language to justify and explain decisions. 'If you are not comfortable, you should open' was a ubiquitous creed. Surgeons kept assessing whether they were beginning to move outside their limits of knowledge or capability or their comfort level. This pointed to a significant aspect of competence relating to calibration. Two essential elements of their comfort level were: (1) whether they could identify structures with 100% certainty and

(2) the perceived likelihood of injury, especially to the common bile duct.[25]

Generally, the staff surgeons and the residents gave similar responses, possibly because the residents were at an advanced stage of their training. There were some differences between those who decided to open and those who would have continued laparoscopically, e.g. expressions of discomfort were higher for 'openers'.

Other studies have shown significant variation in surgeons' ability to estimate the conversion risk in this procedure,[26] with both over- and underestimation found in trainees.[27] Masserwah et al.[28] studied surgeons' risk tolerance and bile duct injuries and found some evidence of a relationship for those with the highest preferences for risk.

Estimating risk is a major component of a surgeon's intra-operative thinking, and it features prominently when surgeons discuss decision making.

> ... that was a risk, I guess, that I was risking – risking what – if I left it, it might cause complications but overall it would be better than going in and risking stabbing the vitreous and having to go in and suck the vitreous out and do the whole thing.
>
> *Ophthalmic surgeon[21]*

Emotion is well known to influence decision making and risk judgements[29,30] and the surgeons' expressions of their level of comfort while judging risk while operating echo pilots' language during in-flight decision making.[31] The relationship between surgeons' personality and risk tolerance has been identified as an important topic, but the samples studied so far have tended to be rather small to draw meaningful conclusions.[32,33]

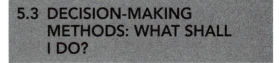

5.3 DECISION-MAKING METHODS: WHAT SHALL I DO?

The second stage of intra-operative decision making is the cognitive process of choosing a course of action (option) to meet the needs of the situation

Table 5.2 Examples of surgeons' dynamic decision making

Decision-making method	Consultant surgeons' statements
Intuitive (recognition primed/ automatic)	'I am under extreme time pressure – there is no time to make decisions – the bleeding must be controlled rapidly and I have 20 minutes before the kidney dies. I tell the anaesthetist immediately as I find the source of bleeding and arrange for it to be clamped. I need to keep the good kidney alive so get some cold saline into the kidney'.
Rule based	'If damage is occurring then you want to stop, especially according to clinical governance guidelines. Part of the expertise lies in doing but the other part is recognizing when you are struggling and knowing that "first do no harm," so I decided to stop and get a second opinion'.
Choice [Analytical]	'There were three options to consider and at this stage we had to balance the potential risk of problems in the post-op phase with the risks of doing something intra-operatively'.
Creative	'None of the usual joints would work so we had to adapt a different one in order to make it fit'.

Source: Flin R et al., *Qual Saf Health Care*, 16:235–239, 2007.

assessment. Studies of dynamic (on-task) decision making[22] suggest that there are four principal methods that experienced practitioners use:

1. *Intuitive:* Recognition-primed/fast automatic selection of single option
2. *Rule based:* Recall rule and the associated actions (i.e. single option)
3. *Analytical:* Slower, more considered choice of option
4. *Creative:* Devise new course of action

As Figure 5.1 illustrates, in the intuitive and rule-based methods only one response option is considered at a time. In the analytical mode, several courses of action are compared simultaneously and one has to be selected. In the creative mode, the situation is sufficiently novel to merit the creation of a new course of action. In some situations, the appropriate course of action may be to do nothing or to observe how the situation develops. There is also the possibility of indecision, failing to make a decision even after realizing that one is required. This is likely to be primarily caused by stress (see Chapter 8), given that indecisiveness would normally be regarded as an undesirable characteristic for a surgeon and therefore ideally 'selected out' during the recruitment process or the early stages of surgical training.

Interviews with surgeons describing challenging situations[5] indicate that these four methods of decision making are used while operating (see examples in Table 5.2). We describe these methods and how they are used by surgeons.

5.3.1 INTUITIVE DECISION MAKING

This mode of decision making has been described by surgeons as 'intuitive',[2] and so that term will be used here. It can also be called 'gut feel' or recognition-primed decision making.[34] Moulton,[17–19] a hepatopancreatobiliary (HPB) surgeon who studies decision making, calls it 'automatic'. In the psychological literature, it is called 'system 1'[35] or as Kahneman[36] (the psychologist who won a Nobel Prize for his work on decision making) labels it, 'thinking fast'. Intuitive decision making is based on a rapid retrieval from memory of a course of action associated with the type of situation that has just been recognized. Thus, the recalled response to resolve this type of situation has been stored with the episodic memories of previous similar occasions of the same type. The situational cues match the memories of previous events stored as patterns or prototypes. It could be recalling a rule (see later) or just remembering a technique used or observed in a previous encounter with this situation. ('When x happens, I know to do *y*'.) In this case, choosing a course of action is likely to be experienced as an automatic process, with little conscious deliberation (and minimal use of working memory) (see Chapter 4). It may be that they are using 'fast and frugal heuristics'[37] – rules of thumb for making rapid decisions.

The term recognition-primed decision making (RPD) has come from field studies of experienced professionals making critical decisions. Klein[34] was investigating how fire commanders compared alternative courses of actions in risky, time-pressured events. He found that they were not in fact always using this decision method, instead 'they were not "making choices", "considering alternatives" or "assessing probabilities". They saw themselves as acting and reacting on the basis of previous experience; they were generating, monitoring and modifying plans to meet the needs of situations. Rarely did the fire commanders contrast even two options. … Moreover, it appeared that a search for an optimal choice could stall the fireground commanders long enough to lose the control of the situation'.[34]

Klein realized that their decision process relied more on situation assessment/classification, which (assuming they recognized the type) was followed by the rapid recall of an appropriate course of action to deal with it (or to buy time). The commanders were not 'optimizing', i.e. they were not striving to find the optimal solution; rather, their aim was to find a satisfactory solution to control the situation. They would mentally check the feasibility of the recalled course of action by imagining how to implement it and thinking whether anything important might go wrong. If they envisaged a problem, then the plan might be modified. Only if they rejected it would they consider another method. The basic RPD model has two variants to encompass: (1) when the situation takes more effort to diagnose, or (2) the decision maker is less sure about the recalled course of action and takes more time to imagine it.

This intuitive method of decision making would be familiar to most experienced surgeons. In interviews[20,21] where general and ophthalmic surgeons recalled a challenging case and answered questions about one key decision, it was found that half of them described intuitive decision making. The focus is on 'reading' the situation to see if it is recognized as a familiar type. Then, if it is identified (i.e. the pattern is matched from memory) a response can be recalled from past experience. Although this might not be the most elegant, economical solution, it should produce a course of action that is workable and satisfactory in the current condition. For instance, a colorectal surgeon doing a sigmoid colectomy realizes that there is too much tension on the anastomosis and so mobilizes the splenic flexure. Here, the surgeon rapidly recognizes the implications of the new pattern of cues and acts accordingly. To the trainee who is observing, these intuitive decisions appear to be automatic reactions requiring minimal cognitive effort.

> Sometimes, the senior surgeon will ask the junior to change positions at the table. Often, apparently suddenly and unexpectedly, the senior, previously at a loss to put the data together, will arrive at an answer, just from feeling the tissues or viewing the situation from a new angle. Although a previously unobtained answer or formulation has appeared, the surgeon is hard put to describe how he got it.[38]

While intuitive decision making is often employed where there is no time pressure, it is particularly appropriate for surgical events requiring immediate action. This type of rapid decision making is required in other risky domains, e.g. police officers determining whether to shoot a suspect[39,40] or pilots in an emergency deciding whether to reject a take-off[41] or, as illustrated later (for an aircraft that had lost all engine power), find an immediate landing site.

> The air traffic controller asked: 'Cactus fifteen twenty-nine, if we can get it to you, do you want to try runway one three?' Patrick was offering us the runway at LaGuardia that could be reached by the shortest path.
>
> 'We're unable,' I responded. 'We may end up in the Hudson.'
>
> I knew intuitively and quickly that the Hudson River might be our only option, and so I articulated it.[42]

The intuitive method is likely to be used by experienced surgeons in relatively familiar situations. It is useful when there is high time pressure and, because less conscious processing in working memory is involved, it may be more resistant to the effects of acute stress and fatigue than other strategies. This is not to suggest that intuitive decision making will always produce the correct answer. Decision errors can still occur if the situation is wrongly assessed and the matched rule for that incorrect situation is retrieved from memory and applied. Novice surgeons need to build up memory banks of stored patterns to use their intuition effectively.

5.3.2 RULE-BASED DECISION MAKING

In some work settings, such as industrial control rooms, extensive use is made of rule-based decision making; the rules will be specified in manuals of standard operating procedures written by equipment manufacturers or subject matter experts. Rule-based decision making involves identifying the situation encountered and remembering or looking up the procedure in a guidance manual to find the steps to be followed. This method does not appear to be frequently used in intra-operative surgery, probably due to the complexity and variability of anatomy and physiological processes across patients. Moreover, surgeons often develop idiosyncratic methods of working that they learn on the job from their surgical trainers. Pauley et al.[20,21] found few examples of general and orthopaedic surgeons describing rule-based decisions. However, as rule-based decision making appears to be used by surgeons on some occasions and, because there are calls for more standardization in surgery,[43] the method is described here.

Rule-based decision making requires more conscious effort than the intuitive method. The decision maker has to actively search his or her memory to retrieve the learned matching rule for the situation ('if x, do y'). Or, as in some industrial settings, a procedures manual or a checklist needs to be located and read to find the appropriate response. (The use of written procedures can be helpful if required to justify your decision after the event, as the protocol can be blamed for an incorrect response.) Rule-based decision making is favoured by novices who can learn standard procedures for frequent or high-risk situations. For instance, the rule for penetrating trauma to the rectum is as follows: above the peritoneal reflection, it can be repaired primarily; below the peritoneal reflection, the surgeon should drain the area and do a diverting colostomy. Procedures are also useful for experts. For example, if a decision rule has been memorized, then that action can be taken if the appropriate event occurs, permitting the operator to react quickly to the situation. With practice, this becomes automatic and when the rule can be retrieved from memory with little conscious effort this mode effectively becomes intuitive decision making. When decisions must be taken rapidly, a checklist can be a helpful aid. A recent study of 17 operating room teams who participated in 106 simulated surgical crisis scenarios found that every team performed better when the crisis checklists were available than when they were not.[44]

Decision errors can still happen in the rule-based mode; the situation could be misjudged or the wrong rule selected (and there is a particular risk of opting for a very familiar one).

5.3.3 ANALYTICAL DECISION MAKING

The other main method of decision making for surgeons when operating can be termed choice or analytical decision making. It requires more conscious thinking about what is to be done, and so it is easier in situations with less time pressure. As with intuitive or rule-based reasoning, the type of situation/problem must first be identified to begin the process. Then, possible courses of action are generated from memory or by asking other team members, or a colleague. These alternatives are simultaneously compared in relation to their component features to determine which one is most appropriate to meet the needs of the situation. Ideally, all the relevant features of the options should be identified and weighted in terms of their match for the situational requirements. There are other labels for this more labour-intensive mode of decision making, such as 'thinking slow'[36] or 'system 2'.[35]

Probability theory and other mathematical devices (decision trees, multi-attribute decision theory and Bayesian modelling) are available to aid the selection of the optimal choice. These are frequently used in medical decision making to determine efficacy and cost-effectiveness of alternative treatments, and there are surgical reports describing the use of these tools[6,45]; typically, they are used preoperatively or post-operatively, e.g. in case comparison studies. A detailed comparison of options requires considerable time, mental effort (concentration) as well as the availability of key information on the situational features and on each option. With this analytical method, the probability of reaching an optimal solution is enhanced because all possible alternatives should be carefully evaluated. Carrying out a rigorous analysis of alternatives requires simultaneous comparison of a significant amount of information, and most people need to write down this information (once it exceeds their working memory capacity). While in the middle of executing a task, this is often not feasible and, in practice, most decision makers use heuristics (shortcuts/rules of thumb) to make comparisons between options. However, these are subject to a range of decision biases: picking the most familiar, choosing the most recently considered and selecting the first one that comes to mind. Croskerry et al.[46,47] explain these biases and how to overcome them in relation to medical diagnosis.

The analytical method, conducted preoperatively when there is ample time to think about a case, should facilitate the faster intuitive decisions that may be needed when the surgeon subsequently carries out the procedure. Pre-thinking or mentally rehearsing what the key decision points may be during an operation, and then considering what alternatives may be available and which of these could be optimal, is what many surgeons do when planning their more unusual or more difficult cases (see Chapter 8). Prior mental preparation can facilitate the more rapid, intuitive decisions when the case is under way, as the 'heavy duty' thinking has already been done. To take a military example, a naval commander described how en route to a conflict zone he thought about the decisions he might have to make once the enemy had been engaged – when there would be little time for reflection, 'much can be gained by maintaining the strategy and the plans derived analytically and thinking through action contingencies

("what-if-ing") to be applied [when reaching the conflict zone] on an RPD [intuitive] basis'.[48]

With analytical decision making, the wrong option can still be chosen, for instance, if the situation was misinterpreted to start with or the most suitable alternatives were not considered or a suboptimal course of action was selected. Surgeons report using analytical decision making while operating,[1,18,20] and trainees are most likely to be taught this method of carefully considering their options when a key juncture in a procedure is reached or an unexpected event arises.

5.3.4 CREATIVE DECISION MAKING

The final method to be described is labelled creative decision making. This is where a new course of action has to be devised 'on the spot' as the situation is unusual and no suitable response is known. This approach appears to be infrequently used in risky, time-sensitive settings, as it requires considerable cognitive effort to devise a novel course of action for an unfamiliar situation. It also means that the course of action has not been tested for the situation in question, thus introducing a level of risk. Airline pilots rarely make decisions in this fashion,[22] although there are notable exceptions with creative components, such as a passenger jet with failed hydraulics being steered using reverse thrust from the engines[49] or the landing on the Hudson River mentioned in Section 5.3.1.[42]

Interview studies with surgeons suggest that this innovative mode is not a method they frequently adopt because of the aforementioned reasons, although they do use it.

> I don't know where I got the idea from but I decided that it would be useful to use a laparoscopic stapling device that we would normally use to divide blood vessels in a laparoscopic surgery and that we would use it here.[15]

Examples from the past can be found for other specialties: in plastic surgery, these include implantation of a toe to create a new thumb after traumatic thumb amputation or performing an abdominoplasty at the time of ventral hernia repair to deal with excess abdominal wall skin. To strictly fit this creative decision category, the course of action should not have been considered in advance. Innovation is obviously of importance to the development of surgery. The point being made here is that intra-operative creative decision making is difficult and can carry significant risk, as by definition it is undertaken without preparation and careful consideration. Cristancho et al.,[15] when discussing surgeons' accounts of this mode of decision making, comment, 'We do not uncritically accept our participants' "positive spin" on their non-standard practices. … Depending on the situation, innovating to improve patient outcomes in one situation may constitute a dangerous migration that threatens patient safety in another'.[15]

5.3.5 COMPARING METHODS OF DECISION MAKING

To summarize, differences in the four methods of dynamic decision making, which can be construed as advantages and limitations, are listed in Table 5.3.

Abernathy and Hamm[1] proposed that about 70% of surgeons tended to use intuitive decision making, with the rest adopting a more analytical mode, but they did not present any data and they appeared to be referring to all clinical decisions

Table 5.3 Comparison of decision methods

Decisions	Advantages	Limitations
Intuitive decisions	Fast; Requires little conscious thought; Can provide a satisfactory, workable option; Useful in routine situations; Reasonably resistant to stress	Requires experience; Could misjudge situation; Risk of confirmation bias; Less likely to use optimal solution (most elegant, economical, etc.); May be difficult to justify
Rule-based decisions	Can be rapid, if rule has been learnt; Gives a course of action that has been determined by experts; Easy to justify as 'following prescribed procedures'; Not necessary to understand the reason for each step; Good for novices	Can be time consuming, if manual has to be consulted; Appropriate procedure/manual may be difficult to locate; Wrong procedure may be selected; Rule may be outdated/inaccurate; May contribute to skill delay; May not understand the reason for each step
Analytical (choice) decisions	Fully compares alternative courses of action; More likely to produce an optimal solution; Can apply decision tools, e.g., staged techniques (e.g. FOR-DEC); Easier to justify	Requires time; Relies on working memory for conscious processing; Not suited to noisy, distracting environments; Can be affected by stress; May cause cognitive overload and stall the decision maker
Creative decisions	Produces solution for an unfamiliar problem; May invent a new solution; Should increase understanding of the problem	Time consuming; Untested solution; Difficult in noise and distraction; Difficult under stress; May be difficult to justify

Source: Flin R et al., *Safety at the Sharp End. A Guide to Non-Technical Skills,* Aldershot, UK: Ashgate, 2008. With permission.

rather than just intra-operative ones. There are questionnaires to assess preferred styles of decision making[51]; however, there is limited evidence on these tendencies for surgeons.

5.3.6 SWITCHING MODES OF DECISION MAKING: 'SLOWING DOWN WHEN YOU SHOULD'

Of these four methods, evidence suggests that surgeons tend to use mainly intuitive and analytical decision modes when making intra-operative decisions. Although they may have a preferred way of thinking, they will often need to switch between decision-making modes during a procedure – 'the trick is in matching the appropriate cognitive activity to the particular task'[52] – and this may be done subconsciously. What is of particular interest is how surgeons learn to do this, especially the mental transition from the more intuitive, automatic mode to a more effortful style of analytical thinking. The following example illustrates how this happens:

Consultant: 'Where's the hole? Can you see it? Well that's no good, if you can't see the whole hole, we can't repair it, can we? If you can't see it, we have to put the clamp on. Another vascular clamp please. Right. Think. Let's just think here. This all started off so nicely, didn't it?'
Registrar: 'I think I can see it'.
Consultant: 'If you can't see it, how are you going to put the graft on it?'
(from an observed case).

Moulton[17-19] conducted a series of insightful studies into surgeons' thinking while executing a procedure. She focused on the fast intuitive mode, which she calls automatic, and the more effortful, analytic method, which requires more conscious processing of both the situational information and the alternative courses of action. What intrigued her was the question of how surgeons switch from one mode to the other, especially when they 'slow down' - moving from intuitive to a more analytical mode. From interviews with 28 surgeons of different specialties and observations of 5 HPB surgeons conducting 29 cases,[18] she found four versions of

the transition from an automatic, intuitive mode ('just know what to do') to a more effortful state. In the most extreme manifestation, 'stopping', surgeons actually stopped the procedure. The operating surgeon might ask a colleague for assistance, look up reports from the patient's file or review imaging. Surgeons frequently used words such as 'regroup' and 'reassess' to describe these moments, reflecting the uncertainty that was often linked to this critical transition. These could be at a juncture that emerged or it was a pre-planned transition, such as orthopaedic surgeons getting ready to divide the pelvis or an HPB surgeon preparing to clamp the portal vein.

In a second type of transition, which Moulton called 'controlling distraction', the surgeon carries on with the procedure but starts to manage the task environment when critical cues are noticed:

The surgeon was assisting the fellow as the liver parenchyma was transected. The situation was relaxed and proceeding uneventfully. The resident, holding a retractor, was telling an unrelated story to the surgical team with the surgeon laughing in response to her story and joining in the discussion. In the operative field, a large hepatic vein was opened suddenly, causing a moderate and steady flow of blood loss. Oblivious to this, the resident continued talking. The surgeon said, 'Wait one minute, [resident name]. Let's just see where we are', as the surgeon and fellow continued operating. Without the situation fully under control, the resident resumed talking. The surgeon said (with some agitation), 'Wait one minute, [name], a bit too much bleeding here.'[18]

In a third version of the transition behaviour, 'focusing more intently', the surgeon did not control the background but instead began to concentrate in a more single-minded fashion on the task, for example, by stopping talking or disengaging from an ongoing conversation. Other team members sometimes recognize cues when a surgeon begins to do this, such as the humming of a particular tune or by stepping out of clogs. In the most subtle manifestation, 'fine-tuning', surgeons were able to continue the procedure and focus on minor events simultaneously, but these were more routine aspects of the cases where there were just moments of slowing down to take particular care.

Her study also found examples of where surgeons did not slow down early enough, described as 'drifting'; this represented surgeons' failure to transition out of the automatic mode when appropriate, resulting in surgical errors or near misses. This may be due to a degree of complacency, especially due to more boring or mundane aspects of a familiar procedure.

> Referring to a recent mishap in the operating room, one surgeon explained, 'It's the routine cases ... it's like the ... bile duct injuries always happened in easy gall bladders, right? That's what happened here. It was an easy case. We were chatting and obviously not being as diligent as we should have been'.[18]

The concept of 'metacognition',[53] knowledge and awareness of your own thinking processes and strategies (thinking about thinking), recently applied in surgery,[54] may be relevant to these transitions when they are consciously enacted.

Having explained the cognitive background to the decision-making process in surgeons, the three elements in the NOTSS category decision making are outlined. It should be noted that NOTSS is an observational system and so only includes behaviours that can be seen for the rater to make inferences about the surgeon's decision making. As with situation awareness, the main indicators of these aspects of decision making will be the surgeon's actions and communication with other team members.

'Considering options' (Table 5.4) is about comparing the merits of alternative courses of action. As explained earlier, in many situations experienced surgeons are able to make rapid decisions in an automatic fashion where a single option has been considered. For more unexpected or challenging situations, or when teaching, the surgeon should ideally be discussing what the problem is and what he or she is considering by way of one or more options. In situations where this is not appropriate, intuitive or rule-based decisions may have to be enacted very quickly without prior consultation. In this case, an explanation can be given to relevant team members after the action has been executed to maintain shared understanding on the task at hand.

The second element in the NOTSS category decision making is 'selecting and communicating option', which focuses on sharing information rather than acting as if working alone (Table 5.5). It is also suggested that the surgeon should have and communicate a backup plan at this point, in case the chosen action fails to work.

The final element is 'implementing and reviewing decisions' (Table 5.6). Having selected a particular course of action, it should be implemented. Perhaps surprisingly, this last essential step can sometimes be omitted, especially under demanding conditions. Trainees in an operating theatre simulator have been observed to make a decision and then fail to carry out the necessary actions. This is probably due to distraction, cognitive overload causing forgetting or becoming mentally 'frozen' with increasing stress.

Following implementation, the surgeon should review the result of the selected course of action: what effect has this had, if any? Is the situation better or worse? Has it caused a new problem? Most

Table 5.4 Behavioural markers for considering options element (from NOTSS)

Good behaviours	Poor behaviours
Recognizes and articulates problems	No discussion of options
Initiates balanced discussion of options, pros and cons with relevant team members	Does not solicit views of other team members
Asks for opinion of other colleagues	Ignores published guidelines
Discusses published guidelines	

Note: Considering options refers to generating alternative possibilities or courses of action to solve a problem. It involves assessing the hazards and weighing up the threats and benefits of potential options.

Table 5.5 Behavioural markers for selecting and communicating option element (from NOTSS)

Good behaviour	Poor behaviour
Reaches a decision and clearly communicates it	Fails to inform team of surgical plan
Makes provision for and communicates 'plan B'	Is aggressive/unresponsive if plan questioned
	Shuts down discussion on other treatment options
	Only does what she/he thinks is best or abandons operation
	Selects inappropriate manoeuvre that leads to complication

Note: Selecting and communicating option refers to choosing a solution to a problem and informing all relevant personnel about the chosen option.

Table 5.6 Behavioural markers for implementing and reviewing decisions element (from NOTSS)

Good behaviour	Poor behaviour
Implements decision	Fails to implement decisions
Updates team on progress	Makes same error repeatedly
Reconsiders plan in light of changes in patient condition or when problem occurs	Does not review the impact of actions
Realizes 'plan A' is not working and changes to 'plan B'	Continues with 'plan A' in face of predictably poor outcome or when there is evidence of a better alternative
Calls for assistance if required	Becomes hasty or rushed due to perceived time constraints

Note: Implementing and reviewing decisions refers to undertaking the chosen course of action and continually reviewing its suitability in light of changes in the patient's condition. It involves showing flexibility and changing plans if required to cope with changing circumstances to ensure that goals are met.

models for training decision making (shown in Section 5.5) explicitly include this critical step, and it is a good idea to include other team members who may be able to offer new information or alternative judgements.

Essentially, a continuous review of intra-operative decisions is required, maintaining an ongoing awareness as to whether the action taken from the last decision is still working as expected. Aviation research has demonstrated how a 'plan-continuation error'[55] can result from failures in the review process. This occurs when there is increasing difficulty in relinquishing the current course of action (the plan), even when the conditions have changed, the level of risk has increased and an alternative course of action might now be more appropriate. One underlying reason for adhering to a course of action in the face of increasing risk is that changing the plan, once it is under way, is likely to increase cognitive workload and stress.

The plan-continuation effect has been researched at NASA with airline pilots,[56] showing that there can be a maintained adherence to the original plan (e.g. to land at the intended destination) even when en route conditions (e.g. deteriorating weather) show increasing risk. Aborting the first plan and working out a new plan would have been the optimal decision. A simulator study indicated that the closer pilots were to their destination, the less likely they were to change their course of action.[57] The task context can influence decision processes, for example, when the situation is 'strong', thus increasing 'goal seduction' – 'the tendency for pilots to continue despite evidence suggesting it is imprudent'.[58] McLennan et al.[59] describe situations where wildfire incident commanders appear to be influenced by sunk cost effects and over-optimistic biases (e.g. continuing to commit crews into a very hazardous environment). These factors, coupled with high motivation to successfully complete the task, may also influence judgements of risk perception or risk tolerance during decision making.

Surgeons can also become 'locked in' to their current plan and be reluctant to abandon it, especially if they have devoted significant time to working it out beforehand.

5.4 FACTORS INFLUENCING INTRA-OPERATIVE DECISION MAKING

As outlined in Chapter 1, the skill of decision making while operating is influenced by a number of variables.[60] The surgeon's level of experience, particularly of the procedure at hand; general expertise in anatomy; procedural techniques, tissue handling; dexterity; as well as intellectual ability will all contribute to the standard of decision making and the range of options available. Work conditions can play an important role, such as workload, equipment, ergonomics, environment, time pressure and organizational culture. It is important to realize that social factors, such as team atmosphere or even being observed by visiting surgeons,[20] can have an influence on intra-operative judgements. Moulton and colleagues described a number of these more subtle pressures, e.g. trainee surgeons endeavouring to preserve an impression of confidence and competence while operating.[61] An interview study across specialties revealed three categories of contextual factors that had this kind of influence, some of which were openly acknowledged ('avowed', e.g. the patient's best interests) and others less so ('unavowed', e.g. teaching pressures, or 'disavowed', e.g. reputation and financial motivations).[62] There are also 'performance-shaping' factors, e.g. stress; fatigue; and physiological states such as hunger, thirst and general well-being. These are discussed in Chapter 8, so they are only briefly considered here.

Under stress, decision making can be more difficult, especially in the more effortful analytical mode. Detrimental effects of acute stress on cognitive processes can be as follows: overselective attention (tunnel vision); reduction of working memory capacity; and slower retrieval from long-term memory, with more reliance on heuristics, such as choosing a familiar option. Shifts in mental strategy, such as speed/accuracy trade-offs, can be observed with people under stress behaving as if they were working under time pressure when in fact there is none.[63] Acute stress does not necessarily have a debilitating effect on decision making; rather, stress may affect, in an adaptive manner, the way information is processed. The more automatic, intuitive mode, which requires less working memory and conscious processing, appears to be less affected by stress[64] and simplified decision strategies (e.g. obtain proximal and distal control of a bleeding vessel; airway/breathing/circulation) may be optimal under such conditions. If procedures can be easily recalled, or checklists located, then a rule-based method of decision making will generally function reasonably well in stressful conditions.

In the Air France fatal accident in which three pilots lost control of an Airbus A330 flying between Rio de Janeiro and Paris,[65] it appears that they may have experienced a 'startle effect',[66] which compromised their decision making. This was probably due to their unfamiliarity with the non-normal state of the aircraft, and the captain had been asleep when the event began to unfold. Surgeons with on-call experience will know how it feels to have to make critical decisions on an unfamiliar problem moments after being woken.

Fatigue (discussed in Chapter 8) can influence the quality of a surgeon's decision making, although it may be less common with working time limitations. Even one night of sleep loss can impair cognitive flexibility, increase perseveration errors and ability to appreciate an updated situation.[67] Petrilli et al.[68] tested the decision-making skills of flight crews who had just flown an aircraft on a long international route compared to crews who had just had 4 days of rest. They handled a 1-hour-long route in the simulator during which a critical decision event occurred. The fatigued crews took longer to implement decisions and were more risk averse, but they engaged in protective behaviours such as cross-checking and picked up minor errors. Thus, self-awareness of tiredness and its associated risks can facilitate compensatory behaviours.

5.5 TRAINING SURGEONS' INTRA-OPERATIVE DECISION MAKING

Surgeons have a long period of training in which they are taught how to operate on increasingly challenging cases and learn to hone their judgement skills. However, they typically receive little formal training in the psychological processes underlying their decision making or on decision-making methods. The Royal Australasian College of Surgeons recently introduced a new 1-day course on clinical decision making, which covers operational decision making and includes stages of decision making,[69] cognitive processes and clinical decisions under stress. Courses on non-technical skills for surgeons (see Chapter 9) typically contain a module on decision making, based on the kind of psychological material discussed in this chapter.

In some operational environments, practitioners are taught a generic process or sequence for analytical decision making. Airline pilots in Lufthansa and Air France learn the acronym FOR-DEC (facts, options, risks and benefits, decision, execution, check),[70] especially for dealing with non-normal or unexpected situations. A similar process has been taught to British Airways pilots – DODAR (diagnosis, options, decision, assign the tasks, review).[71] While experienced surgeons may follow these basic steps intuitively, junior surgeons might find this type of acronym helpful for dealing with more challenging events, especially when there is the risk of a startle effect under stress inhibiting or delaying their decision making.

Another type of generic training for decision making employed in medicine takes a de-biasing approach, endeavouring to teach the risks of residual biases and favoured heuristics. While self-awareness and metacognition can enhance decision quality, this type of training is not a straightforward undertaking given that cognitive bias has been described as a 'normal operating characteristic of the human brain'.[72] Perhaps more practically, awareness of common 'decision traps'[71] that can also snare surgeons (e.g. jumping to conclusions, complacency and lack of communication)

can be increased by revealing these problems from the analysis of surgical adverse events, post-case debriefs or personal feedback from structured observations in the operating room/simulator.

The typical approach in surgery is to teach decision making for specific procedures, often by the trainee first watching a more experienced surgeon who talks through the steps being taken. However, expert surgeons, when relying on a more automatic mode of decision making when performing surgery, can find it tricky to deconstruct their thinking to teach the procedures to trainees or may stop explaining what they are doing when they reach a more demanding part of the procedure.[19] Pugh et al.,[6] when discussing surgeons' intra-operative decision making, note that research on expertise[73] indicates that 'experts are consciously aware of around 30% of the decisions they make during a critical procedure but that different experts are aware of different decisions'.[73] A recent observational study by Bezmer et al.[74] reveals the different ways in which consultant surgeons talk (or not) about their decisions with their trainees.

One method of extracting this information on decision-making processes is cognitive task analysis (CTA),[75] which enables experts to articulate operative steps and decisions in complex procedures to provide a framework which can then be used to identify central teaching points[6] or surgical scripts.[2] For example, Sullivan et al.[76] videotaped three expert colorectal surgeons performing a colonoscopy and then conducted a CTA interview with them to create a 26-step procedural checklist and a 16-step cognitive demands table. The videotape transcriptions were transposed onto the procedural checklist and cognitive demands table to identify steps and decision points that were omitted during traditional teaching. They found that surgeon A described 50% of 'how-to' steps and 43% of decision points. Surgeon B described 30% of steps and 25% of decisions. Surgeon C described 26% of steps and 38% of cognitive decisions. They concluded, 'By using CTA, we were able to identify relevant steps and decision points that were omitted during traditional teaching by all 3 experts'.[76] In a later study, Smink et al.[77] interviewed, again using a CTA (critical decision method), three expert surgeons in laparoscopic appendectomy. They identified 24 operative steps and 27 decision points (only 5 of which were given by all three experts, again indicating the individual variability of techniques). This CTA method can provide a framework to identify key teaching principles to guide intra-operative instruction on decision points during a procedure and how best to respond. It can also be used with less experienced trainee surgeons to reveal their current understanding of the key steps and decisions in a given procedure.

Masterclasses, long favoured in surgery, can teach intra-operative decision making. In one version,[78] 18 cataract surgery experts presented their own video cases in which something had gone wrong, resulting in a complication that taught them valuable lessons (e.g. iris prolapse, incision burn, globe perforation). At critical points during each case, the video was paused at an event: *the nucleus abruptly tilted posteriorly during an attempt at pre-chopping, indicating the presence of a sizeable zonular dialysis. The entire lens appeared to be loose. What now?* The audience made clinical decisions on electronic response pads. Then, two discussants gave management recommendations, before the video of the outcome was shown. The responses were recorded, and significantly different decisions were revealed. These were shown with a transcript of the surgeon's account of what actually transpired, providing valuable material for discussion and decision training.

Medical simulation has advanced rapidly in the last decade,[79] and the range of facilities for surgeons, from simple apps for a smartphone to part-trainers to full operating room suites, is invaluable for practising decision making under controlled conditions. Gaming techniques are being adapted for specific procedures, such as off-pump coronary artery bypass surgery.[80] Even lower fidelity simulation methods for training surgical decision making can be used with paper-based administration, such as tactical decision games in which participants are provided with a scenario and given a few minutes or less to state what actions they would take. This is normally done in a small group setting with a facilitator to ensure that the discussion is non-judgemental.[81] This provides a way of formalizing the 'storytelling' that remains a very powerful, if non-systematic, way for novices to learn the subtleties of their craft from more experienced practitioners, in almost every workplace.[82]

5.6 ASSESSING SURGEONS' INTRA-OPERATIVE DECISION-MAKING SKILLS

Trainee surgeons' decision-making skills may be assessed by written examination, practical skills tests and interviews, which can include situational judgement tests.[83] More senior faculty can be asked to give a summative evaluation of a resident's ability to make intra-operative decisions. Oral examinations (e.g. for board certification in the United States) do attempt to assess decision making, but the extent to which performance in an interview room at 3 PM is an adequate predictor of intra-operative decision making at 3 AM in the middle of a difficult case remains debatable. The introduction of simulator facilities may help to provide more realistic tests of intra-operative decision skills. At the faculty level for qualified surgeons, decision making is rarely, if ever, formally assessed, although in some countries, developments in licensing and revalidation are beginning to address this.

Observations of a surgeon's decision making while operating can be used as an assessment method, with trainers writing reports on judged competence. The behavioural rating systems for non-technical skills, such as decision making, have been designed to assist this process. While the cognitive processes in the head of the surgeon are impossible to observe directly, the surgeons involved in the design of the NOTSS system provided examples of behaviours they would use to make judgements about an operating surgeon's decision-making proficiency. Chapter 10 describes how to use the NOTSS method.

New wearable technologies that can be used by surgeons in the operating room, e.g. eye-trackers,[84] or field-of-view recorders[85] are offering methods of recording aspects of surgeons' behaviour that may help to reveal cognitive processes underlying decision making. These recordings can be used as the basis of a CTA interview after the case has been completed, as shown in studies of fire commanders' decision making. The officers wore helmet-mounted cameras during real fires and rescues, and the videotape was later used for debriefing[86,87] and subsequently can be used for training material.

5.7 SUMMARY

Intra-operative decision making can be conceptualized as a two-stage cognitive process. The first step is situation assessment, defining the situation and judging risk and time. The second step is deciding what to do. Surgeons make decisions in a number of different ways: intuitive, rule based, analytical, and creative. The method of decision making at a given moment will depend on both task factors and the surgeon's level of experience.

REFERENCES

1. Abernathy C, Hamm R. *Surgical Intuition*. Philadelphia, Pennsylvania: Belfus; 1993.
2. Dimick J, Upchurch G, Sonnenday C. *Clinical Scenarios in Surgery: Decision Making and Operative Technique*. Philadelphia, Pennsylvania: Lippincott, Williams & Wilkins; 2012.
3. Stiegler M, Tung A. Cognitive processes in anaesthesiology decision making. *Anesthesiology*. 2014;120:204–17.
4. Flin R, Fioratou E, Frerk C, Trotter C, Cook T. Human factors in the development of complications of airway management: Preliminary evaluation of an interview tool. *Anaesthesia*. 2013;68:817–25.
5. Flin R, Youngson G, Yule S. How do surgeons make intra-operative decisions? *Qual Saf Health Care*. 2007;16:235–239.
6. Pugh C, Santacaterina S, Da Rosa D, Clark R. Intra-operative decision making: More than meets the eye. *J Med Inform*. 2010;44:486–96, 186.
7. Marsh H. *Do No Harm. Stories of Life, Death and Brain Surgery*. London, United Kingdom: Weidenfield & Nicholson; 2014.
8. Campbell G, Watters D. Making decisions in emergency surgery. *ANZ J Surg*. 2013;83:429–33.
9. Association of Surgeons of Great Britain and Ireland. *Emergency Surgery: The Future. A Consensus Statement*. London, United Kingdom: ASGBI; 2007.
10. Cuschieri A. Nature of human error. Implications for surgical practice. *Ann Surg*. 2006;244:642–8.
11. Gawande A, Zinner M, Studdert D, Brennan T. Analysis of errors reported by surgeons at three teaching hospitals. *Surgery*. 2003;133:614–21.
12. Rogers S, Gawande A, Kwaan M, Puopolo A, Yoon C, Brennan T et al. Analysis of surgical errors in closed malpractice claims at 4 liability insurers. *Surgery*. 2006;140:25–33.
13. Flin R. *Sitting in the Hot Seat: Leaders and Teams for Critical Incident Management*. Chichester, England: Wiley; 1996.
14. Zsambok C, Klein G (Eds.). *Naturalistic Decision Making*. Mahwah, New Jersey: Lawrence Erlbaum; 1997.
15. Cristancho S, Apramian T, Vanstone M, Lingard L, Ott M, Novick R. Understanding clinical uncertainty: What is going on when experienced surgeons are not sure what to do? *Acad Med*. 2013;88:1516–21.
16. Cristancho S, Vanstone M, Lingard L, LeBel M, Ott M. When surgeons face intra-operative challenges: A naturalistic model of surgical decision making. *Am J Surg*. 2013;205:156–62.
17. Moulton C, Regehr G, Mylopoulos M, MacRae H. Slowing down when you should: A new model of expert judgment. *Acad Med*. 2007;82:s109–16.
18. Moulton C, Regehr G, Lingard L, Merritt C, MacRae H. Slowing down to stay out of trouble in the operating room: Remaining attentive in automaticity. *Acad Med*. 2010;85:1571–7.
19. Moulton C, Regehr G, Lingard L, Merritt C, MacRae H. 'Slowing down when you should': Initiators and influences of the transition from the routine to the effortful. *J Gastrointest Surg*. 2010;14:1019–26.

20. Pauley K, Flin R, Yule S, Youngson G. Surgeons' intra-operative decision making and risk management. *Am J Surg.* 2011;202:375–81.

21. Pauley K, Flin R, Azuaro-Blanco A. Intra-operative decision making by ophthalmic surgeons. *Brit J Ophthalmol.* 2013;97:1303–7.

22. Orasanu J, Fischer U. Finding decisions in natural environments: The view from the cockpit. In C. Zsambok, G. Klein (1997) (Eds.). *Naturalistic Decision Making.* Mahwah, New Jersey: Lawrence Erlbaum; 1997.

23. Orasanu J. Training for aviation decision making: The naturalistic decision making perspective. In *Proceedings of the Human Factors and Ergonomic Society, 39th Annual Meeting, San Diego.* Santa Monica, California: The Human Factors and Ergonomics Society; 1995.

24. Orasanu J, Dismukes K, Fischer U. Decision errors in the cockpit. In *Proceedings of the Human Factors and Ergonomics Society, 37th Annual Conference.* San Diego, California: The Human Factors and Ergonomics Society; 1993.

25. Dominguez C, Flach J, McDermott P, McKellar D, Dunn M. The conversion decision in laparoscopic surgery: Knowing your limits and limiting your risks. In K. Smith, P. Johnston (Eds.). *Psychological Investigations of Competence in Decision Making.* Cambridge, United Kingdom: Cambridge University Press; 2004. p. 14.

26. Mitchell L, Flin R, Youngson G, Malik M, Ahmed I. Intraoperative surgical decision making—A video study. In H. Chaudet, L. Pellegrin, N. Bonnardel (Eds.). *Proceedings of the 11th Conference on Naturalistic Decision Making, Marseille, France, 21–24 May.* Paris, France: Arpege Science Publishing; 2013.

27. Jacklin R, Sevdalis N, Harries C, Darzi A, Vincent C. Judgement analysis: A method for quantitative evaluation of trainee surgeons' judgments of surgical risk. *Am J Surg.* 2008;195:183–8.

28. Masserwah N, Devlin A, Symons R, Elrod J, Flum D. Risk tolerance and bile duct injury: Surgeon characteristics, risk taking preference and common bile duct injuries. *J Am Coll Surg.* 2009;209:17–24.

29. Damasio A. *Descartes' Error: Emotion, Reason and the Human Brain.* New York: Vintage; 2006.

30. Loewenstein G, Weber E, Hsee C, Welch N. Risk as feelings. *Psychol Bull.* 2001;127:267–86.

31. Mosier K, Fisher U. The role of affect in naturalistic decision making. *J Cogn Eng Decis Making.* 2010;4:240–55.

32. Contessa J, Suarez L, Kyriakides T, Nadzam G. The influence of surgeon personality factors on risk tolerance: A pilot study. *Journal of Surgical Education.* 2013;70:806–12.

33. Tubbs E, Elrod J, Flum D. Risk taking and tolerance of uncertainty: Implications for surgeons. *J Surg Res.* 2006;131:1–6.

34. Klein G. A recognition-primed decision (RPD) model of rapid decision making. In G. Klein, J. Orasanu, R. Calderwood, C. Zsambok (Eds.). *Decision Making in Action.* New York: Ablex; 1993. p. 139.

35. Evans J, Stanovich K. Dual process theories of higher cognition: Advancing the debate. *Perspect Psychol Sci.* 2013;8:223–41.

36. Kahneman D. *Thinking Fast and Slow.* New York: Doubleday; 2011.

37. Gigerenzer G, Goldstein D. Reasoning the fast and frugal way: Models of bounded rationality. *Psychol Rev.* 1996;103:650–69.

38. McPeek B. Intuition as a strategy of medical decision making. *Theor Surg.* 1991; 6:83–4.

39. Gladwell M. *Blink: The Power of Thinking without Thinking.* London, United Kingdom: Penguin; 2005.

40. Mitchell L, Flin R. Decisions to shoot by police officers. *J Cogn Eng Decis Making.* 2007;1:375–90.

41. Harris D, Khan H. Response time to reject a takeoff. *Human Factors and Aerospace Safety.* 2003;3:165–75.

42. Sullenburger C. *Highest Duty.* New York: Harper; 2010. p. 223.

43. NHS England. *Standardise, Educate, Harmonise.* Report of the NHS England Never Events Taskforce. London,

United Kingdom: NHS, Patient Safety Domain; 2014

44. Arriaga A, Bader AM, Wong JM, Lipsitz SR, Berry WR, Ziewacz JE, Hepner DL. Simulation based trial of surgical-crisis checklists. *N Engl J Med.* 2013;368:246–53.

45. Birkmeyer J, Liu J. Decision analysis models: Opening the black box. *Surgery.* 2003;133:1–4.

46. Croskerry P, Singhal G, Mamede S. Cognitive debiasing 1: Origins of bias and the theory of debiasing. *BMJ Qual Saf.* 2013;22:ii58–64.

47. Croskerry P, Singhal G, Mamede S. Cognitive debiasing 2: Impediments to and strategies for change. *BMJ Qual Saf.* 2013;22:ii65–72.

48. Larken J. Military commander—Royal Navy. In R. Flin, K. Arbuthnot (Eds.). *Incident Command: Tales from the Hot Seat.* Aldershot, United Kingdom: Ashgate; 2002. p. 114.

49. Haynes A. United 232: Coping with the 'one chance-in-a-billion' loss of all flight controls. *Flight Deck.* 1992;3(Spring):5–21.

50. Flin R, O'Connor P, Crichton M. *Safety at the Sharp End. A Guide to Non-Technical Skills.* Aldershot, United Kingdom: Ashgate; 2008.

51. Scott S, Bruce R. Decision-making style: The development and assessment of a new measure. *Educ Psychol Meas.* 1995;55:818–31.

52. Croskerry P. The theory and practice of clinical decision-making. *Can J Anaesth.* 2005;52:R1–8.

53. Fleming S, Dolan R, Frith C. Metacognition: Computation, biology and function. *Philos Trans R Soc B.* 2012;367:1280–6.

54. Uemura M, Tomikawa M, Nagao Y, Yamashita N, Kumashiro R, Tsutsumi N. Significance of metacognitive skills in laparoscopic surgery assessed by essential task simulation. *Minim Invasive Ther Allied Tech.* 2014;23:165–72.

55. Orasanu J. Flight crew decision making. In B. Kanki, R. Helmreich, J. Anca (Eds.). *Crew Resource Management* (2nd ed). San Diego, California: Academic Press; 2010.

56. Burian B, Orasanu J, Hitt J. Weather-related decision errors: Differences across flight types. In *Proceedings of the Human Factors and Ergonomics Society Conference.* San Diego, California: The Human Factors and Ergonomics Society; 2000.

57. Orasanu J. Risk behaviours in pilots. Invited address, Quincentennial Conference, Royal College of Surgeons Edinburgh; 2005.

58. Bearman C, Paletz S, Orasanu J. Situational pressures on aviation decision making: Goal seduction and situation aversion. *Aviat Space Environ Med.* 2009;80:556–60.

59. McLennan J, Holgate A, Omodei M, Wearing A. Decision making effectiveness in wildfire incident management teams. *J Conting Crisis Man.* 2006;14:27–37.

60. Sarker S, Chang A, Vincent C. Decision making in laparoscopic surgery: A prospective, independent and blinded analysis. *Int J Surg.* 2008;6:98–105.

61. Jin C, Martimianakis M, Kitto S, Moulton C. Pressures to 'measure up' in surgery. *Ann Surg.* 2012;256:989–93.

62. Leung A, Luu S, Regehr G, Murnaghan L, Gallinger S, Moulton C. 'First do no harm': Balancing competing priorities in surgical practice. *Acad Med.* 2012;87:1368–74.

63. Orasanu J. Stress and naturalistic decision making: Strengthening the weak links. In R. Flin, K. Arbuthnot (Eds.). *Incident Command: Tales from the Hot Seat.* Aldershot, United Kingdom: Ashgate; 1997.

64. Stokes A, Kemper K, Kite K. Aeronautical decision making, cue recognition and expertise under pressure. In C. Zsambok, G. Klein (Eds.). *Naturalistic Decision Making.* Mahwah, New Jersey: Erlbaum; 1997.

65. Bhangu A, Bhangu S, Stevenson J, Bowley D. Lessons for surgeons in the final moments of Air France Flight 447. *World J Surg.* 2013;37:1185–92.

66. Martin W, Murray P, Bates P. Startle, freeze and denial: An analysis of pathological pilot reactions during unexpected events. In *Proceedings of the 65th International Air Safety Seminar.* Washington: Flight Safety Foundation; 2012.

67. Harrison Y, Horne J. One night of sleep loss impairs innovative thinking and flexible decision making. *Organ Behav Hum Dec.* 1999;78:128–45.

68. Petrilli R, Thomas M, Dawson D, Roach G. The decision making of commercial airline crews following an international pattern. In *Proceedings of the Australian Aviation Society Conference.* Sydney, Australia; 2006 Nov.

69. Crebbin W, Beasley S, Watters D. Clinical decision making. How surgeons do it. *ANZ J Surg.* 2013;83:422–8.

70. Hörmann, H.-J. FOR-DEC: A prescriptive model for aeronautical decision making. In R. Fuller, N. Johnston, N. McDonald (Eds.). *Human Factors in Aviation Operations.* Aldershot, United Kingdom: Avebury; 1995.

71. Walters A. *Crew Resource Management Is No Accident.* Wallingford, United Kingdom: Aries; 2002.

72. Croskerry P. Bias: A normal operating characteristic of the diagnosing brain. *Diagnosis.* 2014;1:23–7.

73. Chao C, Salvendy G. Percentage of procedural knowledge acquired as a function of the number of experts from whom knowledge is acquired for diagnosis, debugging and interpretation tasks. *Int J Hum-Comput Int.* 1994;6:221–33, 488.

74. Bezemer J, Murtagh G, Cope A, Kneebone R. Surgical decision making in a teaching hospital: A linguistic analysis. *ANZ J Surg.* 2015; in press.

75. Crandall B, Klein G, Hofmann R. *Working Minds. A Practitioner's Guide to Cognitive Task Analysis.* Cambridge, Massachusetts: MIT Press; 2006.

76. Sullivan M, Ortega A, Wasserberg N, Kaufman H, Nyquist J, Clark R. Assessing the teaching of procedural skills: Can cognitive task analysis add to traditional teaching methods. *Am J Surg.* 2008;195:20–3.

77. Smink D, Peyre S, Soybel D, Tavakkolizadeh A, Vernon A, Anastakis D. Utilization of a cognitive task analysis for laparoscopic appendectomy to identify differentiated intraoperative teaching objectives. *J Surg.* 2012;203:140–5.

78. Chang D. Cataract experts share their surgical mishaps. *Eyenet.* 2012 Feb;45.

79. Riley R. *Handbook of Medical Simulation* (2nd ed). Oxford, United Kingdom: Oxford University Press; 2015; in press.

80. Cowan B, Sabri H, Kapralos B, Moussa F, Christancho S, Dubrowski A. A serious game for off-pump coronary bypass surgery procedure training. In J. Westwood et al. (Eds.). *Medicine Meets Virtual Reality.* Amsterdam, the Netherlands: IOS Press; 2011.

81. Crichton M, Flin R, Rattray W. Training decision makers—tactical decision games. *J Conting Crisis Man.* 2002;8:208–17.

82. Joung W, Hesketh V, Neal A. Using 'war stories' to train for adaptive performance: Is it better to learn from error or success. *Appl Psychol Int Rev.* 2006;55:282–302.

83. Weekley J, Ployhart R. (Eds.). *Situational Judgement Tests.* Washington: Society for Industrial and Organizational Psychology; 2013.

84. Hermen F, Flin R, Ahmed I. Surgeons' eye movements: A literature review. *J Eye Mov Res.* 2013;6:1–11.

85. Muensterer O, Lacher M, Zoeller C, Bronstein M, Kubler J. Google Glass in pediatric surgery: An exploratory study. *Int J Surg.* 2014;12(4):281–9.

86. Omodie M, Wearing A, McLennan J. Head mounted video recording. A methodology for studying naturalistic decision making. In R. Flin, E. Salas, M. Strub, L. Martin (Eds.). *Decision Making under Stress.* Aldershot, United Kingdom: Ashgate; 1997.

87. Cohen-Hatton S, Butler P, Honey R. An investigation of operational decision making in situ: Incident command in the UK Fire and Rescue Service. *Hum Factors.* 2015; in press.

6

Teamwork and communication

PAUL O'CONNOR, IVAN KEOGH AND AUGUSTO AZUARA-BLANCO

6.1 INTRODUCTION

Effective teamwork and communication by surgeons in the operating room (OR) is crucial to patient safety and quality of care. The risks of technical failures in surgery are very well recognized. However, breakdowns in teamwork and communication in OR teams are common and can lead to poor outcomes for patients.[1] Healey et al.[2] found that teamwork failures in cardiothoracic surgery occurred at a rate of 17.4 per hour. Further, when team behaviours, such as co-ordination, backing up others and communicating critical task information at the right time, are infrequent, patients are more likely to experience death or major complications.[3]

Communication failures were the root cause of 54% of the operative/post-operative complication sentinel events reviewed by the Joint Commission in the United States from 2004 to June 2013.[4] In a review of surgical cases in which there was successful litigation, 87% of the failures included a breakdown in communication, most commonly occurring between health care professionals as opposed to those with the patients.[5] It has been found in Canada that there were failures in approximately 30% of the communication exchanges between operating team members.[6]

There is also variability between members of the OR team in how they view their team skills. It has been consistently found that surgeons and anaesthetists rate the team skills of members of their own medical discipline higher than nurses rate the team skills of surgeons and anaesthetists.[7] Therefore, surgeons may not realize that their teamworking and communication skills could be improved.

The following example shows how poor communication and teamworking within an OR team can put a patient at risk.

A failure of teamworking and communication in the operating room

A registrar urologist was carrying out a renal transplant. A junior anaesthetist was present in the OR from the start of the procedure. However, after the incision had been made another more senior anaesthetist came into the OR. Although the surgeon noticed her coming in, he did not speak to her, nor did she speak to him. The surgeon was very focused on the technical aspects of the case. As the procedure progressed, although no vessels were actively bleeding, there was a little bit more blood than would be expected in and around the wound. The surgeon made a mental note of this, assumed that the anaesthetic team was happy for him to continue, put in a few more mops and continued with the procedure.

All of a sudden, from the top of the table he heard a shout, 'Stop! What's going on? We are losing the patient!' The patient's blood pressure had suddenly dropped. A more experienced anaesthetist was called in, and the patient was stabilized and went on to make a full recovery. The surgeon continued with his patient list for that day.

The following morning, the surgeon was called in to see the surgical director as there had been a complaint made against him. The anaesthetist who came in midway through the procedure the previous day said that she thought the surgeon was sexist and racist because he had not spoken to her. The surgeon admitted that he had been remiss in not introducing himself to her as he was very focused on the technical aspects of the surgery. The anaesthetist also acknowledged that she should have introduced herself to him.

This is an example of how a breakdown in communication and teamworking has the potential to contribute to a poor outcome for the patient. Clearly, the lack of communication and teamworking between the surgeon and the anaesthetist was the main causal factor. However, the other members of the OR team could also have alerted the surgeon and anaesthetic team to the higher than expected levels of blood loss.

This chapter discusses the surgeon's skills for enhancing intraoperative teamworking and communication. Although the focus is on the surgeon, the information is also relevant to the other members of the OR team. The chapter is structured using the three elements of the teamwork and communication category in Non-Technical Skills for Surgeons (NOTSS): exchanging information, establishing a shared understanding and co-ordinating team activities. Strategies that surgeons can use to foster effective intraoperative communication are identified. These include the importance of creating a climate for assertiveness and speaking up, and the specific challenges of operating on a conscious patient. Finally, interventions that have been shown to improve teamwork and communication for surgeons, and other members of the OR team, are described, such as briefing, timeouts/checklists, debriefing and team training.

6.2 EXCHANGING INFORMATION

The first element in the NOTSS category of teamwork and communication is 'exchanging information' (Table 6.1) and refers to the exchange of information feedback or response, ideas and feelings between surgeon and other OR team members. These behaviours provide the basis for dynamic team knowledge of ongoing events, allow relationships to be formed, establish predictable behaviour patterns and maintain attention to the task.[8]

Lingard et al.[6] report a study in which they trained observers to record the communication events in 48 surgical procedures. A total of 421 communication events were recorded, of which 129 were categorized as communication failures. These communication failures were categorized

Table 6.1 Behavioural markers for exchanging information element (from NOTSS)

Good behaviour	Poor behaviour
Talks about the progress of the operation	Fails to communicate concerns with others
Listens to concerns of team members	Attempts to resolve problems alone
Communicates that operation is not going to plan	Does not listen to team members
	Needs help from assistant but does not make it clear what the assistant is expected to do

Note: Exchanging information refers to giving and receiving knowledge and information in a timely manner to aid the establishment of shared understanding among team members.

into four different failure types (numbers do not add up to 100% as some events involved multiple communication failures):

1. *Occasion failure (46%):* This refers to a problem in the situation or context of the communication, for example, a surgeon may request for an unexpected instrument at the exact time it is needed, rather than warning the nurses that this was something he or she would require in the future.
2. *Content failures (36%):* This refers to insufficiency or inaccuracy in the information being communicated, for example, a failure to ensure that all in the OR team are aware of a patient's pre-existing medical condition, allergy or medication. An example of the potential for a misunderstanding in eye surgery is provided in the example on the risk of sound-alike words in the next column.
3. *Audience failure (21%):* This refers to gaps in the composition of the group engaged in the communication. For example, the surgeon and the anaesthetist may decide to rearrange the order of the patients for surgery without discussing this with the charge nurse.
4. *Purpose failure (24%):* The purpose of the communication is unclear, not achieved or inappropriate, for example, two of the OR nurses discussing whether the surgeon requires a particular instrument that is not in the standard set. Neither knows, but no one asks the surgeon.

These types of communication failures are not unique to surgeons, or OR teams. Brindley and Reynolds[9] provide an excellent overview of

Risk associated with sound-alike words

In eye surgery, a viscoelastic material is often used to help make the procedure easier and safer. The material keeps delicate tissues apart and avoids the potential for contact that would damage these tissues. There are different types of viscoelastic materials, with different properties and indications and different brand names.

It is common for surgeons to use the term 'visco', a generic term to refer to all types of viscoelastic materials. However, there is also a brand called 'Viscoat', which is only used for special circumstances and can cause some potential (typically minor) problems if used inappropriately.

communication techniques that are commonly used in aviation that they believe have application in a critical care environment. The strategies identified can be grouped into those that foster clear communication and those that improve assertiveness.

6.2.1 STRATEGIES TO FOSTER CLEAR COMMUNICATION

Flying by voice: A good practice in aviation is for the pilot who is carrying out a task to 'say out loud' what he or she is doing. This could be as simple as reporting a change of direction (e.g. 'turning right heading 270'). Articulating the tasks that are being carried out ensures that there is a clear understanding of what is being done, what is being considered and who is doing what. In surgery, 'operating by voice' would simply be when a surgeon describes what he or she is doing (e.g. 'I have placed the tracheostomy tube in the trachea … I will secure it with sutures').

Closed-loop communication: It is common for pilots to use close-loop communication to ensure that tasks are completed, for example, when responding to headings and altitude changes provided by air traffic control:

Air Traffic Control: Shamrock 273. Turn right to heading two seven zero and climb to flight level two niner zero to avoid traffic.
Pilot of Shamrock 273: Roger. Turning right heading two seven zero, and climbing to flight level two niner zero.

Another example is swapping the pilot who is actually flying the aircraft (rather than the pilot who is monitoring) using a positive three-way communication exchange:

Pilot 1: I have the aircraft.
Pilot 2: You have the aircraft.
Pilot 1: I have the aircraft.

In aviation, as both pilots are able to make inputs to the aircraft, it is very important that it is clear which pilot is actually flying the aircraft. This three-way communication exchange may also be good practice when using the dual console da Vinci robotic surgical system (Intuitive Surgical, Sunnyvale, CA, USA). In the dual console version of this system, both surgeons can control the instrument. Therefore, just as in the aviation example, it is very important to know who is controlling the instruments. Although this three-way communication is likely unnecessary in most ORs, closed-loop communication is an important strategy for ensuring good team co-ordination and aiding in team sensemaking. For example,

Surgeon: Can I have everyone's attention, please? I am about to make the incision. Anaesthetics, are you happy for me to proceed?

Anaesthetist: Yes, anaesthetics happy for you to proceed.
Surgeon: Nursing team, are you happy for me to proceed with the incision?
Theatre sister: Yes, the nursing team is happy for you to proceed.
Surgeon: Thank you. Making incision now.

Articulating the tasks that are being carried out so that there is a clear understanding of what is being done, what is being considered and who is doing what is routinely observed in high-performing teams. For example, effective use of closed-loop communication in the OR is particularly important in time-critical situations (e.g. 'put pressure on the bleeding point and tell me when the bleeding stops').

In emergency or time-critical situations, it is important to communicate clearly and succinctly (described in aviation as 'comms-brevity'). Brindley and Reynolds[9] describe this as combating mitigating language (e.g. 'Get i.v access now … Start i.v fluids stat'). Mitigating languages refers to de-emphasizing or 'sugar-coating' what is being said. We mitigate speech to be deferential or polite or when embarrassed or unsure. There is also a need to be sensitive to what others in the team are doing and ensure that the communication is not interfering with the overall goals of the team.

However, it is also important to remain professional in any communication. Rude language and hostile behaviour have been found to impair cognitive performance and negatively impact patient safety and quality of care.[10]

Sterile cockpit: this concept is used to protect the flying team from unnecessary distractions. Typically, during specific sequences of flight – such as when the plane is below 10,000 ft – only flight-related communications are allowed. This ensures that the team can focus on communicating information that relates solely to the flying of the aircraft and sets the tone that operations, and safety, are paramount.

Clarity and precision in communication are also important in high-risk work environments. For example, members of US Navy submarine crews are forbidden from using certain words that can cause confusion or ambiguity (e.g. 'left' and 'right' or 'maximum' and 'minimum'). An example of the potential effect of a lack of precision is an actual wrong-site surgery performed on a young child. The patient was due to have an upper labial frenulum release (division of the labial frenulum). Unfortunately, the electronic patient admission system had only one code for three different types of surgical procedures, all being described as 'tongue tie'. Instead of having the division of her upper labial frenulum, the surgeon erroneously performed a lingual frenectomy (incision of the lingual frenulum under the tongue).[11] Although this was not the only failure of communication in the scenario, the lack of clarity in the admission system was a contributing factor. In the following box, an example of how a procedure was performed on the wrong patient due to a lack of precision is given.

Wrong patient surgery

There were two elderly patients with the same (common) surname and similar first names waiting for cataract surgery in a day case unit.

When the nurse called for the patient, one man walked towards the nurse. The nurse did not seek other verifying information to ensure the identity of the patient (e.g. double-check the name, date of birth and address). In fact, this was the wrong patient and thus the wrong notes led the surgeon to do the cataract operation in the wrong eye using an inappropriate intraocular lens.

The patient was somewhat deaf and went through the whole process without realizing the error. Fortunately, the patient had cataracts in both eyes and the implant was close enough to the one required so that no further surgery was required. This incident led to changes in the procedure carried out in the unit for identifying the correct patient.

6.2.2 COMMUNICATION CHALLENGES OF OPERATING ON A CONSCIOUS PATIENT

There are particular types of surgery in which it is common to operate on conscious patients under local or regional anaesthetic. For example, in ophthalmology the vast majority of operations (e.g. cataract, glaucoma, corneal transplants and retinal surgery) are performed under local anaesthetic. Similarly, abdominal, pelvic and lower limb surgeries are also frequently conducted under epidural anaesthetic. Many operations in low- or middle-resource environments (e.g. East Africa) are also routinely conducted under regional anaesthesia, such as nerve blocks. However, there is a potential negative effect on teamworking and communication between members of the OR team as a result of the presence of a conscious patient who can hear everything that occurs during their procedure.

Wilkinson[12] and Ford[13] found that ophthalmic OR teams would use a range of communication techniques. Of particular relevance was the use of implicit co-ordination techniques that are not necessary when operating on a fully anaesthetized patient. Wilkinson[12] reported that a variety of strategies were used to communicate information between team members during ophthalmic surgery to ensure that the patient did not become alarmed. For example, team members whispered to each other or used gestures or body language to communicate. Some of the consultant surgeons would use code words to communicate with the trainee surgeons (e.g. saying 'well done' to mean 'stop'). The surgeons would also sometimes deliberately use technical language to reduce the information that the patient may understand.

It was also indicated that team communication between team members in ophthalmic surgery was deliberately focused on the procedure, with discussion of case-irrelevant issues kept to a minimum and the surgeon avoiding direct conversation with the patient.[12] The reason provided for this strategy was to ensure that the patient did not nod their head or talk when instruments were in their eye. Nevertheless, despite the lack of active communication with the patient it was felt important to be sensitive to the patient's level of anxiety, especially when this becomes elevated during the surgery such as when the patient senses that something is not going according to plan. This is particularly important during eye surgery due to the effect this can have on the intraocular pressure.[12] A common practice in ophthalmic ORs to allow patients to communicate during surgery under local anaesthetic (e.g. if they have some discomfort) avoiding head movement is to hold a nurse's hand, or a buzzer, and have a pre-planned signal that would lead to a warning to the surgical team. It is possible to make a number of recommendations to address communication and teamworking issues when operating on a conscious or (in some cases) an unconscious patient:

- Standardize code signals. If used, code words or hand signals should be standardized (at least within a unit) to ensure that all members of the OR team are aware of the alternative meaning and can act accordingly using implicit co-ordination.
- Preoperative briefing is essential. It would also seem that operating on a conscious patient is a domain in which a preoperative brief (without the patient being present) is of particular importance. This will ensure that any possible complications can be identified (e.g. diabetes and allergies) and allow the responses to any potential issues to be considered prior to the operation so that the actions do not need to be discussed in detail during the procedure.
- Detect patient anxiety. Manage the potential anxiety that a conscious patient may experience during surgery by telling them their role during the surgery ahead of time and providing reassurance.[14]
- Encourage listening to music. Consideration could be made of encouraging patients to listen to music via headphones (where the headphones do not interfere with the operating field) to mask the communication between the members of the operating team. Music has also been found to significantly lower patients' anxiety levels, heart rate and blood pressure compared to patients who did not listen to music.[15]

6.2.3 SPEAKING UP AND ASSERTIVENESS

Speaking up is defined as an upward voice directed from lower to higher status individuals within and across teams that challenges the status quo, to avert or mitigate errors.[16] Failure to speak up has a negative impact on patient safety and quality of care.[17-21] However, a number of studies across different domains of health care have found that junior personnel are unwilling to speak up or challenge the behaviour of more senior personnel. Moreover, many senior personnel are unaware of this issue.[22-24]

In a survey of Irish surgeons, almost 80% of surgical trainees, but only a third of consultants, reported that junior personnel were frequently or very frequently afraid to express disagreement with more senior personnel.[24] Nurses have also been found to feel constrained in when and what they are able to communicate.[25] Therefore, this creates the dangerous situation in which personnel are afraid to speak up, but seniors are largely unaware of this issue. The overarching reason that has been provided for the failure to speak up is the hierarchy that exists in health care.[22,26] The unwillingness of junior personnel to speak up is a result of having their ideas discounted,[21,22] their fear of appearing incompetent or their unwillingness to offend more senior personnel.[21] A recent study found that surgical trainees were more willing to speak up about an error they observed if the senior surgeon in the room created a culture that encouraged the behaviour.[27]

Brindley and Reynolds[9] present a number of techniques designed to improve assertiveness. Graded assertiveness provides a way for health care professionals to identify how assertive they are being and how their level of assertiveness can be escalated. They provide six levels of assertiveness:

1. Hint: 'Should things look like this?'
2. Preference: 'I think it would be wise to ...'
3. Query: 'What do you think we should do?'
4. Shared suggestion: 'You and I should ...'
5. Statement: 'We need to do the following ...'
6. Command: 'Do it now'

The five-step advocacy approach focuses on advocacy and confirmation to get a piece of information across:

1. Attention getter: 'The patient is desaturating'.
2. State your concern: 'The neck is swelling'.
3. State the problem as you see it: 'Surgical hematoma is compromising the airway'.
4. State a solution: 'We need to open the neck, remove skin clips now'.
5. Obtain agreement: 'Do you agree?'

A similar graded approach to assertiveness is the 'CUSS' mnemonic, which makes use of keywords to aid in the appropriate escalation of concern.

C: 'I am *concerned*'.
U: 'I am *uncomfortable*'.
S: 'This has become a *serious* situation'.
S: 'I think this procedure needs to *stop* at this point'.

The benefit of CUSS is that once remembered it is easier to recall during situations of high stress than other tools, as the mnemonic makes efficient use of cognitive resources that are depleted by acute stress during the very moments when speaking up is required.

Brindley and Reynolds[9] also state that there are times when it may be necessary for team members to be assertive enough to take over control of a situation if it is felt that this is necessary (e.g. 'Intubation has failed … I will secure a surgical airway now'). This is similar to the two-challenge rule used in aviation, where if a co-pilot has not received a satisfactory response to a safety-endangering manoeuvre from the captain then he or she may lawfully take control of the plane.[28]

6.2.4 ACTIVE LISTENING

In addition to creating a culture that empowers juniors to speak up, there is also a need to encourage seniors to listen. There is little sense in teaching junior surgeons to be assertive if their seniors are not willing to listen to them. Listening is an active process and requires effort on behalf of the listener. Even in ideal circumstances, only a small part of

what is heard is actually listened to (usually only about one-third) if the listener is interested; this is even less if the listener is not interested. The earlier part of a communication also tends to be listened to more than the later part – when the listener may be trying to find a place to interrupt. This is described as 'gap searching'.[29] Therefore, it is important that the listener also is engaged in the communication process. Active listening can be encouraged through techniques such as briefings, timeouts and checklists, all of which are discussed in Section 6.4. These methods provide a structured format through which juniors are facilitated to voice an opinion and seniors are encouraged to listen.

6.3 ESTABLISHING A SHARED UNDERSTANDING

The second element in the NOTSS category of teamwork and communication is 'establishing a shared understanding' (Table 6.2), and it concerns the skills required by the surgeon to enable the OR team to work together, anticipate each other's needs, inspire confidence and communicate in an efficient manner.

To discuss how to achieve a shared understanding, it is necessary to discuss two psychological constructs that explain successful teamwork in high-risk industries: shared mental models and team sensemaking. Although these are concepts that are very important for team performance, they have not been systematically investigated in health care.[30]

6.3.1 SHARED MENTAL MODEL

Shared mental models provide the members of a team with a common understanding that then allows them to form accurate explanations and expectations about the task and to co-ordinate their actions and behaviours. Thus, team members can anticipate the needs of the other team members and synchronize their activities. Holding accurate and shared mental models of both the task and the team supports effective co-ordination between team members.

Table 6.2 Behavioural markers for Establishing a shared understanding element (from NOTSS)

Good behaviour	Poor behaviour
Provides briefing and clarifies objectives and goals before commencing operation	Does not articulate operative plan to team
Ensures that the team understands the operative plan before starting	Does not make time for collective discussion and review of progress
Encourages input from all members of the team	Fails to discuss the case beforehand with unfamiliar team members
Ensures that relevant members of team are happy with decisions	Makes no attempt to discuss problems and successes at end of operation
Checks that assistants know what they are expected to do	Fails to keep anaesthetist informed about procedure (e.g. to expect bleeding)
Debriefs relevant team members after operation, discussing what went well and problems that occurred	Appears uncomfortable discussing operative plan if challenged

Note: Establishing a shared understanding refers to ensuring that the team not only has necessary and relevant information to carry out the operation but also understands it and that an acceptable shared 'big picture' of the case is held by all team members.

An example of what it feels like to work in a team in which everyone has a shared mental model comes from an orthopaedic surgeon, 'On a good day, it's as if it's choreographed in the OR – everybody in the right place, at the right time, doing the right thing'. However, if one of the team members has an inaccurate mental model this will lead to co-ordination problems, even if the other members of the team have accurate models.[31] Thus, in a team situation a shared mental model is the extent to which the mental models of team members overlap. It is hypothesized that particularly in fast-moving, or emergency, situations where there is no time to carry out sufficient planning shared mental models are especially important.[32] Mental models provide a set of organized expectations (formed through experience) that team members can use to make predictions about performance in the future. Studies have emerged supporting the utility of shared mental models for team performance.[33,34]

6.3.2 TEAM SENSEMAKING

Team sensemaking is defined as the process by which a team manages and co-ordinates its efforts

to explain the current situation and to anticipate future situations, typically under uncertain or ambiguous conditions.[35] Team sensemaking is required when it is recognized that a shared mental model is no longer accurate. It can be regarded as a response to a situational surprise (e.g. on opening a patient, it becomes clear that the complexity of the operation is greater than expected) and/or failures of expectations (e.g. magnetic resonance imaging scans carried out prior to the surgery suggested that it would be routine). Klein refers to these alarming events as 'tripwires' that indicate that the current plan may have some weaknesses or errors that need to be addressed (e.g. the need to bring in a vascular surgeon and cancel other patients on the list).[36] The first scenario in this chapter in which there was a failure of teamworking and communication in the OR is an example of a failure to recognize a tripwire in which the OR team did not alert the surgeon or anaesthetist to the higher than expected blood loss.

Sensemaking allows practitioners to understand how current accounts of the situation came about and to anticipate future evolutions through a process of fitting data into an explanatory framework.[37]

6.4 CO-ORDINATING TEAM ACTIVITIES

The third and final element in the NOTSS category of teamwork and communication is 'co-ordinating team activities' (Table 6.3). Teamwork requires the surgeon to facilitate co-ordination among all of the members of the OR team. This is especially critical in the OR, where anaesthetists, nurses and surgeons work interdependently in a complex system in which different aspects of patient care are distributed across the OR team. Therefore, to provide safe care the members of the team must work collaboratively.

As can be seen from the behaviours shown in Table 6.3, co-ordinating team activities is concerned with providing support to other team members, sharing workload, accepting individual responsibility, maintaining good working relationships and providing mutual support. Mutual support relates to informational support such as providing advice and information to assist team members to carry out their tasks. This support is particularly important when trainees are part of the OR team. High-performing teams have a climate of openness and trust, where leaders are receptive to alternative views and team members are not afraid to express them.

6.4.1 EXPLICIT AND IMPLICIT CO-ORDINATION

Explicit co-ordination is concerned with the use of verbal communication to actively exchange information with other team members to allow the members of the team to build an accurate shared mental model and engage in team sensemaking. It involves a deliberate effort to co-ordinate the activities of the team and has been found to be appropriate in novel situations and during decision making.[38] For example, if there is an intra-operative complication or a change of plan during the operation. Explicit co-ordination is typically guided by the surgeon and the scrub nurse who will explicitly guide other members of the team.

Implicit co-ordination is less effortful and is concerned with one team member anticipating the needs of another: this can be observed in common and routine procedures (e.g. the scrub nurse opening an additional packet of sutures for the surgeon without being asked to perform the task). Implicit co-ordination requires the team members to have a common understanding of the task including requirements of other team members and the activities that they engage in to support the task. Therefore, a failure in expected implicit co-ordination can be an indicator of the lack of a shared mental model and the need to engage in more explicit co-ordination.

In studies of aviation crews, it has been found that during periods of highly standardized work and high workload there was less reliance on explicit co-ordination, compared to periods in which there was low standardization and low workload.[38] Similarly, anaesthetic teams have also been found to rely on implicit co-ordination in highly standardized scenarios.[39] A high-performing surgical team will be able to use both implicit and explicit communication. A possible strategy for improving implicit co-ordination is to develop a better understanding of the tasks and roles of the

Table 6.3 Behavioural markers for co-ordinating team activities element (from NOTSS)

Good behaviour	Poor behaviour
Checks that other team members are ready to start operation	Does not ask anaesthetist if it is OK to start operation.
Stops operating when asked to by anaesthetist or scrub nurse	Proceeds with operation without ensuring that equipment is ready
Ensures that team works efficiently by organising activities in a timely manner	

Note: Co-ordinating team activities refers to working together with the scrub nurse and anaesthetist to carry out cognitive and physical activities in a simultaneous, collaborative manner.

other team members. A particular intervention that could facilitate this process is cross-training (discussed in Section 6.5.4).

6.4.2 CONFLICT

Research on collaboration in the OR has tended to focus on conflict, the antonym of collaboration. Conflict can be defined as any dispute, disagreement or difference of opinion (for example, related to the management of a patient) involving more than one individual and requiring some decision or action.[40] Unsurprisingly, conflict is prevalent in health care teams. It has been found that conflict occurs during the management of 50–78% of patients, with 38–48% involving doctor–doctor conflict.[41,42] The potential for conflict is arguably particularly high in the OR given the potentially stressful environment, a team of health care professionals who may have overlapping or poorly delineated areas of responsibility and two doctors (possibly of equal seniority) simultaneously caring for one patient.[43] It is interesting to note that OR nurses report seeing themselves as 'keepers of the peace' whose role is to maintain a calm environment to allow surgeons to concentrate on their task.[44]

A distinction can be made between task-related and relationship-related conflicts. Task-related conflict is usually cognitive in nature. This type of conflict focuses on disagreements about decisions and involves differences in viewpoints, ideas and opinions.[45] For example, a disagreement between surgeons regarding exactly how a particular procedure should be carried out. Relationship-related conflict tends to be focused on emotions and is concerned with tensions or clashes of personality related to personal issues or differences.[46] While relationship conflict is associated with poor team performance,[47] the same is not necessarily true of task-related conflict. In fact, a lack of task-related conflict could be detrimental to patient safety as it may mean alternative approaches are not being discussed by the team. Rogers et al.[48] conducted research with OR team members and found that relationship-related and task-related conflicts are tightly connected. As such, they propose that relationship-related conflict should always be carefully managed as it is almost always accompanied by task-related conflict.

6.4.3 CONFLICT RESOLUTION

Katz identifies a number of ways in which a surgeon can manage conflict in the OR[43]:

1. Anticipate conflict.
2. Develop communication skills.
3. Identify the precise source of conflict.
4. Establish rules of conduct.
5. Find a non-judgemental starting point for the discussion.
6. Establish shared standards and goals.
7. Recognize any shared frustrations with the system.
8. If conflict with a colleague is necessary, it should be conducted in a private setting.
9. Have a low threshold for intervention by a third party.
10. If conflict is ultimately irreconcilable, transfer patient care to an uninvolved colleague.

Conflict management is a skill that can be learned, and the most appropriate action will depend on the situation. It has been found that surgical trainees respond to tension in the OR team by withdrawing from communication or mimicking the behaviour of the consultant surgeon. Both responses have negative implications for team performance and may intensify rather than resolve inter-professional conflict.[49] Resolution requires mutual respect among the OR team members, listening to grievances, adherence to the issues, recognition of differences in opinion and acknowledging the emotional aspects of a disagreement.[43]

6.5 INTERVENTIONS TO IMPROVE TEAMWORKING AND COMMUNICATION

6.5.1 BRIEFING

Briefing is crucial to allow team members to develop a shared mental model. In a survey of Irish surgeons, approximately 50% of the respondents indicated that an adequate preoperative brief was seldom completed.[24] All of the team members, regardless of seniority, should attend the brief; the briefing should (obviously) be carried out before the operation begins, and the brief should follow a formal and predictable structure. Generally, a senior member of the team should lead the briefing. However, it is important that input is encouraged, and accepted, from all other team members. All of the pertinent information relating to the task should be discussed including both technical and non-technical issues. Two-way verbal communication should be used.

6.5.2 TIMEOUTS AND CHECKLISTS

Two types of timeouts are described in the surgical literature. The first, and the one gaining wide acceptance, if not universal application, is the initiation and first step involved in the World Health Organization (WHO) safety checklist. (This is also referred to by some as a briefing, although for most surgeons the briefing relates to discussions had by all staff prior to the subsequent operating list and its patients collectively, whereas the timeout relates specifically to the case in question.)

The second type of timeout relates to a cessation/pause in the procedure mid-task, usually to re-evaluate the ongoing situation. This kind of mid-task timeout can be particularly effective during a period of high stress. If unexpected complications occur, experienced surgeons stop what they are doing and try to gain time (e.g. by putting pressure on bleeding).[50] This pause allows the surgeon to mentally stand back from the situation, reassess, make a decision and prepare for how to continue (see also Chapter 5 on slowing down). It can also be an opportunity to engage with other members of the team to develop a shared mental model of what is going on (e.g. discuss the blood loss with the anaesthetist and develop a plan for how to continue with the operation). This reassessment helps to avoid the likelihood of tunnel vision and over-focusing on a particular task to the detriment of others.

Checklists are widely used as memory aids in high-risk work domains such as aviation, nuclear power generation and the maritime industry. These are workplaces in which deviations from a checklist are uncommon. Although it is recognized that it is not possible to have a checklist for every activity performed in the OR, the use

of checklists is becoming more commonplace. For example, in a survey completed by 469 UK cataract surgeons, 93% reported using a surgical checklist.[51] Checklists are particularly relevant as a tool to improve the performance of routine tasks to ensure that specific steps are not being missed. Checklists are also helpful in highly stressful situations in which it is easy to miss a step if working from memory alone.

A specific checklist that has particular relevance in improving teamworking and communication in the OR is the WHO surgical checklist. The WHO surgical checklist is a tool for structuring a briefing prior to starting a procedure. Recognizing the risk to surgical patients, the WHO published guidelines to improve patient safety in the OR.[52] Based on these guidelines, a 19-item checklist was designed with the goal of reducing the rate of major surgical complications.[53]

Initial evaluations of the effects of the WHO surgical checklist were overwhelmingly positive. In a meta-analysis of three before and after studies evaluating the effect of the WHO surgical checklist, there was a 43% decrease in risk of operative death and a 37% decrease in risk of complications.[54] The WHO checklist has also been found to positively influence the safety culture of OR personnel.[55] However, despite the benefits of the WHO checklist for patient safety, in some cases the practical implementation of the checklist has been found to be less than universal,[56] and to decay over time.[57] In a study carried out in Ontario, Canada, no differences were found in risk of death or surgical complications as a result of the implementation of the surgical checklist.[58] Possible reasons provided for the lack of an effect in this study included the following: it is not the ticking off of the items on the checklist that is important but performing the action it calls for, full implementation of the checklist is difficult, hospitals need help in implementing the checklist, not all surgeons will use the checklist and full implementation of the checklist takes time.[59]

To improve compliance with the checklist process, it is important that all members of the OR team are involved such that it is a true multidisciplinary intervention and that the checklist is initiated prior to the anaesthetizing of the patient. Surgeons must openly demonstrate support for checklist adherence. Giving the job of initiating the checklist to the circulating nurse reduces the likelihood of diffusion of responsibility whereby a person is less likely to take responsibility for action or inaction when others are present. However, the circulating nurse must be supported in this role by other members of the OR team, particularly those in more senior positions. For example, visible leadership has been found to be the most important factor in implementing teamwork-training techniques and principles in a health care setting.[60]

Training has been found to be effective in raising the frequency of implementation of surgical checklists from 8% to 97%.[61] However, there is a need for continued reinforcement of safety initiatives such as the implementation of the checklist. A one-off training programme will have limited effectiveness. It is recommended that each department has a designated 'checklist champion' who is responsible for providing training and reinforcing the use of the checklist in the OR.[62]

6.5.3 DEBRIEFING

A team debriefing occurs after a task, such as an operation, has been completed. The purpose is to review how the task went from both a technical and a non-technical perspective to include what went well, what did not go well and how things could be improved in the future. It is easy for a team to fail to debrief after a task, particularly if everything went according to plan. Often, the last thing people want to do after completing a procedure is to spend time discussing their performance, especially if that performance was routine, normal and successful. Interestingly, in a survey of Irish surgeons on attitudes to teamworking and communication no trainee surgeon stated that an adequate postoperative briefing was conducted, compared to 19% of consultant surgeons.[24] Therefore, it is likely that debriefing and feedback is particularly important for juniors who are interested in learning and improving their future performance. Taking the time to carry out a debriefing following an event is something that should be emphasized to foster learning. During a debriefing, the senior team members are crucial in ensuring that an effective debriefing is completed. This is particularly important if there was a catastrophic event. However,

even if the operation did proceed as expected, and particularly if some members of the team are trainees, a debriefing is important.

Tannenbaum et al.[63] identified eight behaviours which should be exhibited during a debriefing, and these are relevant for the lead surgeon:

1. An effective briefing environment should be one in which team members feel comfortable admitting when they were confused or made a mistake. Therefore, to encourage this behaviour the surgeon should model this behaviour during the briefing.
2. To optimize learning in debriefing, team members should show acceptance of feedback from others and so the surgeon must also demonstrate this acceptance of feedback.
3. The feedback should relate to task-focused feedback as opposed to person-focused feedback. Critiques of particular team members should be avoided. Feedback should be focused on behaviours which should be changed instead of personal attacks on individual team members.
4. The feedback should provide specific, constructive suggestions, as opposed to vague negative feedback. This type of feedback will help identify and summarize areas of improvement for both individuals and the team.
5. All team members should be encouraged to participate in debriefings. Surgeons should guide and facilitate team debriefs rather than simply lecturing the team members.
6. Ensure that the non-technical and technical aspects of performance are discussed. Team members do not necessarily understand the specific teamwork behaviours related to their performance of a task.
7. Refer to prior briefings and team performance when conducting subsequent debriefs. This provides a sense of continuity, reliability and consistency.
8. Tell the individual team members or the team as a whole when they demonstrate an improvement in performance.

It is recognized that conducting a thorough debriefing after a case is extremely challenging as this can be a time of high workload for the OR team. The surgeon will have paperwork to complete (e.g. OR notes), the anaesthetist may be in the recovery room with the patient and the nurses may be cleaning the OR and preparing for the next case. However, as with the surgical checklist, there is a growing body of evidence that shows that briefings and debriefings are effective in reducing morbidity and mortality in surgery.[64] There may also be efficiency benefits that far outstrip the 5 minutes it takes to conduct a team debrief. The challenge is being able to 'pause' and fit in the debriefing before beginning the next case.

6.5.4 TEAM TRAINING

Crew Resource Management (CRM) training, described in Chapter 2, is a set of instructional strategies designed to improve teamwork in operational environments by applying well-tested tools (e.g. performance measures, exercises and feedback mechanisms) and appropriate training methods (e.g. simulators, lectures and videos) targeted at specific content (i.e. teamwork knowledge, skills and attitudes). It has been used for more than three decades in commercial aviation, and in recent years there has also been a large proliferation of CRM training in the medical community for improving performance in both critical and routine situations.

An example of a study of a CRM training intervention for OR teams is reported by McCulloch et al.[65] They note that 9 hours of didactic and interactive teaching based on an aviation CRM model was delivered to 54 members of the OR team. Training was provided in the following topics: safety, situation awareness, error management, self-awareness, communication and assertiveness, decision making and briefing and debriefing. The initial training was delivered by civil aviation CRM trainers, and this training was then followed by 3 months of twice-weekly coaching. It was found that non-technical skills and attitudes improved after the training and that operative technical errors and non-operative procedural errors decreased. However, considerable cultural resistance to adoption was encountered, particularly among medical staff. Also, debriefing and challenging authority seemed more difficult to introduce than other parts of the training.

A systematic review of 12 studies of the application of team training with OR teams concluded that there were statistically significant before and after improvements in teamwork behaviours, and in some secondary outcomes (e.g. complication rates).[66] It is important to recognize that a single training course, completed once in a career, is unlikely to result in a sustained cultural shift. There is a need for continuous reinforcement of good teamwork behaviours in the OR, as well as the involvement of other members of the OR team.

A meta-analysis of the effect of CRM training in health care found there were considerable variations in the length and content of the training (e.g. inclusion of simulation or not).[67] Although the majority of the studies (except for two) were single site, there was variation in the number, specialty, type of health care provider and seniority of the training participants. Overall, participants liked this type of training and there was a large effect of the training on knowledge, a small effect of training on attitudes and a large effect of training on behaviour. Although the evidence for an effect on organizational outcomes (e.g. mortality) in the meta-analysis was largely unsupported, there are examples in the literature in which this type of training has had organizational level impacts. To illustrate, a study of the Veteran's Administration Medical Team Training (designed on the CRM principles described earlier) showed an 18% reduction in annual mortality where hospitals that had received the training were compared to those where the training had not been carried out.[68]

Another team-training strategy that would seem to have relevance to improving team performance in the OR is called cross-training. This training strategy has not been widely applied in health care. Cross-training can be defined as an instructional strategy in which each team member is trained in the duties of his or her teammates.[34] There are three levels of cross-training, which differ in the depth of information provided.[69] These levels are described as positional clarification, positional modelling and positional rotation:

- Positional clarification aims to provide team members with a general understanding of the role and responsibilities of each member of the team. Discussions, lectures and demonstrations can be used to provide this level of knowledge.

- Positional modelling provides the team members with a greater level of understanding. The duties of each team member are discussed and observed. This technique results in the team members knowing about both the duties of each team member and how these relate to the other members of the team. The training consists of observing teammates in a simulated situation.
- Positional rotation provides team members with direct, hands-on practice of their colleagues' specific tasks and how the tasks interact. Although the aim is not for team members to become experts in the other roles, they should reach a basic competence level for specific tasks carried out by their teammates that demand high degrees of cooperation and interdependency.

For an OR team, it is suggested that an improved understanding of the roles will have a positive effect on both explicit and implicit co-ordination. It is likely that there would be particular benefits to trainees of any discipline in gaining some more knowledge of each other's roles.

6.6 CONCLUSION

It is irrefutable that poor teamworking and communication have a negative effect on patient safety and quality of care. Surgeons should reflect on their own communication and consider where some of the techniques for effective communication reviewed in this chapter could be integrated into their own practice. For senior surgeons there is a need to be open to the opinions of others, and junior surgeons should practice speaking up. Surgeons should identify when explicit co-ordination is necessary to build an accurate team mental model and be sensitive to the tripwires that indicate that things may not be going to plan.

Briefing, timeouts/checklists, debriefing and team training can have a positive effect on patient safety and performance. However, there is also evidence that the impact of these interventions decays over time as they cease to be used as frequently and rigorously as when they were first introduced. The challenge to those who work in and with OR teams is to ensure that these interventions lead to lasting and sustained improvements in teamwork and communication.

REFERENCES

1. Flin R, Mitchell L (Eds.). *Safer Surgery*. Aldershot, UK: Ashgate Publishing, Ltd.; 2009.
2. Healey AN, Sevdalis N, Vincent CA. Measuring intra-operative interference from distraction and interruption observed in the operating theatre. *Ergonomics*. 2006;49(5–6):589–604.
3. Mazzocco K, Petitti DB, Fong KT, Bonacum D, Brookey J, Graham S et al. Surgical team behaviors and patient outcomes. *Am J Surg*. 2009;197(5):678–85.
4. Commission TJ. Sentinel Event Data Root Causes by Event Type 2004—June 2013. 2013 [March 12, 2014]. Available from: http://www.jointcommission.org/assets/1/18/Root_Causes_by_Event_Type_2004-2Q2013.pdf.
5. Morris JA, Jr., Carrillo Y, Jenkins JM, Smith PW, Bledsoe S, Pichert J et al. Surgical adverse events, risk management, and malpractice outcome: Morbidity and mortality review is not enough. *Ann Surg*. 2003;237(6):844–51.
6. Lingard L, Espin S, Whyte S, Regehr G, Baker GR, Reznick R et al. Communication failures in the operating room: An observational classification of recurrent types and effects. *Qual Saf Health Care*. 2004;13(5):330–4.
7. Wauben LS, Dekker-van Doorn CM, van Wijngaarden JD, Goossens RH, Huijsman R, Klein J et al. Discrepant perceptions of communication, teamwork and situation awareness among surgical team members. *Int J Qual Health Care*. 2011;23(2):159–66.
8. Kanki BG, Palmer MT. Communication and crew, resource management. In E. Wiener, B. Kanki, R. Helmreich (Eds.). *Cockpit Resource*

Management. San Diego, California: Academic Press; 1993. pp. 99–136.

9. Brindley PG, Reynolds SF. Improving verbal communication in critical care medicine. *J Crit Care*. 2011;26(2):155–9.

10. Flin R. Rudeness at work. *BMJ*. 2010;340:c2480.

11. Madden E. Prof Corbally vindicated in high court decision. *Irish Med Times*, November 27, 2013.

12. Wilkinson J. Non-technical skills in ophthalmic surgeons. MSc thesis. Aberdeen, United Kingdom: University of Aberdeen; 2012.

13. Ford R. Playing our roles in the operating theatre: The impact of the awake patient on training complex surgical procedures. MSc thesis. London, United Kingdom: Imperial College; 2010.

14. Thorp JM, Kennedy BW, Millar K, Fitch W. Personality traits as predictors of anxiety prior to caesarean section under regional anaesthesia. *Anaesthesia*. 1993;48(11):946–50.

15. Mok E, Wong KY. Effects of music on patient anxiety. *AORN J*. 2003;77(2):396–7, 401–6, 9–10.

16. Bienefeld N, Grote G. Silence that may kill: When aircrew members don't speak up and why. *Aviat Psych Appl Hum Fact*. 2012;2(1):1–10.

17. Reader T, Flin R, Lauche K, Cuthbertson BH. Non-technical skills in the intensive care unit. *Br J Anaesth*. 2006;96(5):551–9.

18. Pronovost PJ, Thompson DA, Holzmueller CG, Lubomski LH, Dorman T, Dickman F et al. Toward learning from patient safety reporting systems. *J Crit Care*. 2006;21(4):305–15.

19. Leonard M, Graham S, Bonacum D. The human factor: The critical importance of effective teamwork and communication in providing safe care. *Qual Saf Health Care*. 2004;13(Suppl 1):i85–90.

20. Burke CS, Salas E, Wilson-Donnelly K, Priest H. How to turn a team of experts into an expert medical team: Guidance from the aviation and military communities. *Qual Saf Health Care*. 2004;13(Suppl 1):i96–104.

21. Sutcliffe KM, Lewton E, Rosenthal MM. Communication failures: An insidious contributor to medical mishaps. *Acad Med*. 2004;79(2):186–94.

22. Belyansky I, Martin TR, Prabhu AS, Tsirline VB, Howley LD, Phillips R et al. Poor resident-attending intraoperative communication may compromise patient safety. *J Surg Res*. 2011;171(2):386–94.

23. Reader T, Flin R, Cuthbertson BH. Communication skills and error in the intensive care unit. *Curr Opin Crit Care*. 2007;13(6):732–6.

24. O'Connor P, Ryan S, Keogh I. A comparison of the teamwork attitudes and knowledge of Irish surgeons and U.S. Naval aviators. *Surgeon*. 2012;10(5):278–82.

25. Lingard L, Garwood S, Poenaru D. Tensions influencing operating room team function: Does institutional context make a difference? *Med Educ*. 2004;38(7):691–9.

26. Walton MM. Hierarchies: The Berlin Wall of patient safety. *Qual Saf Health Care*. 2006;15(4):229–30.

27. Salazar MJB, Minkoff H, Bayya J, Gillett B, Onoriode H, Weedon J et al. Influence of surgeon behavior on trainee willingness to speak up: A randomized controlled trial. *J Amer C Surg*. 2014; 219(5):1001–7.

28. Pian-Smith M, Simon R, Minehart RD, Podraza M, Rudolph JW, Walzer T et al. Teaching residents the two-challenge rule: A simulation-based approach to improve education and patient safety. *Simulat Healthcare*. 2009;4(2):84–91.

29. Flin R, O'Connor P, Crichton M. Safety at the sharpend: Training non-technical skills. Aldershot, England: Ashgate Publishing, Ltd.; 2008.

30. Manser T. Teamwork and patient safety in dynamic domains of healthcare: A review of the literature. *Acta Anaesthesiol Scand*. 2009;53(2):143–51.

31. Converse SA, Cannon-Bowers JA, Salas E (Eds.). Team member shared mental models: A theory and some methodological issues. *Proceedings of the Human Factors Society, 35th Annual Meeting, San Francisco, CA*. Human Factors Society; 1991.

32. Cannon-Bowers J, Salas E, Converse S. Shared mental models in expert team decision making. In J. Castellan (Ed.). *Current Issues in Individual and Group Decision Making*. Hillsdale, New Jersey: Lawrence Erlbaum Associates; 1993. pp. 221–46.

33. Blickensderfer E, Cannon-Bowers JA, Salas E. Theoretical bases for team self-correction: Fostering shared mental models. *Adv Int St*. 1997;4:249–79.

34. Volpe CE, CannonBowers JA, Salas E, Spector PE. The impact of cross-training on team functioning: An empirical investigation. *Hum Factors*. 1996;38(1):87–100.

35. Klein G, Wiggins S, Dominguez CO. Team sensemaking. *Theor Issues Ergonomics Sci*. 2010;11(4):304–20.

36. Klein GA. *The Power of Intuition*. New York: Doubleday; 2004.

37. Crandall B, Klein GA, Hoffman RR. *Working Minds: A Practitioner's Guide to Cognitive Task Analysis*. Cambridge, Massachusetts: MIT Press; 2006.

38. Zala-Mezo E, Wacker J, Kunzle B, Bruesch M, Grote G. The influence of standardisation and task load on team co-ordination patterns during anaesthesia inductions. *Qual Saf Health Care*. 2009;18(2):127–30.

39. Grote G, Zala-Mezö E, Grommes P. Effects of standardization on co-ordination and communication in high workload situations. *Linguistische Berichte Sonderheft* (Linguistic Reports Special Issue). 2003;12:127–55.

40. Studdert DM, Mello MM, Burns JP, Puopolo AL, Galper BZ, Truog RD et al. Conflict in the care of patients with prolonged stay in the ICU: Types, sources, and predictors. *Intensive Care Med*. 2003;29(9):1489–97.

41. Burns JP, Mello MM, Studdert DM, Puopolo AL, Truog RD, Brennan TA. Results of a clinical trial on care improvement for the critically ill. *Crit Care Med*. 2003;31(8):2107–17.

42. Breen CM, Abernethy AP, Abbott KH, Tulsky JA. Conflict associated with decisions to limit life-sustaining treatment in intensive care units. *J Gen Intern Med*. 2001;16(5):283–9.

43. Katz JD. Conflict and its resolution in the operating room. *J Clin Anesth*. 2007;19(2):152–8.

44. Riley RG, Manias E. Governance in operating room nursing: Nurses' knowledge of individual surgeons. *Soc Sci Med*. 2006;62(6):1541–51.

45. Simons TL, Peterson RS. Task conflict and relationship conflict in top management teams: The pivotal role of intragroup trust. *J App Psy*. 2000;85(1):102–11.

46. Janss R, Rispens S, Segers M, Jehn KA. What is happening under the surface? Power, conflict and the performance of medical teams. *Med Educ*. 2012;46(9):838–49.

47. De Dreu CKW, Weingart LR. Task versus relationship conflict, team performance, and team member satisfaction: A meta-analysis. *J App Psy*. 2003;88(4):741–9.

48. Rogers D, Lingard L, Boehler ML, Espin S, Klingensmith M, Mellinger JD et al. Teaching operating room conflict management to surgeons: Clarifying the optimal approach. *Med Educ*. 2011;45(9):939–45.

49. Lingard L, Reznick R, Espin S, Regehr G, DeVito I. Team communications in the operating room: Talk patterns, sites of tension, and implications for novices. *Acad Med*. 2002;77(3):232–7.

50. Wetzel CM, Kneebone RL, Woloshynowych M, Nestel D, Moorthy K, Kidd J et al. The effects of stress on surgical performance. *Am J Surg*. 2006;191(1):5–10.

51. Kelly SP, Steeples LR, Smith R, Azuara-Blanco A. Surgical checklist for cataract surgery: Progress with the initiative by the Royal College of Ophthalmologists to improve patient safety. *Eye (Lond)*. 2013;27(7):878–82.

52. World Health Organization World Alliance for Patient Safety. *WHO Guidelines for Safe Surgery*. Geneva, Switzerland: WHO; 2008.

53. Haynes AB, Weiser TG, Berry WR, Lipsitz SR, Breizat AH, Dellinger EP et al. A surgical safety checklist to reduce morbidity and mortality in a global population. *N Engl J Med*. 2009;360(5):491–9.

54. Borchard A, Schwappach DL, Barbir A, Bezzola P. A systematic review of the effectiveness, compliance, and critical factors for implementation of safety checklists in surgery. *Ann Surg.* 2012;256(6):925–33.

55. Helmio P, Blomgren K, Takala A, Pauniaho SL, Takala RS, Ikonen TS. Towards better patient safety: WHO Surgical Safety Checklist in otorhinolaryngology. *Clin Otolaryngol.* 2011;36(3):242–7.

56. Gueguen T, Coevoet V, Mougeot M, Pierron A, Blanquart D, Voicu M et al. Deployment of the checklist 'Patient safety in the operating room' in two Lorraine hospitals. Performances and difficulties. *Ann Fr Anesth Reanim.* 2011;30(6):489–94.

57. Paugam-Burtz C, Guerrero O. French surgical checklist in a universitary hospital: Achievements one year after implementation. *Ann Fr Anesth Reanim.* 2011;30(6):475–8.

58. Urbach DR, Govindarajan A, Saskin R, Wilton AS, Baxter NN. Introduction of surgical safety checklists in Ontario, Canada. *N Engl J Med.* 2014;370(11):1029–38.

59. Leape LL. The checklist conundrum. *N Engl J Med.* 2014;370(11):1063–4.

60. France DJ, Leming-Lee S, Jackson T, Feistritzer NR, Higgins MS. An observational analysis of surgical team compliance with perioperative safety practices after crew resource management training. *Am J Surg.* 2008;195(4):546–53.

61. Sewell M, Adebibe M, Jayakumar P, Jowett C, Kong K, Vemulapalli K et al. Use of the WHO surgical safety checklist in trauma and orthopaedic patients. *Int Orthop.* 2011;35(6):897–901.

62. O'Connor P, Reddin C, O'Sullivan M, O'Duffy F, Keogh I. Surgical checklists: The human factor. *Pat Saf Surg.* 2013;7(1):14.

63. Tannenbaum SI, Smith-Jentsch KA, Behson SJ. Training team leaders to facilitate team learning and performance. In J.A. Cannon-Bowers, E. Salas (Eds.). *Making Decisions Under Stress: Implications for Individual and Team Training.* Washington, DC: American Psychological Association; 1998. pp. 247–70.

64. Wahr JA, Prager RL, Abernathy JH, 3rd, Martinez EA, Salas E, Seifert PC et al. Patient safety in the cardiac operating room: Human factors and teamwork. A scientific statement from the American Heart Association. *Circulation.* 2013;128(10):1139–69.

65. McCulloch P, Mishra A, Handa A, Dale T, Hirst G, Catchpole K. The effects of aviation-style non-technical skills training on technical performance and outcome in the operating theatre. *Qual Saf Health Care.* 2009;18(2):109–15.

66. Gillespie BM, Chaboyer W, Murray P. Enhancing communication in surgery through team training interventions: A systematic literature review. *AORN J.* 2010;92(6):642–57.

67. O'Dea A, O'Connor P, Keogh I. A meta-analysis of the effectiveness of team training in healthcare domains. *J Postgrad Med.* 2014;90(1070):699–708.

68. Neily J, Mills PD, Young-Xu Y, Carney BT, West P, Berger DH et al. Association between implementation of a medical team training program and surgical mortality. *JAMA.* 2010;304(15):1693–700.

69. Blickensderfer E, Cannon-Bowers JA, Salas E. Cross training and team performance. In J.A. Cannon-Bowers, E. Salas (Eds.). *Making Decisions Under Stress: Implications for Individual and Team Training.* Washington, DC: American Psychological Association; 1998. pp. 299–311.

7

Leadership

CRAIG MCILHENNY, SARAH HENRICKSON PARKER AND GEORGE G YOUNGSON

7.1 INTRODUCTION

A leader leads by example, not by force.

Attributed to Sun Tzu

Safe surgical practice relies on the performance of a surgical team and surgeons rely on the operating room team to deliver high-quality and safe surgical care to their patients, often under difficult circumstances. Good leadership has been identified as a key variable for the optimal functioning of these teams and is one of the main reasons for the success or failure of team-based working. The fundamental importance of front-line leadership in health care teams is thus becoming increasingly recognized as vital for patient safety. This acknowledgement is in line with other high-hazard industries, such as commercial aviation, where leadership has long been identified as a key

to safe performance. High-reliability organizations understand the impact of good leadership on their safety culture, staff adherence to safety policy and feeling safe to speak up about safety concerns.[1]

Despite a clear need for excellent intra-operative leadership, and the emphasis placed on this skill as an essential ingredient for safe patient care, the behaviours associated with good surgical leadership are not well defined or formally taught. The goal of this chapter is to discuss how the Non-Technical Skills for Surgeons (NOTSS) taxonomy can be used as a framework to describe good leadership behaviours in the operating room, and ultimately to provide useful guidance for practising surgeons to better understand and improve intra-operative leadership be it their own or for helping develop leadership in their trainees. Within this discussion, the good leadership behaviours contained within the NOTSS leadership category are examined. The wider leadership literature is referred to where appropriate, and a practical and useable body of knowledge on the leadership skills that can be used to improve the safe delivery of surgical care within the operating room is provided. The chapter does not provide an exhaustive examination of leadership styles (for a full explanation of leadership style in the wider context and further leadership theory discussion, the study by Yukl[2] can be referred to). Included in this chapter is a brief discussion on the Surgeons' Leadership Inventory (SLI), which details intra-operative leadership behaviours.

To best illustrate the principles being discussed, and to emphasize the practical importance of leadership, case studies of surgeons' leadership in the operating room are presented throughout the chapter.

7.2 LEADERSHIP IN NOTSS

Leadership is a subject that is gaining increasing recognition for its role in patient safety, but defining good leadership is not as straightforward as may first appear. Although the concept of leadership, and the proliferation of leadership courses, is now gaining prominence in medical training programmes, most of these courses are aimed at strategic or organizational leadership. The skills needed for effective leadership of an operating room team are very different from the managerial skills of an organizational leader. The focus for front-line leaders is on accomplishment of task goals and ensuring the team is functioning adequately.[3] A significant amount of research has examined these two dimensions and concluded that ensuring both optimal task and team performance is an essential skill for a front-line leader.

In the NOTSS taxonomy, the leadership category involves the surgeon leading the entire team in the operating room and providing a clear direction and goal; it involves demonstrating the highest standards of clinical practice, care and technical expertise and also being considerate and supportive of other team members. The leadership category emphasizes that one of a surgeon's main responsibilities is to maximize team performance and ensure safe and effective team functioning, in addition to completion of the surgical task. While

leadership taxonomies in other high-risk industries have clearly identified team-building behaviours to be a crucial part of safety leadership, surgeons may, on occasion, focus their leadership behaviours more on the surgical task than the team.[4]

This finding may reflect the fact that surgeons are often working with different team members or do not see themselves as the leader of the entire operating room team but rather only of the team doing the actual operation.[4] Unlike many other designated team leaders, surgeons are not usually working with a consistent team and are not in a positional leadership role, such as a supervisor, for the multidisciplinary operating room team. These circumstances, therefore, require a different type of leadership than that is typically described in popular leadership texts or seminars. Being the technical expert plus the individual who can influence the team to be in attendance, be co-ordinated and be engaged in supportive team behaviour requires special skills.

The NOTSS framework, moreover, is useful for teaching the essential skills of leadership to trainee surgeons and by providing a rating system that can be used to assess both personal individual leadership behaviours and leadership behaviours of other surgeons. As with all of the NOTSS categories, leadership is subdivided into three elements: setting and maintaining standards, supporting others and coping with pressure. These elements have indicative behaviours that demonstrate good or poor behaviours within each element. The taxonomy is designed to be used within the operating room and to relate directly to the observable behaviours of the surgeon in question.

7.3 SETTING AND MAINTAINING STANDARDS

Surgeons need to set the standards for behaviour within their operating room and demonstrate these by adhering to good surgical practice and attention to technical skills and also by expressing positive attitudes towards wider clinical codes of good practice and by following theatre checklists and protocols (Table 7.1). The surgeon who displays these leadership skills will be rewarded with

Table 7.1 Behavioural markers for setting and maintaining standards element (from NOTSS)

Good behaviours	Poor behaviours
Introduces self to new or unfamiliar members of theatre team	Fails to observe standards (e.g. continues even though equipment may be contaminated or inadequate)
Clearly follows theatre protocol	Breaks theatre protocol
Requires all team members to observe standards (e.g. sterile field)	Shows disrespect to the patient

Note: Setting and maintaining standards refers to supporting safety and quality by adhering to acceptable principles of surgery, following codes of good clinical practice and following theatre protocols.

a more positive attitude towards safety within the team.[5] A lack of such behaviours or, even worse, the demonstration of opposing attitudes or behaviours will provide a hidden curriculum for the rest of the team, especially surgeons in training, that positive behaviours regarding safety are not necessary for consultant surgeons. The rest of the team will quickly follow suit in letting standards slip, and very rapidly 'normalisation of deviance' occurs with lack of compliance with protocols and best practice becoming the norm within that operating room and being seen as acceptable behaviour.[6,7] This drift towards non-adherence is especially risky because it is difficult to detect. However, this type of slow deterioration with respect to standards is important for leaders to be aware of and to monitor. Drift can be quietly insidious to an organization's safety efforts. Instituting communication standards alongside clinical performance standards may help to mitigate some of the risk.

Standard setting should continue throughout the surgical procedure and beyond. What may seem like minor aspects of performance are crucially important in maintaining a high standard within the operating room. These small but vital aspects of how the surgeon as leader deals with the process of care acts as a demonstration of how the team should act. Seemingly small details such as how thoroughly to scrub and what to do if the sterile field is accidentally breached, in addition to the attention paid to standards in other members of the team, are also vital. As stated by Lt. Gen. David Morrison, 'the standard you walk past is the standard you accept'.[8] If a team member regularly transgresses boundaries or provides a lesser degree of attention to detail and safety without challenge,

then this will degrade overall team performance and requires address.

In addition to maintaining standards within the bounded domain of the operating room, as a surgical leader one should aim to permeate this same high standard in the wider surgical environment. The provision of safe and reliable surgical care requires that within the whole domain of care delivery a positive safety culture is consistently maintained. The most important factor in achieving patient safety at a wider systems level, outside individual operating rooms, is overt and visible commitment from surgical leaders to foster an environment that supports and expects safe and reliable care. This same standard must accompany the surgeon into the operating room and be part of the operative procedure.

Positive role modelling of safe behaviours should not be underestimated and is essential at an organizational level as well as at a front-line level. The direct effects of a leader's modelling of safe and unsafe behaviours and their reinforcement of subordinates' behaviour through monitoring and control have been well defined in other high-reliability industries. In an investigation of supervisors' self-reported involvement in safety activities in 100 manufacturing workplaces in Canada, Simard and Marchand[9] found higher rates of involvement in supervisors working in safe compared with unsafe plants. Specifically, they showed that supervisor participatory leadership behaviours, wherein a leader is personally involved in safety activities alongside the workers he or she supervises, were related to an increase in occupational safety. Other researchers have investigated subordinates' perception of safety behaviours of their supervisors and reported a positive correlation with safety outcomes, such as accident rates, attitudes and risks.[10] In a survey study of 429 workers in high-risk companies in Spain, Tomas et al.[11] found that supervisor response to safety had a strong relationship with both worker attitude and safety behaviour. These findings show that leadership behaviours and styles that emphasize safety improve safety outcomes and that the leaders must create an environment in which safety is valued.[12] Therefore, it is crucial that positive leadership behaviours towards patient safety and the pursuit of excellent care are emphasized at both a managerial level and a workplace level.

7.3.1 PREOPERATIVE BRIEFING AS A LEADERSHIP TOOL

One example of setting standards is the use of preoperative briefings as a leadership tool. Most hospitals have adopted some form of universal protocol or World Health Organization checklist.[13] These tools provide detailed information about the patient, procedure and equipment required for a successful operation. However, these briefings can also be used as opportunities to establish expectations and set standards for the team. As has been discussed at length in the literature,[5,14–16] speaking up behaviour is critical to patient care. However, some team members may still feel hesitant to communicate with their team for fear of reprisal or because of the assumption that the leader is aware of the situation and has chosen to pursue a certain care path.[17] The briefing is the surgeon's opportunity for communication directly with the team, as set out in Chapter 6, and to provide a positive role model around the subject of patient safety from the beginning of the surgery. The consultant can set the tone for the entire day with this briefing and encourage a climate of psychological safety to ensure that all team members feel empowered to speak up (see Chapter 6).

Airline captains who are rated as excellent team members by their subordinates engage in more teamwork and communication behaviours in the first few moments of a new crew than captains who are technically equal but receive lower teamwork ratings.[18] This suggests that simple leadership behaviours such as reviewing crew members' roles and identifying, commenting on and

engaging crews in discussion about the unique characteristics of the task ahead can move a team from a list of names to a bounded social system. Captain Sullenberger, the pilot of the 'miracle on the Hudson' flight, greets his first officers at the pre-flight briefing by telling them that the left-hand seat in the cockpit is assigned on the basis of seniority and not ability and so they should speak up if any unsafe behaviour is noted.[19] Likewise, a simple sentence to the effect of 'if anyone sees myself or another team member doing something unsafe please speak up' at the end of the safety briefing helps flatten hierarchies and encourages assertive safety behaviour on the part of the whole surgical team (Chapter 6). Positive role modelling in this regard, which is carried further and echoed at each surgical preoperative pause, and post-operative debrief, emphasizes the focus on safety and then becomes the norm for the operating team.

When there is effective leadership of the checklist process, the quality of surgical care shows marked improvement. The Surgical Checklist Implementation Project shows that patients are more likely to receive correct antibiotic prophylaxis and appropriate deep venous thrombosis prophylaxis when the surgeon leads the checks. In addition, teamwork (communication, co-ordination, leadership and situational awareness) is better when the surgeon leads, when all team members are present and paused and when more information is shared; there are fewer equipment problems when all team members are present for the checks and post-operative complications are reduced significantly when all three parts of the checklist are used (i.e. including the sign-out) (Report of the NHS England Never Events Taskforce, February 2014). These data suggest that the surgeon's leadership of the process has significant positive effects. The checklist is a tool to help standardize and optimize the team's engagement and to ensure focus. In addition to the final front-line safety check, there is an added benefit of the checklist in that it requires all team members to be present. The checklist's usefulness as a final safety check may be augmented if it is used to ensure that all team members are physically and mentally present, aware and ready to proceed, rather than using the checklist as a perfunctory task check (Box 7.1).

BOX 7.1: Clinical scenario 1

A patient is about to undergo a ureteroscopy and laser fragmentation of a ureteric stone and is anaesthetized in the operating room. Two members of the operating room team are distracted by discussing what equipment is needed for the first case on the next day's operating list. The surgeon interrupts the team members and brings their attention back to the impending timeout. He asks for their full attention, emphasizing the importance to the patient of this crucial preoperative safety check. The patient's penicillin allergy is highlighted correctly at the timeout and the team confirms that ciprofloxacin will be used as antibiotic cover for the procedure. After the timeout, the surgeon thanks everyone for their full input. At the debriefing, the surgeon leads the team in a discussion about the importance of full attention for the timeout for all team members and ways that they can learn from today's lapse.

7.4 SUPPORTING OTHERS

The second element within the NOTSS leadership category is that of supporting others (Table 7.2). In addition to setting and maintaining standards within the operating room, it is a vital aspect of leadership that the consultant surgeon takes into account the needs of others within the operating room team. The perceived role of surgeons has now transcended that of exclusively possessing high levels of technical skill, and it rightly now includes the necessity of incorporating non-technical skills, such as effective leadership, to maximize safe surgical task performance and also to ensure effective team functioning in the completion of this task. Although there can be more than one task-specific leader in the operating room (e.g. anaesthetist or scrub nurse at certain points), the surgeon is the focal point for creating a safe working environment and ensuring that surgical goals are realized effectively, efficiently and safely.[20]

Effective teamworking is a vital and integral component in the delivery of safe surgical care. In 1999, the Institute of Medicine report on medical error[21] concluded that there is a need to 'promote effective team functioning' as one of the five principles for creating safer hospital systems. The current literature identifies that high levels of teamworking within the surgical team translates into better outcomes for patients, and so effective leadership of that surgical team is essential to minimize adverse outcomes from surgical interventions (Chapter 6). A notable challenge of working with teams within the surgical domain is their fluidity and diversity. Within the surgical environment, professionals with different training and backgrounds are expected to function optimally within a high-risk and very dynamic environment that is littered with error traps. Although surgeons may be well trained in the technical aspects of surgical performance, little or no formal training in leadership of operating teams is received. For truly effective teamworking to occur, the surgeon must apply leadership to both completion of the task and functioning of the team.

7.4.1 LEADERSHIP INCLUDES BOTH TASK- AND TEAM-FOCUSED BEHAVIOURS

Studies have shown that surgeons generally do not engage in team-building behaviours as would be expected.[22] Indeed, surgeons do not display leadership skills to the degree that may be expected. Measurement of leadership skills in an operating room team has found that of all the non-technical skills measured, leadership scores are the lowest among the team.[23] Moreover, both surgeons and anaesthetists score lower in leadership than nurses within the team. It is likely, therefore, that surgeons do not perceive their role to involve building the team in the same way that the team leadership literature describes. The surgeon is the leading technical expert and may consider his or her role to only accomplish the technical task, rather than build positive team climate and develop group cohesion. This may be in part explained by the fact

Table 7.2 Behavioural makers of supporting others element (from NOTSS)

Good behaviours	Poor behaviours
Modifies behaviour according to trainee needs	Does not provide recognition for tasks performed well
Provides constructive criticism to team members	Fails to recognize needs of others
Ensures delegation of tasks is appropriate	Engages in 'tunnel vision' approach to technical aspects of operation
Establishes rapport with team members	Shows hostility to other team members (e.g. makes sarcastic comments to nurses)
Gives credit for tasks performed well	

Note: Supporting others refers to providing physical, cognitive and emotional help to team members; judging different team members' abilities; and tailoring one's style of leadership accordingly.

that leadership and other non-technical skills have not yet been fully integrated into surgical training and most surgical training programmes as yet do not specifically address this competency, but this may also derive from the fact that surgeons automatically assume leadership roles without necessarily identifying leadership functions and responsibilities. Therefore, they are on occasion ill-prepared for this duty.

7.4.2 LEADERSHIP SHOULD BE FLEXIBLE AND DISTRIBUTED

For an operating room team to be effective, leadership must be adaptive, flexible and dynamic. Flexible leadership focuses on the leader's ability to balance competing demands and tradeoffs among different performance determinants, i.e. demonstrating ability to recognize what team members need and responding appropriately to a team's changing task conditions. To be most effective, the leader should adapt his or her behaviour based on the context and the urgency being faced during the operation.

A related leadership concept applicable to surgery is shared or distributed leadership. Shared leadership is 'a dynamic, interactive influence process among individuals in groups for which the objective is to lead one another to the achievement of group or organisational goals or both. This process often involves peer, or lateral, influence and at other times involves upward or downward hierarchical influence'.[24] According to this approach, multiple members of the team may enact leadership informally at appropriate stages of the operation even if a formal leader is present. This

concept of shared leadership has been described in current surgical leadership research. Surgeons tend to regard leadership in the operating room as entirely their own responsibility but can recognize leadership as a shared responsibility between the surgeon, anaesthetist and nursing team leader.[25] While there is limited empirical research on shared leadership in surgeons, anaesthesia team performance has been related to sharedness of leadership, suggesting that the higher performing teams share more, whereas one member of the team leads significantly more in lower performing teams.[26]

This model of shared leadership is useful in low-urgency and low-risk situations. In these conditions, and where the junior members' skills are thought to be appropriate, the senior leaders can delegate leadership of the team to their juniors.[27] This enables effective training of the junior members of staff's non-technical skills and gives them experience in leading both the team and the task. If the situation changes, and becomes more urgent or risky, then the leadership role should be rapidly reclaimed by the senior leader. This delegation of leadership and the plan for when and how the leadership should revert to the consultant should be explicitly discussed at the preoperative team briefing.

The positive effects of shared leadership on team performance are particularly impressive when interdependence and complexity of tasks are high (see the study by Friedrich et al.[28] for a review). Furthermore, shared forms of leadership are effective in teams operating in extreme or safety-critical situations (e.g. firefighting or medical action teams) because as levels of complexity, time pressure and task load rise, exclusively vertical leadership structures can fail as even the most competent formal leader can no longer cope with the significant leadership task load. The leader may thus serve as a bottleneck rather than a funnel. Although funneling and allocating information as needed is important, it is also necessary that one leader does not stifle decision making during emergency situations. Additionally, in such time-critical situations, if the formal leader is also a technical expert complete concentration on the problem-solving tasks therefore requires a reliance on others to maintain the leadership functions.[24,29]

As leader of the team, the operating surgeon needs to be able to judge different team members' abilities and then allocate tasks accordingly, also taking the context of the current situation into account. This explicit allocation of roles is often taken as implicit at best within surgical teams, but this is essential for optimizing team performance and providing backup behaviours. Being seen to recognize individual team members' competencies and to delegate appropriately and explicitly within that team is a very positive leadership and team-building behaviour. Ensuring that there are limited assumptions about individual team members' capabilities is helpful practice. Many industrial accidents can be traced back to assumptions about team members' capabilities or their understanding of the task. Providing good constructive feedback to team members and giving credit for tasks performed well signify positive behaviours in this element and help build team rapport and improve team functioning.

An example of good leadership in this element includes modification of behaviour according to trainees' needs. It also includes how to establish a rapport with the team, and again the preoperative briefing is the ideal time to establish this rapport, especially when most operating room team membership is temporary to the extent of changing within the same day or even occasionally within the same surgical case. Changes to a patient's condition or to team membership make it crucial to ensure that delegation of tasks is appropriate, that tasks are in fact delegated to individuals rather than to the operating room team at large and that such delegation is repeated as required.

Parker et al.[25] have demonstrated that surgeons tend to address requests to the operating room in general rather than to an individual in particular, making us all familiar with the surgical request 'will somebody get me the …?'. Although this may be useful, in most cases it leads to repeated requests or delays because no individual team member was identified as being allocated that task or request, with subsequent failure of task execution.

7.4.3 LEADERSHIP AND LEGAL RESPONSIBILITY

Though shared and flexible leaderships are required, the ultimate legal responsibility for the safety of the patient may or may not be held by the surgeon depending on the jurisdiction of practice. For example, in the United States the attending surgeon is in legal charge of the operating room, surgery and fate of the patient. This legal precedent for 'who is in charge' was set in 1949, in the case of *McConnell v. Williams*.[30] The Pennsylvania Supreme Court established a judicial precedent regarding surgeons' liability in medical malpractice cases that was subsequently followed by most courts throughout the United States. The 'captain of the ship' doctrine, as it became known, established that a surgeon was responsible for any negligent conduct in the operating room just as the captain of a ship is responsible for the actions of its crew. In its strictest interpretation, the captain of the ship indicates that the surgeons are held liable for negligence even if they are entirely free of negligence themselves.

The situation in the legal systems of the United Kingdom is significantly different, however, and surgeons (both senior and junior), while they have a 'duty of care' to their patients, are regarded as the 'servants' of the hospital authorities, who are hence automatically ('vicariously') liable for any negligent actions. The senior surgeon would only be legally liable if he or she could be shown to be personally negligent, by failing to supervise a junior surgeon adequately or letting him or her do something he or she did not have the skill or experience to do. It should be borne in mind, however, that consultant surgeons remain fully responsible for all patients under their duty of care.

7.4.4 LEADERSHIP MUST SUPPORT SPEAKING UP BY TEAM MEMBERS

An essential leadership element of supporting the operating room team is to emphasize that patient safety is the responsibility of every team member. Everyone on the team, from the surgeon to the anaesthetist, nurse and surgical technician, should feel empowered to speak up about potential safety concerns. The surgeon, as a leader of the team, is instrumental in supporting every member of the team to speak up to promote a safe environment for both current and future procedures. One of the greatest barriers to speaking up is the hierarchy or authority gradient that can exist within an operating theatre (Chapter 6).

The terms hierarchy, authority gradient and status asymmetry refer to the established, or even the perceived, distribution of power within a team. Concentration of power in one person leads to a steep gradient, whereas a more democratic and inclusive style of leadership with involvement of other team members results in a shallow gradient. This concept of authority gradient was introduced in medicine as far back as 1999 in the US Institute of Medicine report *To Err Is Human*,[21] but little has been written or acknowledged in the medical literature regarding the impact of authority gradients in medical care. Despite what surgeons may perceive, the surgical workplace is still a largely hierarchical system, with clear delineations between professions and seniority and with a clear and strict chain of command in most surgical specialties.

As the leader of the operating room team, it is therefore important to think about how hierarchy and leadership styles can affect team function, and ultimately affect patient safety. Cultivation of a steep authority gradient means that expressing concerns, questioning decisions or even simply clarifying instructions will require considerable determination. These steep authority gradients can act as barriers to team involvement, reducing the flow of feedback, halting cooperation and preventing creative ideas for threat analyses and problem solving. Only the most assertive, confident team members may feel able to challenge authority and raise safety concerns.

Therefore, the most effective leaders are those who consciously establish a team hierarchy that ensures that the task is executed safely and appropriately and also ensure a working climate where junior team members are confident enough to raise concerns, question decisions and offer solutions. Reducing the risks that arise from inappropriate authority gradients means raising personal and team awareness, learning some communication tactics such as briefing or asking the team for feedback explicitly and applying those skills during routine and emergency operations. It is also essential, after each of these stages, to openly discuss any issues that have arisen and to feed these back to the team.

Surgeons who effectively overcome authority gradients have teams that function better and are more able to learn new surgical procedures effectively and safely.[5] These teams, in which members speak up with observations, concerns and questions, are better able to learn new techniques than those in which members are reluctant to voice what they are thinking. Thus, effective leadership emphasizes safety and motivates the team and acts in ways that downplay power difference (noting their own fallibility or elevating others' importance).

The ideal time to address the issue of authority gradients and to cultivate this atmosphere of patient safety is during the preoperative briefing. An appropriate and comprehensive pre-task briefing allows clarification of roles, responsibilities, capabilities, limitations and boundaries in both normal and abnormal conditions. During this briefing, an active leadership role should be adopted by the operating surgeon and positive behaviours illustrated.

Authority gradients, however, may not always be viewed negatively. Most teams require some degree of authority gradient; otherwise, roles can become blurred and decision making can become slow and ineffective. Shallow gradients are good for team building and generating solutions when either the nature of the problem is unclear or the remedy is neither routine nor obvious. Steep gradients can be appropriate in a crisis, where immediate action is required and a 'command/control' approach is required (Box 7.2).

BOX 7.2: Clinical scenario 2

A patient is about to undergo a laparoscopic cholecystectomy and is anaesthetized in the operating room. The floor nurse knows that the patient has an allergy to cephalosporins and hears the anaesthesiologist say during the safety pause that she is going to administer cephazolin. The nurse speaks up about the allergy to protect the patient from an allergic reaction. The surgeon has previously encouraged this behaviour by creating a supportive environment, and he always specifically states at the preoperative briefing that all members of the team should speak up if they see anything that they consider unsafe. The surgeon thanks the nurse for speaking up to protect the patient. At the end of the day, the incident is brought up by the surgeon and discussed at the team debriefing to learn from the incident and prevent its recurrence.

The surgeon in this scenario is demonstrating supporting others within the team. His thanking the nurse and discussing the incident in a non-judgemental manner at the debriefing creates an environment of psychological safety in which team members feel able to discuss potential safety issues without fear of reprisal or ridicule.

7.5 COPING WITH PRESSURE

The third element in the NOTSS leadership category is coping with pressure (Table 7.3). The practice of surgery is unpredictable with a potential for high-risk situations to arise rapidly. Although the majority of surgical procedures progress without major difficulties, certain portions of even routine elective surgery can be intense and stressful. The operating surgeon plays an important role in leading the team through such situations, and this need for effective leadership comes at a time when there are increasing calls on the surgeon's personal resources. The literature on exact behaviours that a leader should utilize in non-routine situations is inconsistent, but it does seem that flexibility while updating mental models and openly and rapidly exchanging information with the rest of the operating room team are critical.[29,32] In addition, quick decision making based on expert (often front-line) feedback is also important. As a situation becomes more complex, a leader must engage differently with the team than they would during a routine situation. As a team's task becomes more dynamic, researchers have argued that leadership must keep pace. For an operating surgeon faced with an intra-operative crisis, this places unique demands on them, with the need to balance an increased need for technical input into the operation with their team's need for increased leadership in a time of crisis.

In general, in cases where the situation becomes more urgent or complex the surgeon's and the team's workload usually increases greatly and a more directive and active leadership may be required.[33] Yun et al.[34] studied surgical trauma teams and demonstrated that effective treatment of the most severely injured patients requires the most experienced team member to take up a more direct leadership role and to make direct decisions. They also reported that it is usually the senior surgeon in trauma teams who takes a more directing leadership role in high-stress situations, thereby shifting the team to a more hierarchical structure. On the other hand, when no complicated treatment is necessary and workload is low, effective leaders use more empowering leadership strategies with a flatter hierarchy, inviting input and feedback from the rest of the team. This empowering strategy enables the leadership role to shift between team members depending on the condition of the patient. This is consistent with the case being delegated to the trainee when risk is low but leadership quickly coming back to the attending surgeon with resultant steepening of the hierarchy if a crisis develops.

To date, research has shown that surgeons within the intra-operative environment do not seem to adjust their leadership in these non-routine situations as literature on similar leaders in other action

Table 7.3 Behavioural markers for coping with pressure element (from NOTSS)

Good behaviours	Poor behaviours
Remains calm under pressure	Suppresses concern over clinical problem
Emphasizes urgency of situation (e.g. by occasionally raising voice)	'Freezes' and displays inability to make decisions under pressure
Takes responsibility for the patient in emergency/ crisis situation	Fails to pass leadership of case when technical challenge requires full attention
Makes appropriate decision under pressure	Blames everyone else for errors and does not take personal responsibility
Delegates tasks in order to achieve goals	Loses temper
Continues to lead team through emergency	

Note: Coping with pressure refers to retaining a calm demeanour when under pressure and emphasizing to the team that one is under control of a high-pressure situation and adopting a suitably forceful manner if appropriate without undermining the role of other team members. 'The mood in the OR depends on the surgeon. The surgeon sets the tone. You know surgery can be the most relaxing thing in the world, when things go smoothly.' Cardiac surgeon quoted in Millman M.[31]

team settings might suggest. Rather than increase their leadership behaviours, the surgeons tend to become more focused on the clinical task at hand.[4] This reaction is entirely reasonable, especially if the situation creates risk for the patient, as the surgeon is the technical expert in mitigating and controlling the surgical crisis. However, from a leadership perspective this greater focus on the surgical task means that additional leadership mechanisms are necessary to maintain team performance and ensure optimal communication and interaction across team members at this critical time.

This reaffirms the concept of shared leadership discussed earlier. Although the surgeon is still the leader in a crisis situation, it is often the leading surgeon's technical skills that are called on to improve the situation, leaving him or her in a position of being potentially unable to lead the team effectively. In these situations, many surgical teams share leadership in an implicit fashion. The anaesthetist may take over and direct and co-ordinate the team members while the surgeon is focused on the surgical task. However, unlike typical shared leadership theory[24] these shifts in leadership may not be made explicit among the surgical team. Recognizing that formal leadership is infrequently established during surgery, post-surgery discussions often reveal the assumption, by both surgeons and anaesthetists, that the surgeon was the de facto leader. In general, leadership in operating rooms is very seldom handed over through an explicit verbal exchange but team behaviour changes as task

requirements change (such as an unexpected equipment malfunction or unexpected difficult patient anatomy). As might be expected during these situations, the lead surgeon may again be expected to become more directive in communication style, and at times nursing or anaesthetic colleagues will assume leadership over certain tasks or the operating room team. Anecdotally, this type of dynamic leadership shift has been regularly seen but has been seldom documented.[29]

7.5.1 ROLE DEFINITION AND LEADERSHIP

As described earlier, lack of explicit expression of leadership leading to an absence of team leadership is an inherent danger particularly in crisis situations. An important role of the leader is therefore that of ensuring role definition within the surgical team, and this includes the role of the leader at particular stages of the surgical procedure. Several studies, mainly performed in resuscitation or cardiac arrest teams, have examined the relevance of unambiguous leadership behaviour to effective team performance. Teams without instantly recognizable leadership are associated with lower levels of effectiveness and poorer quality of teamwork. For this reason, leadership must be unambiguous, comprehensible and visible to team members.

Identification of the leadership role is important to gain control and avoid confusion within a team.[35] Conflicts in assuming the role of the leader between the emergency physician and the anaesthetist in emergency departments produce problems in team co-ordination,[36] and the negative effects of shared leadership between two senior team members have been previously highlighted: 'Both gave orders which at times contradicted and countermanded each other'. All of the aforementioned findings imply that unambiguous leadership behaviour and explicit communication are essential. However, structuring and guiding should not be equated with autocratic leadership behaviour, which can have negative effects on team motivation and effectiveness, and an effective balance between role definition, delegation and collaboration is needed.

Good leadership behaviours in crisis situations include clear delineation of the leadership roles at different stages of the operation, both routine and non-routine. Again, the ideal time to perform this explicit leadership role allocation is as part of the preoperative surgical team briefing when the surgeon should explicitly discuss the leadership role at different stages of the surgery and also if a crisis develops. This discussion should include an exploration of any unexpected situation that may arise, a definition of the crisis and a clear definition of roles for both leadership and team in this situation.

Continuation into the intra-operative phase allows the surgeon to indicate that there is a stressful situation developing or a known difficult operative phase approaching. Notifying the team that this is an important portion of the procedure may assist the team in coping with the extra demands of that stressful situation. Exemplary leadership will also involve keeping composed even in the most difficult of times. In general, team members will appreciate that declaration of intensity of the situation and will respond to the surgeon's composure by maintaining their own. As the situation changes, the requirements for the team also change. There may be periods where explicit leadership is needed (e.g. prior to the beginning of surgery or during an emergency) or periods where explicit leadership is unnecessary because of the expertise of the team. If the surgeon can recognize the situational requirements as well as the requirements of the team members, and adjust their style accordingly, leadership may be optimized.

Another leadership requirement relates to the appreciation that demands affect not only the surgeon but also the other members of the operative team and the timing of such demands may be different for different team members. Different members of the team will have differing task loads at different phases of the operation, and the task load frequently fails to coincide across the individuals.[37] The closure of the wound is traditionally seen as the moment when the operating surgeon begins to relax and chat with other members of the team, but a good surgical leader will recognize that this is a crucial operative phase for the scrub nurse as his or her workload increases as the instrument and needle count is performed. Good leadership consists of realization of this increased workload on another team member and supporting him or her in this role, in this case by minimizing distraction in this crucial phase of the surgery.

When the surgery is going to plan, the good surgical leader will distribute leadership as appropriate and support his or her trainee leading the operation, but when the situation changes and becomes more expedient leadership must quickly and explicitly move back to the consultant surgeon. It needs to be clearly communicated to the team that this has happened and that the consultant is again the leader and is taking full responsibility for that patient and that situation. It may also be appropriate at that stage to explicitly delegate leadership to the designated individual within the operating room team such as the consultant anaesthetist, as discussed at the briefing, if the surgeon has to direct all of his or her attention and cognitive ability to remedy the surgical crisis. The need for reallocation or return of leadership, if previously delegated, makes it clear to the team who is now controlling the team and is taking full responsibility for that patient.

Within this element of the NOTSS leadership taxonomy, the ability of individual surgeons to deal with increased task load and leadership load at a time of crisis is considered. Surgeons should not only cope but also be seen to cope with this vastly increased demand on leadership capabilities. A surgeon who buckles under pressure and begins to demonstrate negative behaviours under stress is counterproductive to effective team functioning at a time when effective leadership is most

---

BOX 7.3: Clinical scenario 3

During the performance of a right inguinal hernia repair, injury to the femoral vein occurs. Significant bleeding ensues. The surgeon remains calm and composed while she gains temporary control of the bleeding and asks the team to obtain the proper instruments to complete the vascular repair. Composure on the part of the surgeon promotes composure in the entire operating room team. While waiting for the equipment, the surgeon relays to the team that she will be focused on the task and that the anaesthesiologist will lead the rest of the team until the vascular repair is completed. Roles within the team are reallocated to best deal with this surgical crisis, and the nursing team leader calls the operating room manager to let him know that the next case will be delayed.

---

required. The surgeon who freezes physically and, perhaps more importantly, freezes cognitively under stress; the surgeon who apportions blame when something goes wrong, or complications develop; or indeed the surgeon who suppresses or minimizes concerns over an obvious problem or adverse outcome all risk losing both the support and the respect of their team. Ill temperament and loss of composure are poor leadership behaviours. In emergency situations, emphasis of the urgency of the situation, for instance, may be achieved by vocal tone and volume; however, the margins between assertive behaviour and demonstration of abusive personality can be blurred. Rosenstein and O'Daniel[38] report that disruptive behaviour such as shouting and the use of abusive language is still observed in operating theatres, and this increases frustration and stress and stifles further communication and inter-professional collaboration. This behaviour has a profoundly negative effect on teamworking and communication often at a time when it is most crucial to optimize the outcome of the patient (Box 7.3).

7.6 SURGEONS' LEADERSHIP INVENTORY (SLI)

The three-element structure of leadership found in NOTSS has been discussed in detail in Sections 7.3, 7.4 and 7.5. Though this structure is valuable for a high-level understanding of intra-operative leadership, for some purposes a more detailed, in-depth analysis is required. To fill this gap, a group of researchers at the University of Aberdeen, UK,

developed the SLI. The SLI offers a detailed bottom-up approach to understand intra-operative leadership utilizing the elements discussed in NOTSS and also providing additional components, expanding the three-element structure to an eight-element structure. In addition, the SLI requires each leadership behaviour throughout a case to be examined, rather than having one overall leadership score for the entire case. This tool provides a detailed 'mapping' of leadership across an operation, allowing a finer grained assessment and feedback.

The SLI was developed based on a review of the literature, expert focus groups and observations ($n = 29$) and was then tested in situ and via video observations ($n = 29$). The final taxonomy, the SLI, included eight elements: maintaining standards, making decisions, managing resources, directing, training, communicating, supporting others and coping with pressure (Table 7.4). The three NOTSS elements of maintaining standards, supporting others and coping with pressure are all present. The additional five elements were added based on the feedback from the focus groups that more nuance is required to describe leadership in detail throughout an operation. Decision making, resource management, directing and training were specifically identified as critical skills for intra-operative leaders. Communicating, though often included as a separate non-technical skill, was listed by expert panellists as a part of leadership. Excellent communication skills are a part of being a good leader; therefore, communication was included in the final taxonomy.

To test the SLI, videos of live operations were coded according to the taxonomy. In-depth analysis of the impact of surgical stage on leadership was

Table 7.4 The Surgeon's Leadership Inventory (SLI)

Element	New definition of surgeon's leadership elements
Maintaining standards	Supporting safety and quality by adhering to acceptable principles of surgery, following codes of good clinical practice and enforcing operating room procedures and protocols by consistently demonstrating appropriate behaviours (i.e. asking for help when required).
Making decisions	Seeking out appropriate information and generating alternative possibilities or courses of action, synthesizing the information, choosing a solution to a problem and letting all relevant personnel know the chosen option. Making an informed and prompt judgement based on information, clinical situation and risk and continually reviewing its suitability in light of changes in the patient's condition.
Managing resources	Assigning resources (people and equipment) depending on the situation or context, delegating tasks appropriately to team members and ensuring the team has what it needs to accomplish the task.
Directing	Clearly stating expectations regarding accomplishment of task goals; giving clear instructions; using authority where required, demonstrating confidence in both leadership and technical ability.
Training	Instructing and coaching team members according to goals of the task, modifying own behaviour according to team's educational needs, identifying and maximizing educational opportunities.
Supporting others	Judging the capabilities of team members, offering assistance where appropriate, establishing a rapport with team members and actively encouraging them to speak up.
Communicating	Giving and receiving information in a timely manner to aid establishment of a shared understanding among team members. Asking for information, speaking appropriately for the situation. Asking for input from team members.
Coping with pressure	Showing flexibility and changing plans if required to cope with changing circumstances to ensure that goals are met; anticipating possible complications and communicating them to staff; adopting a forceful manner if appropriate without undermining the role of other team members.

Source: Henrickson Parker S, Flin R, McKinley A, Yule S, *Am J Surg*, 2013;205(6):745–51.

conducted. Elements of surgeons' leadership differed before and after a specific point in the operation, the 'point of no return' (PONR). Maintaining standard behaviours differed before and after the PONR, but no significant differences were found for any of the other eight elements. Throughout the operations observed, most leadership behaviours were directed towards the trainee surgeon. There were no significant differences in quality of leadership before and after the PONR.[4]

In a subset of the videos, an unexpected event occurred. These videos were matched with operations of the same type in which an event did not occur, and the operating surgeon's intra-operative leadership was compared, revealing differences in training and supporting behaviours. However, because of the extremely small sample size, these results should be interpreted with some caution. This analysis again showed that the surgeon most often leads the surgical trainee, not other members of the team.

These studies provide a first step towards identifying the important behaviours and a basis on which to measure and potentially improve surgeons' intra-operative leadership. The SLI was created using multiple methods (literature review, observations and focus groups) and then found to be reliable and relatively easy to use in the live setting. This allows for a more granular feedback mechanism when using the SLI for training and also creates the opportunity for more detailed understanding of leadership as it evolves throughout an operation.

The results of the final study showed that surgeons' intra-operative leadership may be reactive, situation based and often transactional in nature. Whether or not this type of leadership is optimal within the operating room setting has yet to be determined. In comparison to the existing literature on action teams,[33,39] it would appear that surgeons' intraoperative leadership could be improved.

7.7 CONCLUSION

Leadership is now recognized as a critical skill for surgeons and for patient safety. The NOTSS taxonomy provides a structured framework with which to demonstrate, teach and assess the leadership skills of the surgeon in the operating theatre environment. The three main non-technical skills for leaders within the NOTSS leadership category are those of maintaining standards, supporting others and coping with pressure. Utilizing this framework enables the surgeon to improve the functioning of the surgical team and to enhance patient safety. Maintaining and role modelling a high standard within the operating room enables the surgeon to encourage the desired behaviours related to team functioning and patient safety. The second element of supporting others within the team is crucial to ensure clarity of role within the team for effective task completion and promoting a culture of psychological safety within the team so that all team members feel safe to speak up to challenge an unsafe practice or behaviour. The last element is that of coping with pressure, and this ensures a calm and collected atmosphere within the theatre at all times, even in times of crisis. A calm surgeon means a calm operating theatre team that works efficiently, smoothly and safely even under crisis conditions.

Leadership within the operating theatre is crucial for safety but should not be confused with command authority or bullying behaviour, even in times of crisis. Although it should be clear that the surgeon is in overall charge, a flexible approach to leadership is most effective, and the leadership role can be delegated to junior team members when conditions are suitable. As the surgeon in charge of the operating room team, it is your responsibility to oversee this flexible approach to leadership and explicitly state who is the leader during the differing phases of the surgical procedure. Likewise, if a crisis situation does develop, remember that as the surgeon you may need exclusive focus on the task, and in these situations obvious delegation of the leadership role should again be carried out.

Overall, the most powerful behaviour a leader can display is that of role modelling of what ought to happen in the operating room. Surgeons can discuss the importance of leadership and non-technical skills at length; but if these principles are not modelled on actual illustrative behaviours, or if practised behaviours run contrary to the spoken word, then an engaged, highly co-ordinated and safety conscious team will be difficult to produce.

REFERENCES

1. Carroll JS, Rudolph JW. Design of high reliability organizations in health care. *Qual Saf Health Care.* 2006;15(Suppl 1):i4–9.
2. Yukl G. *Leadership in Organizations* (8th ed). Upper Saddle River, New Jersey: Prentice-Hall, Inc.; 2012.
3. Northouse P. *Leadership: Theory and Practice* (6th ed). Chicago, Illinois: Sage Publications; 2012.
4. Parker SH, Flin R, McKinley A, Yule S. Factors influencing surgeons' intraoperative leadership: Video analysis of unanticipated events in the operating room. *World J Surg.* 2014 Jan;38(1):4–10.
5. Edmondson AC. Speaking up in the operating room: How team leaders promote learning in interdisciplinary action teams. *J Manag Stud.* 2003;40(6):1419–52.
6. Amalberti R, Vincent C, Auroy Y, de Saint Maurice G. Violations and migrations in

health care: a framework for understanding and management. *Qual Saf Health Care.* 2006 Dec;15(Suppl 1):i66–71.

7. Vaughan D. *The Challenger Launch Decision: Risky Technology, Culture, and Deviance at NASA* (1st ed). Chicago, Illinois: University of Chicago Press; 1997.

8. Morrison D. The standard you walk past is the standard you accept. Australia: Address to the closing plenary session at the global summit to end sexual violence in conflict. [Accessed March 23, 2015.] Available from: http://www.army.gov.au/Our-work/Speeches-and-transcripts/Message-from-the-Chief-of-Army.

9. Simard M, Marchand A. The behaviour of first-line supervisors in accident prevention and effectivenss in occupational safety. *Safety Sci.* 1994;17(3):169–85.

10. Zohar D. A group-level model of safety climate: Testing the effect of group climate on microaccidents in manufacturing jobs. *J Appl Psychol.* 2000;85(4):587–96.

11. Tomas JM, Melia JL, Oliver A. A cross-validation of a structural equation model of accidents: Organizational and psychological variables as predictors of work safety. *Work Stress.* 1999 Mar;13(1):49–58.

12. Hofmann DA, Morgeson FP. The role of leadership in safety. In J. Barling, M.R. Frone (Eds.). *The Psychology of Workplace Safety.* Washington DC: American Psychological Association; 2004. pp. 159–80.

13. Haynes AB, Weiser TG, Berry WR, Lipsitz SR, Breizat AH, Dellinger EP et al. A surgical safety checklist to reduce morbidity and mortality in a global population. *N Engl J Med.* 2009;360(5):491–9.

14. Dayton E, Henriksen K. Communication failure: basic components, contributing factors and the call for structure. *Jt Comm J Qual Patient Saf.* 2007; Jan;33(1):34–47.

15. Lingard L, Espin S, Whyte S, Regehr G, Baker GR, Reznick R et al. Communication failures in the operating room: An observational classification of recurrent types and effects. *Qual Saf Health Care.* 2004 Oct 1;13(5):330–4.

16. Espin S, Lingard L, Baker GR, Regehr G. Persistence of unsafe practice in everyday work: An exploration of organizational and psychological factors constraining safety in the operating room. *Qual Saf Health Care.* 2006;15(3):165–70.

17. Pian-Smith MC, Simon R, Minehart RD, Podraza M, Rudolph J, Walser T et al. Teaching residents the two-challenge rule: A simulation-based approach to improve education and patient safety. *Simuation Healthc.* 2009;4(2):84–91.

18. Ginnett RC. Crews as groups: Their formation and their leadership. In E.L. Wiener, B.G. Kanki, R.L. Helmreich (Eds.). *Cockpit Resource Management.* Orlando, Florida: Academic Press; 1993. pp. 71–98.

19. Sullenberger CB, Zaslow J. *Highest Duty: My Search for What Really Matters.* New York: Harper Collins Publishers; 2009.

20. Giddings AE, Williamson C. *The Leadership and Management of Surgical Teams.* London: Royal College of Surgeons of England; 2007 June.

21. Kohn LT, Corrigan JM, Donaldson MS. *To Err Is Human – Building a Safer Health System.* T.K. Linda, S. Molla, J.M.C. Donaldson (Eds.). Washington DC: National Academy Press; 2000.

22. Henrickson PS, Yule S, Flin R, McKinley A. Surgeons' leadership in the operating room: An observational study. *Am J Surg.* 2012;204(3):347–54.

23. Sevdalis N, Lyons M, Healey AN, Undre S, Darzi A, Vincent CA. Observational teamwork assessment for surgery: Construct validation with expert versus novice raters. *Ann Surg.* 2009 Jun;249(6):1047–51.

24. Pearce CL, Conger JA. *Shared Leadership: Reframing the Hows and Whys of Leadership.* Thousand Oaks, California: Sage Publications (CA); 2002.

25. Henrickson Parker S, Flin R, McKinley A, Yule S. The Surgeons' Leadership Inventory (SLI): A taxonomy and rating system for surgeons' intraoperative leadership skills. *Am J Surg.* 2013;205(6):745–51.

26. Künzle B, Zala-Mezö E, Wacker J, Kolbe M, Spahn DR, Grote G. Leadership in anaesthesia teams: The most effective leadership is shared. *Qual Saf Health Care*. 2010 Dec;19(6):e46.

27. Marsch SC, Muller C, Marquardt K, Conrad G, Tschan F, Hunziker PR. Human factors affect the quality of cardiopulmonary resuscitation in simulated cardiac arrests. *Resuscitation*. 2004;60(1):51–6.

28. Friedrich TL, Vessey WB, Schuelke MJ, Ruark GA, Mumford MD. A framework for understanding collective leadership: The selective utilization of leader and team expertise within networks. *Leadersh Q*. Elsevier, Inc. 2009 Dec;20(6):933–58.

29. Künzle B, Kolbe M, Grote G. Ensuring patient safety through effective leadership behaviour: A literature review. *Saf Sci*. Elsevier, Ltd. 2010 Jan;48(1):1–17.

30. Murphy EK. 'Captain of the ship' doctrine continues to take on water. *AORN J*. 2001;74(4):525–8.

31. Millman M. *The Unkindest Cut. Life in the Backrooms of Medicine*. New York: Morrow; 1976.

32. Henrickson Parker S, Yule S, Flin R, McKinley A. Towards a model of surgeons' leadership in the operating room. *BMJ Qual Saf*. 2011;20(7):570–9.

33. Klein KJ, Ziegert JC, Knight AP, Xiao Y. Dynamic delegation: Shared, hierarchical, and deindividualized leadership in extreme action teams. *Adm Sci Q*. 2006;51:590–621.

34. Yun S, Faraj S, Sims HP. Contingent leadership and effectiveness of trauma resuscitation teams. *J Appl Psychol*. 2005 Nov;90(6):1288–96.

35. Cooper S, Wakelam A. Leadership of resuscitation teams: 'Lighthouse Leadership.' *Resuscitation*. 1999;42(1):27–45.

36. Flin R, Maran N. Identifying and training non-technical skills for teams in acute medicine. *Qual Saf Heal Care*. 2004;13(Suppl 1):i80–4.

37. Wadhera R, Henrickson Parker S, Burkhart H, Greason K, Neal J, Levenick K et al. Is the 'sterile cockpit' concept applicable to cardiovascular surgery critical intervals or critical events? The impact of protocol-driven communication during cardiopulmonary bypass. *J Thorac Cardiovasc Surg*. 2010;139(2):312–9.

38. Rosenstein AH, O'Daniel M. A survey of the impact of disruptive behaviors and communication defects on patient safety. *Jt Comm J Qual Patient Saf*. 2008 Aug;34(8):464–71.

39. Kolbe M, Burtscher MJ, Manser T, Künzle B, Grote G. The role of co-ordination in preventing harm in healthcare groups: Research examples from anaesthesia and an integrated model of co-ordination for action teams in health care. In M. Boos, M. Kolbe, P. Kappeler, T. Ellwart (Eds.). *Co-ordination in Human and Primate Groups*. Heidelberg, Germany: Springer; 2011. pp. 75–92.

Performance-shaping factors

SONAL ARORA, IAN FLINDALL AND GEORGE G YOUNGSON

8.1 INTRODUCTION

There is a wide range of factors, beyond those already outlined in Chapter 1, which may affect a surgeon's personal well-being on a day-to-day basis and therefore may, directly or indirectly, influence surgical performance. These can be called performance-shaping factors.

Self-calibration of 'personal status' has been used in aviation in relation to pilot fitness for flying, employing the I'M SAFE mnemonic[1] to run a check on well-being status and how it is holding up on the day. I'M SAFE represents the following:

I: Illness
M: Medication (e.g. antihistamines for a coryzal illness and coping with a 'runny nose' behind a surgical mask)
S: Stress (personal relationships and time pressures)
A: Abuse – substance/alcohol (or its after-effects)

F: Fatigue
E: Emotion (rudeness, anger, aggression and personal grief), or E for eating (impact of hypoglycaemia)

All these factors can have an influence on technical and non-technical aspects of surgical performance. Moreover, due note should be taken of their potential effect on the performance of other members of the team. However, one hallmark of surgical expertise is consistency in performance and an ability to accommodate the external (and internal) pressures that apply during an operation. As outlined in Chapters 4 and 5, the cognitive skills of situation awareness and decision making are particularly susceptible to potential disruption from stress and fatigue. The more challenging the operative environment, the greater the dependency on the competence of the surgeon and the greater the need for a resilient and responsive performance, if a good outcome is to be had for the patient.

As has been already outlined, the Non-Technical Skills for Surgeons (NOTSS) system is restricted to those cognitive and behavioural aspects of surgical performance that can be directly or indirectly observed and rated. The skills relating to coping with fatigue and stress should be covered in non-technical skills training, but they have not been directly integrated into the NOTSS taxonomy as a category. There is, however, an element termed 'coping with pressure' within the leadership category of NOTSS. The reason why the skills for coping with stress and fatigue are not more explicitly included is that their effects can be difficult to observe, particularly when experienced at low levels of intensity. Moreover, there is a strong and understandable propensity to minimize their effect (that being easier said than done). Nonetheless, their deleterious effect on performance may be reflected in the demonstration of the cognitive and social skills and thus be indirectly identified. The same rationale was applied in the design of the NOTECHS taxonomy for airline pilots, as described in Chapter 2.

This chapter explores the particular threats posed by excessive stress and fatigue and also examines the potential for sustaining performance under challenging conditions. How these personal factors can shape surgical performance by their effect on both technical and non-technical skills is described, as is the relevant research on stress and fatigue. The use of non-technical skills in coping with their detrimental effects is also outlined.

8.2 STRESS IN SURGERY

Numerous factors contribute to the high prevalence of stress in surgery.[2,3] These can be divided into personal factors, patient factors and environmental factors. From a personal perspective, training and work hours are long and arduous, requiring a significant time commitment as well as personal sacrifices. In addition, dealing with critically unwell patients, complex pathologies and high-stakes decision making can all take a toll. The advent of newer technologies such as laparoscopic or robotic surgery, although designed to improve patient care, has led to protracted

learning curves that both new and more senior surgeons must master. In addition, the operating environment itself is also dynamic, time-pressured, noisy and rife with interruptions and distractions, leading to further pressure.[3] Ironically, however, a sense of isolation has also been reported, perhaps partly because surgeons are required to simply cope with stress, because the clandestine culture in surgery is one where 'surgeons don't get stressed, they just get on with it'.[4] As a result, surgeons have acknowledged that many have been left to contend with this on their own – either by 'trial and error' or by whatever other means possible – sometimes resulting in aberrant behaviours such as substance abuse and mental health problems[5,6] (Figure 8.1).

8.2.1 IMPACT OF STRESS ON PERFORMANCE

Although a certain degree of stress may help facilitate task execution, anything beyond this compromises performance. This idea that performance is best when the subject is in some optimal stress or arousal state, above or below which efficiency of performance decreases, is known as the Yerkes–Dodson law.[7] This follows most surgeons' perceptions that a small amount of stress can actually help them perform better but excessive levels compromise skills. Studies suggest that laparoscopic procedures can trigger higher stress levels and consequently impaired performance compared with open surgery.[8,9] This may be because of the nature of the technology involved, as well as the reliance on other team members to ensure the case progresses. Other studies have highlighted how the presence of stressors, such as distractions and interruptions, correlates with poorer performance in terms of impaired manual dexterity and increased error.[4] This is of significant concern given evidence to suggest that the operating theatre is flush with distractions.[3,10]

8.2.2 NON-TECHNICAL SKILLS AND STRESS

Few studies have evaluated the impact of stress on surgeons' non-technical performance. The majority of these studies have been conducted in

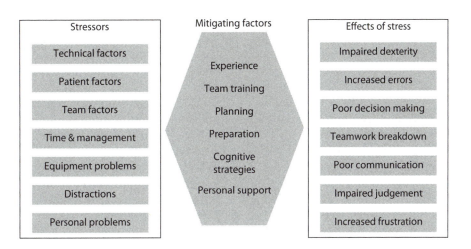

Figure 8.1 Causes and effects of stress in surgery

the simulation setting or have been self-reported. Undre et al.[11] studied the effect of bleeding (stressor) in a simulated scenario on teamwork and found that this significantly impaired surgeons' leadership and decision-making abilities. Conversely, Moorthy et al.[12] found a significant impact of stress on non-technical skills (particularly decision making) in their simulated study, albeit the surgeons were more experienced. This suggests that experience does play a role in mitigating some of the adverse effects of stress and this is supported by other studies, which have identified the fact that experienced surgeons are subject to less stress and consequently generally perform better in the operating theatre than their less experienced counterparts.[13,14] Qualitative studies have also highlighted how stress can impair a surgeon's judgement and communication, which then leads to a cascade effect that impairs teamwork.[4,5]

The systems view of surgery[15] acknowledges that patient outcome is not purely a function of illness severity and the surgeons' technical skill. Rather, non-technical skills, such as communication, teamwork, decision making, situation awareness and leadership, are equally important determinants of outcome. However, all of these skills can be compromised by stress. As such, the ability to recognize, prevent or mitigate stress is a crucial component of a surgeon's non-technical competence. To effectively manage stress, however, it is first important to understand its basis and its relationship to human performance.

8.2.3 STRESS TYPES

In most circumstances, stress can be defined as bodily processes that result from psychological or physical demands placed on a person. These demands are denoted as 'stressors', and when they outweigh an individual's perceived ability to cope the situation of stress or distress arises. In contrast, eustress is when the demands of a situation match the individual's ability to cope. There are several theories and models of stress, but two well-accepted ones are the 'systemic stress approach' and the 'psychological stress approach'. According to the former theory, developed largely by Selye,[16] stress is a state manifested by a syndrome that consists of all the non-specifically induced changes in a biologic system. In contrast, the psychological approach to stress regards it as a relationship between an individual and his or her environment. It is therefore a function of how an individual perceives a situation (primary cognitive appraisal) and his or her coping abilities (secondary cognitive appraisal), which determine whether stress is experienced.[17]

Specific patterns of primary and secondary appraisals lead to different kinds of stress. Three types are distinguished: harm, threat and challenge. Harm refers to the (psychological) damage or loss that has already happened. Threat is the anticipation of harm that may be imminent. Challenge results from demands that a person feels confident about mastering. After the acute event has been appraised by the individual, meaning and emotions are generated. Then, a behaviour called coping ensues. Most approaches in coping research follow Folkman and Lazarus, who define coping as the cognitive and behavioural efforts made to master, tolerate or reduce external and internal demands and conflicts among them.[17,18] Coping includes attempts to reduce the perceived discrepancy between situational demands and personal resources.

Several types of coping have been identified.[18] The following are of particular relevance:

1. Problem-focused coping, which is actively altering the external person–environment relationship. Problem-focused coping is when the individual focuses attention on situation-specific objectives and allows a sense of mastery and control in working towards attaining that particular goal. Strategies include gathering more information or evaluating the pros and cons of options.

> I had tried several times to get the bleeding to stop from the parenchyma of the spleen but once I thought about my options, I concentrated on using all the haemostatic aids and asked the anaesthetist to tell me that the patient was not coagulopathic … I got the bleeding to finally stop.

2. Emotion-focused coping, which is altering the personal meaning of or how the person feels about the problem. This type of coping involves positive reappraisal, which involves cognitively reframing typically difficult thoughts in a positive manner. Strategies include self-control, seeking support and minimizing emotional response.

> Although we were losing blood, I took a deep breath and tried to remain calm and not become alarmed about the situation. I told myself to be confident that the technique I had used before would sort it out.

8.2.4 MEASURING STRESS

Although the amount of stress cannot be quantified directly, measures can be used to approximate it by looking at the physiological (objective) and psychological (subjective) effects of stress.

Objective measures include cardiac indices such as heart rate and heart rate variability. These detect changes in cardiac activity resulting from the endogenous catecholamine release as part of the normal physiological response to stress. Other physiological measures include salivary cortisol and skin conductance level. Studies using these metrics have highlighted how they change during stressful episodes in the operating theatre.[10,15,19] These measures have been shown to be both valid and reliable and can be carried out relatively non-intrusively, efficiently and effectively using widely available technology.[15]

Subjective assessment of stress typically involves participants self-reporting the amount of stress that they experience. This is particularly important because the perception of stress psychologically is more likely to affect responses and coping.[20] Methods for this can involve capture of a surgeon's perceptions using qualitative interviews, questionnaires or validated scales, such as the State Trait Anxiety Inventory or the Perceived Stress Scale.[21] Regarding the former, a short six-item version has been validated for use in the operating theatre and demonstrated to have high levels of concurrent validity compared to objective indices. Its concise nature makes it particularly suitable for the busy setting of an operating theatre.[15]

However, a focus on any isolated measure may give an oversimplified view of what is a complex, multifactorial and dynamic picture. For instance, studies that have used skin conductance level, heart rate and salivary cortisol as proxy measures for stress could not attribute a rise in these measurements to solely increased mental demand, as they may very well be a result of the physical nature of surgery. Likewise, relying on self-reporting introduces bias due to a lack of insight or the surgeon's reluctance to admit to stress. The way forward for stress measurement research is to use a toolbox incorporating both subjective and objective measures.

8.2.5 STRATEGIES FOR REDUCING STRESS IN SURGERY

Although some stressors (e.g. distractions) can be reduced by changes to operating theatre environment and practices, for other stressors this is not possible: patients will still be critically ill, colleagues may be inexperienced and rapid decisions with serious consequences may need to be made, often under time pressure. This is all in addition to personal pressures such as career problems, relationship issues and financial issues. Thus, the recognition and management of stressful situations is imperative to high quality and safe surgery. As highlighted previously, stress is experienced when perceived resources are outweighed by perceived demands.[17] Possibilities for overcoming this include reducing external demand (primary stress management) or improving the perceived ability to cope by optimizing personal resources (secondary stress management).[20]

With respect to reducing demands, it is important to address those disruptions found in the operating room environment and to identify those other stressors that can be minimized. This includes addressing equipment problems and poor teamwork resulting from miscommunication or unfamiliarity with team and hierarchical barriers, as pointed out in Chapters 6 and 7 where strategies to counteract some of these problems involve some introduction of predictability into the operative setting by including briefings and checklists. Briefings in particular provide an opportunity for the entire surgical team to plan the list and any required equipment, thereby anticipating and pre-empting potential problems that can trigger stress levels. However, the success of these interventions in reducing stress is dependent on how they are implemented. Simply having a briefing and ticking boxes on a checklist are not enough. In fact, this can introduce a false sense of security and complacency or in fact may be a source of irritation to others and provoke a negative response. It is crucial therefore that briefings and checklists are utilized in the spirit with which they were intended so that they can truly have their best effect on both stress levels and patient safety.

Secondary stress management techniques include increasing perceived resources available. This can be done by providing surgeons an opportunity to experience task-related stress, for example, through simulation, and become accustomed to stress and practise its management. While previous generations of surgeons experienced their

training in coping with pressure through working (excessively) long duty hours and repeated exposure to many different clinical situations, an obvious alternative is simulation-based stress management training. Simulation offers a safe, realistic training environment in which trial and error can occur without risk to patient safety and with the opportunity for structured, systematic feedback on performance. Structured experience of simulated crises before encountering them in a real operating setting could function as a 'preconditioning' mechanism – known to alter a person's approach to psychological challenges. Wetzel et al.[22] describe such a simulation-based stress management training programme and report that participants found it both useful and practical in learning how to cope more effectively in the operating room. Outside health care, simulation-based crisis management modules have been widely used in the aviation industry as part of Crew Resource Management training[23] (see Chapter 2). Lessons learnt in the context of the aviation industry could be applied to surgery with evidence highlighting that these programmes are well received from trainers and trainees alike, which is important if the surgical culture surrounding stress is to change.[5,22]

Another less resource-intensive possibility for preconditioning is mental rehearsal or mental practice. Mental practice can be defined as 'the cognitive rehearsal of a task in the absence of overt physical movement' where the systematic use of mental imagery is employed to rehearse an action or skill symbolically prior to the actual performance.[24] By providing exposure to the contents of the task, surgeons can experience what it feels like to perform the task in their mind. This can reduce stress through providing stress inoculation or by increasing the perceived ability (resources) to cope with task demands. Evidence for the use of mental practice as a technique to modify stress can be found in the sports psychology literature. Studies here have shown that imagery can be used to reduce the symptoms of performance anxiety[25] and that it can help performers to change their perceptions of stress from debilitative (or threatening) to facilitative.[26] Mental practice also improves cognitive skills and leads to measurable physiological change.[4,26]

8.3 FATIGUE

The lack of consensus within the scientific community and thus the inability to create an agreed on definition of fatigue and its causation[27,28] is an inherent problem in the detection and management of fatigue within society in general and surgery in particular. Fatigue is typically defined as 'extreme and persistent tiredness, weakness or exhaustion – mental, physical or both'.[29] It can be acute or chronic and can be triggered by stress, medication, overwork, illness or disease. Epidemiological studies have indicated that 20–24% of the US population have reported fatigue, whereas the prevalence rate of fatigue was found to be 18% in the United Kingdom.[30–32] The unfortunate use of nomenclature such as 'tiredness' has proved detrimental for the advancement of fatigue research. Without an agreed on use of terms, in-depth discussions are difficult. At present, tiredness can sometimes be used inaccurately but synonymously with fatigue. Tiredness is ultimately a non-scientific term that can encompass fatigue but also separate conditions such as sleep deprivation. One can be fatigued but not sleep deprived, and vice versa. Fatigue is also different from burnout. Burnout can be defined as 'the exhaustion of physical or emotional strength as a result of prolonged stress or frustration'.[33] This state of exhaustion is closely related to chronic fatigue, whereas acute fatigue, by definition, resolves with rest or decrement in the intensity of the task. When fatigue is combined with the phenomenon of absenteeism and a negative work-related state of mind, employees are considered to be experiencing burnout. The scale of magnitude of burnout among surgeons in the USA has already been documented and has been noted to be more prevalent than was previously acknowledged.[34]

Acute fatigue, however, is a normal and reversible phenomenon that resolves after a period of rest or through a reduction in the intensity of the task performed (mental or physical). At a single point in time, whether the fatigue is acute or chronic does not negate the importance that the individual is physically or mentally impaired. Within a working environment, individuals who are in a state of acute mental fatigue are at a higher risk of errors, placing their safety, that of their colleagues and patients at risk. Perceived work-based fatigue is recognized in industry to reduce productivity, and more recently it has been gaining recognition within the health care profession for its detrimental effect on staff performance.

8.3.1 FATIGUE IN HEALTH CARE

Subjective fatigue is well documented among health care workers. A US survey reported greater fatigue in 43% of residents who perceived they had made a medical error in a single year of training.[35] In a study of emergency service workers, 55% of the respondents were classified as fatigued while at work,[36] with 17.8% documenting an injury in the previous 3 months, which is 1.9 times higher than that for a non-fatigued worker. The odds of a fatigued worker having perceived that safety had been compromised were 3.6:1 compared to a non-fatigued worker, whereas the odds of a medical error or adverse event occurring in a fatigued worker were 2.2 times higher. A separate study found doctors had increasing subjective fatigue if their work limit exceeded 60 hours per week[37] with 19% suggesting they had performed a medical/surgical error when fatigued. A higher incidence of injury has been found in health care professionals who work over 60 hours per week.[38] This evidence reinforces the fact that workers who are in an acute state of mental fatigue are at a higher risk of errors, placing their safety; the safety of their colleagues; and, in the medical profession, patients at risk. Subjective assessments rely on an individual's perception of fatigue. A person can be fatigued without insight.

The accumulation of frequent, repetitive exposures to trauma and high levels of stress can lead to compassion fatigue. This is receiving increased recognition within health care workers. Society is frequently critical about the lack of empathy by health care staff, so it appears that compassion fatigue is a problem.[39] The increasing expectations of a critical society may have little insight into what is likely a presenting symptom of mental fatigue of the carer, and it is quite feasible that a significant proportion of complaints concerning staff behaviour and attitudes are as a result of fatigue. Resulting litigation payouts combined with physical fatigue-related errors has significant cost implications related to compensation claims.

In a systematic review of patient safety and empirical working hours by the Jefferson Medical College Duty Hours Review Group,[40] laboratory studies of performance on clinical simulations and tests of cognitive and fine motor skills in the sleep deprived state suggested that limits on duty hours should have strong positive effects on patient safety. The US Accreditation Council for Graduate Medical Education has twice recommended reductions in work time for medical trainees due in part to concerns about fatigue,[41] whereas in Europe work hour limitation policy has been implemented through the European Working Time Directive. Although measurable effects from the impact of duty hour regulations on patient safety have been difficult to demonstrate, the World Health Organization (WHO) has identified fatigue as a leading factor in occurrence of medical error and injury in health care.[42] Worker fatigue has large cost implications that range from sick leave to negligence claims attributed to medical errors. In the UK, the National Health Service Litigation Authority's bill for 2011–2012 was documented to have increased to £1.2 billion,[43] and some costs can be attributed to fatigue-related error. Therefore, a fatigue reduction plan can reduce errors, improve patient and staff safety and reduce complaints from patients regarding lack of empathy and caring.

Studies on trainees, in particular, show that extended work hours significantly increase fatigue and impair performance and public safety.[44] Traditional 24-hour on-call shifts demonstrate 36% more serious preventable adverse events (compared to a 16-hour shift pattern). Doctors have also been found to have twice the number of attentional failures[45] at night and a 61% increase in needle stick/sharp injury after 20 hours of work.[46] There are five times the number of serious diagnostic errors and a 300% increase in fatigue-related serious adverse events causing patient death.[47] In the fatigued state, doctors display a 1.5–2 standard deviation deterioration in performance compared to baseline measurements for clinical and non-clinical tasks.[48]

8.3.2 WHY IS FATIGUE IMPORTANT?

Higher cognitive processes are a limited resource (see Chapter 4). Tasks that involve a high mental workload can have an impact on and cause the temporary depletion of these processes. Prolonged, low-stimulus and monotonous tasks can also cause an effect. It is this resource depletion that creates the symptoms of mental fatigue.

Overall, fatigue causes reduced effectiveness through compromised problem solving, memory lapses and impaired communication with slow or faulty information processing and judgement.[49] Reduced motivation, irritability, impaired communication with indifference and loss of empathy[50] can be displayed. The focus and attention of an individual can be significantly impaired by fatigue through reduced vigilance, which can be demonstrated by the increase in lapses of attention.[51] Mental fatigue results in increased distractibility and irritability and thus leads to stimulus-driven attention response[52] and loss of goal-directed attention. The decrements in cognition have significant implications for patient and staff safety within the operating room environment.

8.3.3 FATIGUE AND NON-TECHNICAL SKILLS

After the implementation of work hour limitations in the United States, the Joint Commission assessed the impact of fatigue on health care workers.[53] They concluded that fatigue was still caused by extended hours or insufficient sleep that contributed to errors at work. Concerns were also raised regarding patient safety at 'hand-off' (handover), a process at risk of error that is heightened when fatigued. However, a review of the effects of fatigue on surgeon performance and surgical outcomes concluded that there was little evidence to inform on the effect of fatigue on surgical performance.[54] This assessed 16 studies out of the 823 initially reviewed. It found that less experienced surgeons were more susceptible to making errors when sleep deprived compared to their senior counterparts. Other causes for fatigue, such as time-on-task effects, were not addressed in the review. Most of the evidence uses virtual reality to assess performance without correlating to the clinical setting. Additionally, as outlined in Chapters 4 and 5, fatigue generally will be an element that contributes to performance shaping in a prejudicial fashion and therefore will compromise both situation awareness and decision making without necessarily culminating in a surgical error.

In this aspect, a simulation study also suggested that surgical proficiency was significantly impeded in the fatigued state among junior- and senior-level residents.[55] There were an increased number of cognitive errors and decreased psychomotor efficiency and overall task performance in the fatigued condition. Again, cognitive skills were more impaired than psychomotor skills. A possible explanation for this involves the aspect of working memory applied to the task. Procedural memory is the unconscious memory of skills and performance of tasks, for example, surgical knot tying. These sensorimotor behaviours are deeply embedded for experienced surgeons to the point that no conscious effort is required and they are able to automatically perform the task. Thus, fatigue may not cause as significant an impairment in psychomotor tasks in more experienced subjects compared to inexperienced colleagues due to reduced cognitive recall requirements.

8.3.4 DETRIMENTAL EFFECTS OF FATIGUE OR THE BENEFICIAL EFFECTS OF CONTINUITY OF CARE?

The beneficial effects of care experienced by a patient under the continuous care of a single named surgeon result from the intimate knowledge of the presentation, history, diagnosis and surgical management of the patient. Teams that have a reduced frequency of handoff/handover to the care of others experience an obligate increase in their working hours, and they may advocate that patients benefit from this process. Acknowledging that points of transition are particularly susceptible to introduction of errors, in the case of complex patients (where the handoff requires significantly more information to be relayed by shift-based teams) the risk of error increases, thereby reducing efficiency and safety. Yet, with prolonged duty hours there is the increased risk of fatigue-induced

error and, although it is difficult to identify the precise point of trade-off between these two models, there needs to be a balance between frequency of handoff-induced errors and errors through lack of shared situational awareness of a patient's condition.

The alternative model is based on not 'how we can reduce the frequency of handoff' as fatigue-induced error must be reduced. Instead, the question should be 'what extra patient safety measures can be implanted to reduce the risk of adverse events in high risk patients?'. Explicit recognition of the prejudicial effects of fatigue itself in affecting communication during the handoff process is also required.

8.3.5 FATIGUE AND CHECKLISTS

Fatigue risk management strategies are analogous to (or a subset of) a safety management system[56] that systematically and comprehensively addresses the risk of fatigue using formal assessment processes (see Chapter 11). Checklist systems are used to reduce error-related effects by stimulating the recall of specific aspects of a procedure, thus improving safety.[57] Evidence from cognitive psychology demonstrates that a cued response will improve recollection[58] compared to free recall of information.[59]

The use of cues for information recall is one feasible strategy for fatigue management. Cues need not be specific but can interrogate generic aspects of a patient's care, for example, past medical history. However, with increased generality there is increased risk of an unsuccessful cue. When fatigued, cues are arguably of increased relevance; however, the system is only as good as operator compliance to the checklist protocol. Some checklist protocols remove the need for recall of information, with the worker being forced to check the system in the presence of a colleague.

The 'Swiss cheese model of accident prevention'[60] described in Chapter 2 can be used as part of prevention of fatigue-related error. It consists of multiple layers of processes and procedures that constitute mitigating defences and barriers against an error, prior to it producing a negative effect. A checklist can certainly be considered as one layer of this model (see Figure 2.3).

8.3.6 STRATEGIES FOR MANAGING FATIGUE

As costs of medical negligence claims rise[43] and public (and media) concern for mistakes made by surgeons mounts, a multifaceted approach to the management of fatigue becomes increasingly important. As health care worker fatigue is linked to patient safety, it has been recommended that health care organizations examine processes at high risk of error, especially where these areas of risk are compounded by fatigue.[53]

Much of the research literature on fatigue focuses on the sleep-deprived state and uses cognitive assessments involving well-documented cognitive tasks. Examples have included word recollection tasks in emergency department doctors[61] and vigilance and reaction time as part of a battery of cognitive tests in year 1–qualified doctors.[62] Fatigue studies frequently imply sleep deprivation studies that are typically laboratory based or performed around shift work. However, acute mental fatigue produced through high mental workload can also cause impairment in working memory,[63] and this is of particular relevance in high-demand situations such as operative surgery. Indeed, the effect of fatigue on performance has been compared to the effects of alcohol intoxication, where one night of sleep deprivation produced performance impairment greater than is currently acceptable in the United Kingdom for alcohol intoxication and a loss of 2 hours of sleep produced a performance decrement on psychomotor tasks equivalent to drinking 3–4 units of alcohol.[64]

When fatigued, medical staff may attempt to maintain performance and reduce errors through legalized stimulants such as caffeine, chocolate and nicotine.[65] Short 'naps' are also an evidence-based measure to maintain performance.[66] It is notable, however, that in the United Kingdom shift work has curtailed such measures by removal of amenities that would facilitate tactical napping.[67]

Legal stimulants to counteract fatigue are not without their side effects. For example, caffeine may induce tremor and has gut-stimulant effects that may adversely influence a physician's ability to work. Moreover, in high doses it is recognized to have serious risks to health.[68] The recently popularized 'energy drinks' have also raised health concerns if drunk in significant volumes due to the high levels of caffeine and sugar content in them. Some products also contain unregulated quantities of taurine or ginseng.

The use of 'off label' wake-enhancing medication, for example, modafinil, has been documented in professional groups.[69] Its extent of use in the medical profession is unknown. Modafinil has been demonstrated to improve performance in the sleep-deprived (fatigued) state.[70] Neuropharmacological intervention as a fatigue amelioration strategy has documented use in the military[71] and professional groups (including doctors).[72,73] Critically, albeit under simulated conditions, modafinil has improved attentional performance[74] and decision making in fatigued (sleep-deprived) doctors performing non-clinical cognitive tasks.[75] There are significant moral and medicolegal consequences to the use of wake-enhancing medication that are yet to be addressed.

Within current health care, fatigue is rarely the focus for interventional safety strategies. Work hour restrictions cannot be the single intervention for fatigue management. A multifaceted approach is required to address this pervasive problem. Research into strategies that detect and limit procedural time-on-task effects is essential. Adequate facilities must be provided for sufficient breaks, relaxation and nutrition. Work hour restrictions are important but require effort to provide a shift system that limits circadian effects and provide sufficient recuperation time. Staff should be educated on fatigue reduction and be responsible for adequate rest when on leave, along with the limited and conscientious use of legal stimulants when experiencing subjective fatigue.

Education to promote fatigue self-awareness and recognition of fatigue in colleagues is a simple but essential aspect of fatigue management. Acknowledgement of fatigue allows for compensatory strategies to be implemented if an alert member of staff is unavailable. Preoperatively, this may include the reordering of an operative list or the conscious attempt to maximize the ergonomics of a procedure to minimize operative fatigue. Cognitive strategies could include repetition or rehearsal of important steps or management strategies for unexpected complications. One of the principal aspects of the WHO Preoperative Safety

Checklist[76] is to prevent gross errors by (possibly) a fatigued operating room team by forcing the individuals to verify key aspects of the case, for example, the site of an operative procedure. Intra-operatively, the surgeon can apply similar principles to check that the planned step is correct through repeated checks until satisfied. At safe points during a procedure, a short break can be implemented prior to a cognitively demanding step, thus allowing staff to re-cooperate and re-focus on the next difficult aspect of the procedure.

Maintaining communication with operating room team members throughout the procedure is of paramount importance for fatigue management, allowing informed staff to maintain focus ensuring a smooth operation. An analysis of malpractice claims found 42% to be related to communication failure.[77] Predominantly, these fatigue countermeasures focus on addressing the decrement in vigilance associated with fatigue by promoting a conscious action by the surgeon. Many of these measures could arguably be deemed good surgical practice and if practised in the alert state may become 'second nature' and be implemented when fatigued.

8.4 CONCLUSION

Some are of the view that the hazards of fatigue are overstated and the modifications made to pre-empt its potentially deleterious effect constitute a significant threat to continuity of care and therefore to the management of patients. Others would add to that by indicating that the reduction to experiential learning caused by the reduction in duty hours to protect against fatigue results in depleted experience with resultant lack of confidence affecting the judgement and decision-making processes of the operating surgeon, as well as potentially prejudicing the opportunity for acquisition of technical skills. The effects of fatigue and stress on the performance of the experienced surgeon are possibly less pronounced than they are on the performance of those in training and acquiring surgical skills. There are also individual differences in response, but these conditions do affect all surgeons and that effect

is predominantly on the non-technical skills set. Both stress and fatigue adversely affect innovative thinking and flexible decision making, as well as reducing the ability to cope with unforeseen rapid changes. This, in turn, reduces the ability to adjust plans when new information becomes available and there is a tendency to adopt more rigid thinking and accept lower standards of performance, all of which are elements contained by the NOTSS taxonomy and relevant to operative surgery.

This chapter itemizes the effects produced by both fatigue and stress and discusses what can be done by surgeons to address them. Although tolerance of these effects varies from individual to individual and needs to be contextualized in relation to the level of experience of the surgeon, type of surgery and time of operative surgery, both states are real and should be acknowledged as shaping the performance of the operating surgeon.

REFERENCES

1. Flight Fitness: The 'I'm Safe' Checklist. *FAA Medical Certification*. Pilot Medical Solutions, Incorp. [Accessed March 25, 2015.] Available from: http://www.leftseat.com/imsafe.htm.
2. Arora S, Sevdalis N, Nestel D, Woloshynowych M, Darzi A, Kneebone R. The impact of stress on surgical performance: A systematic review of the literature. *Surgery*. 2010;147(3):318–30.
3. Arora S, Hull L, Sevdalis N, Tierney T, Nestel D, Woloshynowych M et al. Factors compromising safety in surgery: Stressful events in the operating room. *Am J Surg*. 2010;199(1):60–5.
4. Arora S, Sevdalis N, Nestel D, Woloshynowych M, Tierney T, Kneebone R. Managing intra-operative stress: What do surgeons want from a crisis training programme? *Am J Surg*. 2009;197(4):537–43.
5. Wetzel C, Kneebone R, Woloshynowych M, Nestel D, Moorthy K, Kidd J et al. The effects of stress on surgical performance. *Am J Surg*. 2006;191(1):5–10.
6. Shanafelt TD, Balch CM, Bechamps G, Russell T, Dyrbye L, Satele D et al. Burnout

and medical errors among American surgeons. *Ann Surg.* 2010;251:995–1000.

7. Yerkes RM, Dodson JD. The relation of strength of stimulus to rapidity of habit formation. *J Comp Neurol Psychol.* 1908;18:459–82.

8. Berguer R, Smith WD, Chung YH. Performing laparoscopic surgery is significantly more stressful for the surgeon than open surgery. *Surg Endosc.* 2001;15:1204–7.

9. Bohm B, Rotting N, Schwenk W, Grebe S, Mansmann U. A prospective randomized trial on heart rate variability of the surgical team during laparoscopic and conventional sigmoid resection. *Arch Surg.* 2001;136:305–10.

10. Sevdalis N, Forrest D, Undre S, Darzi A, Vincent C. Annoyances, disruptions, and interruptions in surgery: The Disruptions in Surgery Index (DiSI). *World J Surg.* 2008;32:1643–50.

11. Undre S, Koutantji M, Sevdalis N, Gautama S, Selvapatt N, Williams S et al. Multidisciplinary crisis simulations: The way forward for training surgical teams. *World J Surg.* 2007;31:1843–53.

12. Moorthy K, Munz Y, Adams S, Pandey V, Darzi A. A human factors analysis of technical and team skills among surgical trainees during procedural simulations in a simulated operating theatre. *Ann Surg.* 2005;242:631–9.

13. Hassan I, Weyers P, Maschuw K, Dick B, Gerdes B, Rothmund M et al. Negative stress-coping strategies among novices in surgery correlate with poor virtual laparoscopic performance. *Br J Surg.* 2006;93:1554–9.

14. Arora S, Tierney T, Sevdalis N, Aggarwal R, Nestel D, Woloshynowych M et al. The imperial stress assessment tool (ISAT): A feasible, reliable and valid approach to measuring stress in the operating room. *World J Surg.* 2010;34(8):1756–63.

15. Vincent C, Moorthy K, Sarker S, Chang A, Darzi A. Systems approaches to surgical quality and safety. *Ann Surg.* 2004;239:475–82.

16. Selye H. The evolution of the stress concept. *Am Scientist.* 1973;61(6):692–9.

17. Lazarus RS, Folkman S. *Stress, Appraisal and Coping.* New York: Springer;1984.

18. Lazarus RS. Coping theory and research: Past, present, and future. *Psychosom Med.* 1993;55:234–47.

19. Czyzewska E, Kiczka K, Czarnecki A, Pokinko P. The surgeon's mental load during decision making at various stages of operations. *Eur J App Phys Occup Phys.* 1983;51:441–6.

20. Lazarus RS. *Stress and Emotion: A New Synthesis.* New York: Springer 1999.

21. Marteau TM, Bekker H. The development of a six-item short-form of the state scale of the Spielberger State-Trait Anxiety Inventory (STAI). *Br J Clin Psychol.* 1992;31(Pt 3):301–6.

22. Wetzel CM, George A, Hanna GB, Athanasiou T, Black SA, Kneebone RL et al. Stress management training for surgeons – A randomized, controlled, intervention study. *Ann Surg.* 2011;253(3):488–94.

23. Helmreich RL, Merritt AC, Wilhelm JA. The evolution of Crew Resource Management training in commercial aviation. *Int J Aviat Psych.* 1999;9:19–32.

24. Driskell JE, Copper C, Moran A. Does mental practice enhance performance? *J App Psych.* 1994;79:481–92.

25. Page SJ, Sime W, Nordell K. The effects of imagery on female college swimmers' perceptions of anxiety. *Sport Psych.* 1999;13:458–69.

26. Weinberg R. Does imagery work? Effects on performance and mental skills. *J Imagery Res Sport Phys Activ.* 2008;3(1):1–21.

27. Hardy G, Shapiro D, Borrill CS. Fatigue in the workforce of national health service trusts: Levels of symptomatology and links with minor psychiatric disorder, demographic, occupational and work role factors. *J Psychosom Res.* 1997;43(1):83–92.

28. Pigeon W, Sateia M, Ferguson RJ. Distinguishing between excessive daytime sleepiness and fatigue: Toward improved detection and treatment. *J Psychosom Res.* 2003;54(1):61–9.

29. Dittner A, Wessely S, Brown RG. The assessment of fatigue: A practical guide for clinicians and researchers. *J Psychosom Res.* 2004;56(2):157–70.

30. Chen MK. The epidemiology of self-perceived fatigue among adults. *Prev Med.* 1986;15(1):74–81.

31. Kroenke K, Price RK. Symptoms in the community. *Arch Intern Med.* 1993;153(21):2474–80.

32. Pawlikowska T, Chalder T, Hirsch SR, Wallace P, Wright DJ, Wessely SC. Population based study of fatigue and psychological distress. *BMJ.* 1994;308(6931):763–6.

33. Felton JS. Burnout as a clinical entity – Its importance in health care workers. *Occ Med.* 1998;48(4):237–50.

34. Shanafelt TD, Boone S, Tan L, Dyrbye LN, Sotile W, Satele D et al. Burnout and satisfaction with work-life balance among US physicians relative to the general US population. *Arch Intern Med.* 2012;172(18):1377–85.

35. West CP, Tan AD, Habermann TM, Sloan JA, Shanafelt TD. Association of resident fatigue and distress with perceived medical errors. *JAMA.* 2009;302(12):1294–300.

36. Patterson PD, Weaver MD, Frank RC, Warner CW, Martin-Gill C, Guyette FX et al. Association between poor sleep, fatigue, and safety outcomes in emergency medical services providers. *Prehosp Emerg Care.* 2012;16(1):86–97.

37. Cammu H, Haentjens P. Perceptions of fatigue – and perceived consequences – among Flemish obstetricians-gynaecologists: A survey. *Eur J Contracept Reprod Health Care.* 2012;17(4):314–20.

38. Dembe AE, Delbos R, Erickson JB. Estimates of injury risks for healthcare personnel working night shifts and long hours. *BMJ Qual Saf.* 2009;18(5):336–40.

39. Markwell AL, Wainer Z. The health and well-being of junior doctors: Insights from a national survey. *Med J Aust.* 2009;191(8):441–4.

40. Caruso J, Veloski J, Grasberger M, Boex JR, Paskin DL, Kairys JC et al. Systematic review of the literature on the impact of variation in residents' duty hour schedules on patient safety. Report of ACGME by the Jefferson Medical College Review Group. 2009. [Accessed August 17, 2014]. Available from: https://www.acgme.org/acgmeweb /Portals/0/PDFs/Jefferson_Medical_College _Duty_Hours_Review[1].pdf.

41. Nasca TJ, Day SH, Amis ES. The new recommendations on duty hours from the ACGME Task Force. *N Engl J Med.* 2010; 363(2):e3.

42. World Alliance for Patient Safety. WHO Safety Curriculum for Medical Schools. 2009; pp. 1–258. [Accessed October 1, 2014]. Available from: http://whqlibdoc.who .int/publications/2009/9789241598316_eng .pdf.

43. House of Commons Committee of Public Accounts. *Whole of Government Accounts 2009–10.* Sixty seventh report of session 2010–2012. pp. 1–40. [Accessed October 1, 2014]. Available from: http://www .publications.parliament.uk/pa/cm201012 /cmselect/cmpubacc/1696/1696.pdf.

44. Lockley SW, Barger LK, Ayas NT, Rothschild JM, Czeisler CA, Landrigan CP et al. Effect of healthcare provider work hours and sleep deprivation on safety and performance. *Jt Comm J Qual Patient Saf.* 2007;33(Suppl 11):7–18.

45. Lockley SW, Cronin JW, Evans EE, Cade BE, Lee CJ, Landrigan CP et al. Effect of reducing interns' weekly work hours on sleep and attentional failures. *N Engl J Med.* 2004;351(18):1829–37.

46. Ayas NT, Barger LK, Cade BE, Hashimoto DM, Rosner B, Cronin JW et al. Extended work duration and the risk of self-reported percutaneous injuries in interns. *JAMA.* 2006;296(9):1055–62.

47. Barger LK, Ayas NT, Cade BE, Cronin JW, Rosner B, Speizer FE et al. Impact of extended-duration shifts on medical errors, adverse events, and attentional failures. *PLoS Med.* 2006;3(12):487.

48. Philibert I. Sleep loss and performance in residents and nonphysicians: A meta-analytic examination. *Sleep.* 2005;28(11):1392–402.

49. Patient Safety Advisory Group. Health care worker fatigue and patient safety. *Sentinel Event Alert.* 2011;48:1–4.

50. Friesen MA, White SV, Byers JF. Chapter 34. Handoffs: Implications for nurses. In Hughes RG, (Ed.) *Patient Safety and Quality: An Evidence-Based Handbook for Nurses,* Volume 2. 2008. Rockville, MD: Agency for Healthcare and Policy. pp. 285–332.

51. Lee I, Bardwell WA, Ancoli-Israel S, Dimsdale JE. Number of lapses during the Psychomotor Vigilance Task as an objective measure of fatigue. *J Clin Sleep Med.* 2010;6(2):163–8.

52. Boksem MAS, Meijman TF, Lorist MM. Effects of mental fatigue on attention: An ERP study. *Brain Res Cogn Brain Res.* 2005;25(1):107–16.

53. Joint Commission. The Joint Commission alert: Action urged to fight health care worker fatigue 2011; pwrnewmedia.com. pp. 1–3. [Accessed October 1, 2014.] Available from http://www.pwrnewmedia.com/2011/joint_commission/sea_fatigue/.

54. Sturm L, Dawson D, Vaughan R, Hewett P, Hill AG, Graham JC et al. Effects of fatigue on surgeon performance and surgical outcomes: A systematic review. *ANZ J Surg.* 2011;81(7–8):502–9.

55. Kahol K, Leyba MJ, Deka M, Deka V, Mayes S, Smith M et al. Effect of fatigue on psychomotor and cognitive skills. *Am J Surg.* 2008;195(2):195–204.

56. Lerman SE, Eskin E, Flower DJ. Fatigue risk management in the workplace. *J Occup Env Med.* 2012;54(2):231–58.

57. Davidoff F. Checklists and guidelines: Imaging techniques for visualizing what to do. *JAMA.* 2010;304(2):206–7.

58. Hunt RR, Smith RE. Accessing the particular from the general: The power of distinctiveness in the context of organization. *Mem Cognition.* 1996;24(2):217–25.

59. Winter L, Uleman JS. When are social judgments made? Evidence for the spontaneousness of trait inferences. *J Pers Soc Psychol.* 1984;47(2):237–52.

60. Reason J. *Human Error.* Cambridge, United Kingdom: University Press; 1990.

61. Machi MS, Staum M, Callaway CW, Moore C, Jeong K, Suyama J et al. The relationship between shift work, sleep, and cognition in career emergency physicians. *Acad Emerg Med.* 2012;19(1):85–91.

62. Orton DI, Gruzelier JH. Adverse changes in mood and cognitive performance of house officers after night duty. *BMJ.* 1989;298(6665):21–3.

63. Tanaka M, Mizuno K, Tajima S, Sasabe T, Watanabe Y. Central nervous system fatigue alters autonomic nerve activity. *Life Sci.* 2009;(84):235–9.

64. Dawson D, Reid K. Fatigue, alcohol and performance impairment. *Nature.* 1997;388:235.

65. Bonnet MH, Arand DL. The use of prophylactic naps and caffeine to maintain performance during a continuous operation. *Ergonomics.* 1994;37(6):1009–20.

66. Takahashi M. The role of prescribed napping in sleep medicine. *Sleep Med Rev.* 2003;7(3):227–35.

67. Varughese GI. Junior doctors' shifts and sleep deprivation – Please make on-call rooms available to doctors at night. *BMJ.* 2005;331(7515):515.

68. Sepkowitz KA. Energy drinks and caffeine-related adverse effects. *JAMA.* 2013;309(3):243–4.

69. Sahakian B, Morein-Zamir S. Professor's little helper. *Nature.* 2007;450:1157–9.

70. Repantis D, Schlattmann P, Laisney O, Heuser I. Modafinil and methylphenidate for neuroenhancement in healthy individuals – A systematic review. *Pharmacol Res.* 2010;62(3):187–206.

71. Greely H, Sahakian B, Harris J, Kessler RC, Gazzaniga M, Campbell P et al. Towards responsible use of cognitive-enhancing drugs by the healthy. *Nature.* 2008;456:702–5.

72. Wise J. Cognitive enhancers are set to change workplaces. *BMJ.* 2012;345:e7538.

73. McBeth BD, McNamara RM, Ankel FK, Mason EJ, Ling LJ, Flottemesch TJ et al. Modafinil and zolpidem use by emergency medicine residents. *Acad Emerg Med.* 2009;16(12):1311–7.

74. Gill M, Haerich P, Westcott K, Godenick KL, Tucker JA. Cognitive performance following modafinil versus placebo in sleep-deprived emergency physicians: A double-blind randomized crossover study. *Acad Emerg Med.* 2006;13(2):158–65.

75. Sugden C, Housden CR, Aggarwal R, Sahakian BJ, Darzi A. Pharmacological enhancement of performance in doctors. *BMJ.* 2010;340:c2542.

76. Haynes AB, Weiser TG, Berry WR, Lipsitz SR, Breizat AS, Dellinger EP et al. A surgical safety checklist to reduce morbidity and mortality in a global population. *N Engl J Med.* 2009;360(5):491–9.

77. Somville F, Van Sprundel M, Somville J. Analysis of surgical errors in malpractice claims in Belgium. *Acta Chir Belg.* 2010;110(1):11–8.

PART III

Implementation and improvement

9

Training methods for non-technical skills

STEVEN YULE, NIKKI MARAN, AKIRA TSUBURAYA AND AJIT K SACHDEVA

9.1 INTRODUCTION

This chapter provides an overview of surgical education and training with respect to non-technical skills, focusing on the needs of both trainees and established surgeons. It is written with surgeons who have particular interests in education and curriculum design in mind.

For individual surgeons to perform effectively as part of a team in the operating room (OR), they must be proficient in the non-technical skills discussed in the earlier chapters. This requires deliberate practice and training in non-technical skills; this has not been commonplace in surgical training across the world to date, which has tended to focus primarily on technical skills and medical knowledge. As non-technical skills training programmes are beginning to be introduced, educators have a number of pertinent questions: what are the most effective training techniques to achieve this? How to develop a curriculum? And perhaps most crucially, how do you demonstrate that training can improve non-technical skills and enhance outcomes for surgical patients?

The purpose of this chapter is to provide guidance on developing training designed to improve the non-technical skills of surgical trainees and practising surgeons. A general framework for training development will be presented, emphasizing that designing effective training in non-technical skills is a systematic and scientific process. This chapter therefore outlines the main stages required to conceptualize, design, implement, reinforce and evaluate non-technical skills training to enhance surgical performance. There are major resources and time limitations in surgical training and continuing education, similar to other high-risk professions; thus, focus on efficiency and effectiveness is paramount.

For decades, surgical training has followed the apprenticeship model. Considered as a form of coaching, a surgeon-teacher taught and assessed an individual trainees' surgical skills. However, there has been criticism that the traditional assessment of surgical skills is commonly associated with competency determination based on inadequate metrics.[1,2] Moreover, the traditional apprenticeship model focuses mainly on technical skills at an individual level without much emphasis on non-technical skills.

This is now changing as a number of regulatory bodies for accreditation and certification in surgery and professional organizations are now emphasizing the need to focus on non-technical skills education during surgical training. These include the Accreditation Council for Graduate Medical Education (ACGME), the American College of Surgeons (ACS) and the Surgical Council on Resident Education (SCORE). The American College of Surgeons/Association of Program Directors in Surgery (ACS/APDS) Surgery Resident Skills Curriculum includes several modules on teamwork, and non-technical skills were recently included in the SCORE Curriculum. In addition, the ACGME includes 'interpersonal and communication skills' and 'professionalism' as two of six core competencies, requiring accredited general surgery residency programmes to cover these domains.[3] This activity is all based on the increasing evidence that team training interventions in non-technical skills help in reducing communication failures[4] and decrease surgical morbidity and mortality.[5,6] A recent systematic review of training in this area found that a number of instructional strategies for non-technical skills had been studied but evidence of effectiveness was moderate at best.[7] The general advice is that training in and assessment of non-technical skills should begin as early as possible in surgical training to reduce the adoption of negative behaviours. In addition, regular refresher training and content focusing on advance skills for practising surgeons should be made available.

9.2 TRAINING DESIGN AND DEVELOPMENT FOR NON-TECHNICAL SKILLS

Developing a training course may seem daunting, but it can be tackled by breaking the task into a number of discrete stages. For the purpose of structuring this chapter, we propose a model of non-technical skills development that defines the stages of delivering a successful course in non-technical skills. This is the model we developed to structure simulation training at the Neil and Elise Wallace STRATUS Center for Medical Simulation at Brigham & Women's Hospital/Harvard Medical School in Boston, Massachusetts. It is typical of the majority of training models in the literature.[8] Figure 9.1 provides an overview of the model, which comprises four stages, as follows:

1. Needs assessment: what is the problem to be addressed? What underpinning concepts will be addressed? What are the needs of learners? What level of proficiency or experience do they already have? What are the specific aims and objectives of the training? What is the learning gap to be addressed?
2. Training development/instructional design: how will the training be designed? What methods and modalities will be used? How long will the training take? Who will teach? What are the qualifications and teaching skills of the faculty?
3. Implementation: what will happen to learners on the days of the course? If taught online or virtually, how will the material be shared with learners? How will faculty ensure that participants learn what they need to? If debriefing is involved, which technique will be used? How will didactic, interactive, discussion and practical sessions build on one another?
4. Evaluation: how will it be demonstrated that the training met the needs of learners? How will effectiveness of the training/transfer to the workplace be shown? How will the training be deemed worthwhile and valuable for time and money invested?

The aim of this chapter is to address these questions and provide either answers or further discussion of topics that will help surgical educators develop curricula.

The need for training in non-technical skills has prompted a number of approaches, some mirroring technical skills training paradigms, others

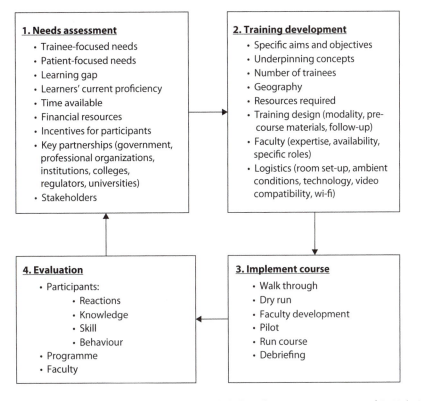

Figure 9.1 Model to develop training for non-technical skills. (Illustration courtesy of S. Yule.)

adapting models from other industries and some built specifically from the ground up. Contextually appropriate training that is developed for a particular organization works best.[9] This is because many well-intentioned training programmes fail not because the content is inappropriate but because it has not been designed specifically for the group of learners to be trained. Training courses may fail to meet the needs of trainees or organizational priorities for other reasons as well. For example, confusing structure, lack of specific measurable aims and objectives and poor faculty development are reasons for failure. Many of these problems stem from an underappreciation of the role of robust evaluation in the process of curriculum development. It may seem unusual to start with a description of the assessment of training before topics such as needs assessment and implementation are described. But all too often, evaluation is treated as an afterthought in non-technical skills training design – something that can be addressed with a short survey of user attitudes or knowledge. However, learner assessment and course evaluation are essential parts of training because they help to demonstrate that the training has met specific pre-defined goals; has been a useful investment of time and money; and, above all, has been effective in changing awareness, knowledge, behaviours or skills of participants. When there is increasing pressure on training time and resources, it is imperative to have data on the effectiveness of the training programme. To do that, it is of course important to know the specific desired outcomes of the training.

9.3 EVALUATION

The aim of evaluation is to provide data that help faculty, sponsoring societies and governing bodies determine the extent to which a training programme achieves its goals. There are two fundamental rules when undertaking evaluation:

1. The evaluation must include assessment of all levels of intended impact. Just as the training course is likely to have impact at different levels (individual, team and organizational), the evaluation must also be focused at different levels.
2. Learning and behaviour change are different. There is a difference between evaluating whether people learned the intended material and content of the course (evaluation of learning) and whether the training made a difference in subsequent performance (evaluation of transfer).[10] Some people argue that the effectiveness of the training programme can also be evaluated independently of these, for example, by studying return on investment, or return on expectation.

These different levels of evaluation mean that different methods and techniques are required.

9.3.1 KIRKPATRICK'S LEVELS OF EVALUATION

Most training evaluation studies can be based on Kirkpatrick's training evaluation framework, which proposes four distinct levels of evaluation: reactions, learning, behaviour and results (Figure 9.2):

1. The first level, reactions, measures trainees' affective responses to the training. These are the most commonly collected evaluation data because the trainees are usually in a captive place at the end of the course and complete an immediate post-course evaluation form, often using pencil and paper or an electronic survey (Table 9.1). Questions at this level tend to focus on the perceptions of the trainees.
2. The second level, learning, focuses on whether the training resulted in an impact on knowledge, skills or attitudes. This is usually measured through faculty assessments, tests, surveys, or self assessments.

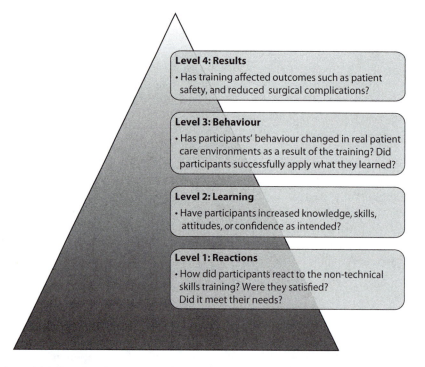

Figure 9.2 Kirkpatrick's four-level training evaluation model, amended for training surgeons' non-technical skills.

3. The third level, behaviour, focuses on whether participants change their behaviour in the workplace as a result of the training. Usually, self-assessment surveys are not suitable to assess this; however, it may be valid to ask co-workers to complete an inventory assessing the behaviour of the trainee post course. Alternatively, third-party observations of teamwork behaviours during routine patient care may be used. It is important to note that studies that assess behaviour during training cannot be classified as behaviour change according to Kirkpatrick's framework. In this sense, level 3 assessment of behaviour change can be likened to assessing the transfer of training, i.e. did the training make a meaningful difference to behaviour in the workplace? Relatively few studies of non-technical skills training gather these types of data, but two studies from a recent review of coaching did collect follow-up data 3–6 months after the intervention period to determine the sustainability of the impact of coaching on surgical performance.[11,12]

Table 9.1 Data collection strategies for the four stages of Kirkpatrick's training evaluation model

Evaluation level	Data collection strategies
Results	Workplace survey
	Adverse event reports
	Assessing change in other outcomes (efficiency, resources and innovation)
Behaviour	Peer observation
	Surgical trainer assessment
	Third-party (independent) assessor
	360° appraisal
Learning	Self-assessments
	Participants' learning portfolio
	Knowledge test
	Skills test
Reactions	Mid-training survey
	Post-training attitude survey
	Discussion forum

4. The final level, results, is concerned with whether the training has affected process or outcomes, such as better quality and patient safety, reduced adverse events, decreased costs or high return on investment. Examples of this include annual patient satisfaction surveys, adverse event rates, length of hospital stay, patients' insurance claims, staff retention and employee satisfaction survey results.

Much has been said about the comparison between Crew Resource Management (CRM) training in aviation and health care. Clearly, the cockpit and OR are different environments, but the principle of evaluating training to assess impact is common to both. As the profession with the most established training in non-technical skills as part of CRM training, aviation is a useful industry to examine with respect to how we may evaluate surgical non-technical skills training. Using Kirkpatrick's (1976) framework for evaluating training, Salas et al.[13] reviewed 58 published accounts of CRM training to determine effectiveness within aviation. They concluded that CRM training generally produced positive reactions, enhanced learning and promoted desired behavioural changes. However, direct evidence for impact on safety records (level 4 impact) was not clear.

9.4 INTEGRATING NON-TECHNICAL SKILLS TRAINING INTO SURGICAL TRAINING

There are several options for integrating non-technical skills into surgical curricula. Currently, there are stand-alone courses for surgeons to develop their skills, and for surgeons to learn how to assess others' non-technical skills. As we will see later in Section 9.5, there have been several efforts to develop simulation and classroom-based courses in non-technical skills aimed mainly at medical students and surgical trainees. These typically complement technical skills training. This is important to emphasize certain skills such as communication, leadership and situation awareness. In time, non-technical skills content may be embedded in technical skills training, negating the need for specific courses, but this is a work in progress.

An important recent advance in this area has been the addition of two modules to the SCORE curriculum in 2014 covering 'social skills' and 'cognitive skills' within the interpersonal and communication skills section.

A recent systematic review highlighted a total of nine empirical investigations of situation awareness training[14]; and a number of studies were found to incorporate non-technical skills training in simulated environments for minimally invasive surgery and open surgery. Other training courses are focused primarily on training non-technical skills alone, albeit within the context of team dynamics in the OR.

9.4.1 TECHNICAL SKILLS TRAINING CURRICULA

Surgical training programmes often offer inanimate and animate labs in which basic technical skills, critical response and team skills and more advanced surgical procedures (open and laparoscopic) are taught. In the United Kingdom, the syllabus and assessment tools are overseen by the Intercollegiate Surgical Curriculum Programme (ISCP) (www.iscp.ac.uk). In the United States, surgical residents follow a national curriculum presented via SCORE and draw on content from the ACS/APDS Surgery Resident Skills Curriculum. The ACS/APDS Surgery Resident Skills Curriculum was jointly developed by the ACS and the Association of Program Directors in Surgery (APDS) and includes three phases. Phase 1 includes 20 modules that address basic surgical skills. Phase 2 includes 15 modules that address advanced skills and procedures, and phase 3 includes 10 modules that address team-based skills (https://www.facs.org/education/program/apds-resident).

Surgeons in training also follow the Fundamentals of Laparoscopic Surgery (FLS) curriculum which was originally developed by the Society of American Gastrointestinal and Endoscopic Surgeons (SAGES) and is now a joint program of SAGES and ACS. As residents progress through training, they also tend to participate in animate laboratories focusing on minimally invasive procedures and participate in more complex procedures, such as laparoscopic Nissen, common bile duct exploration and hernia repair, using hybrid simulation.

9.4.2 NON-TECHNICAL SKILLS TRAINING CURRICULA

Formal training in these skills for trainees is at an early stage and is not comprehensive or universal. However, things are changing. The ACS/APDS modules on team-based skills were released in 2009 and the modules on non-technical skills were added to the SCORE Curriculum in 2014. These two non-technical skills modules on cognitive skills (situation awareness and decision making) and social skills (communication, teamwork and leadership) were developed by Douglas Smink, Alexandra Briggs and Steven Yule at Brigham & Women's Hospital/Harvard Medical School in Boston.

In the United Kingdom, there has been steady progress in the development and rollout of training in non-technical skills, particularly by the Royal College of Surgeons of Edinburgh, since the inception of Non-Technical Skills for Surgeons (NOTSS). The NOTSS masterclass has been run by the Patient Safety Board of the Royal College of Surgeons of Edinburgh for consultant surgeons and senior trainees to teach identifying and assessing non-technical skills. For the needs of the early years of a surgical trainee, e-learning modules introducing the concepts of non-technical skills have also been developed by the Patient Safety Board. This group also developed 'NOTSS in a box', an e-learning package for surgical trainers focusing on assessing surgical trainees. This is available through the college website and also the ISCP to help support a national assessment trial. There is also a non-technical skills module as part of the ChM (Master's in Surgery) offered through the Edinburgh Surgical Sciences Qualification in trauma, orthopaedic surgery, and general surgery. The Royal Australasian College of Surgeons offers NOTSS courses roughly every month, in collaboration with RCSEd, and other groups around the world are formulating this type of training. This continued evolution of non-technical skills featuring in syllabi and curricula points to the value being placed by colleges and other educational bodies on the importance of this skill set as an integral component of intra-operative performance. Expanding the faculty who can teach this subject and developing a strategic approach for embedding training on non-technical skills in the curricula of all surgical specialties in the United Kingdom is the next stage.

The possibility of future assessment of non-technical skills in trainees is under active consideration by the ISCP with some form of formative assessment being a likely product of that review in the near future. Creating benchmarks for non-technical skills for each training level is required to ensure that residents obtain the appropriate level of skill as they progress.

9.5 TRAINING MODALITIES

In this section, we see how technical simulation is now commonplace in surgical training programmes. However, non-technical skills are also starting to be addressed in national training programmes, and this has resulted in the challenge of creating appropriate curricula that allow 'serious games' to be integrated into training of surgeons of the future. Training is not merely for trainees though, and we explore advances in non-technical skills training for practising surgeons and their teams; these often also involve simulation. Finally, the complex issue of training evaluation and transfer of learning is explored.

9.5.1 SIMULATION TRAINING FOR INDIVIDUAL SURGEONS

With the understanding that it is no longer acceptable to achieve clinical proficiency by practising on patients,[15] simulation constitutes one of the fastest growing training approaches to emerge in recent years. Simulated learning environments provide a safe environment to make mistakes, practise technical skills to competence and proficiency and gain initial experiences of complex technical challenges before seeing them in patients. The technology allows training to be learner centred and does not place patients at risk. Reduced working hours and advances in technology have aided this growth, but more importantly the requirement for all surgical residencies in the United States to have access to a simulation centre for training and accreditation of simulation centres by the ACS is shaping the future of surgical training. This sets the tone for the future of training and places simulation-based learning as one of the core modalities for developing the surgical workforce of the future. Figure 9.3 shows an example of a simulated OR used for training in non-technical skills.

These modalities range from ultra-realistic high-fidelity mock ORs with the capability to recreate surgical emergencies for a fully immersive learning experience to simple box trainers to allow surgeons to hone and master the knowledge, judgement and technical skills required of basic laparoscopic surgery. Standardized patients are also employed to prepare and assess residents' interpersonal and communications skills and professionalism.

In a recent systematic review, two studies[14] showed that simulation-based surgical team crisis training has construct validity for assessing situational awareness in surgical trainees in minimally invasive surgery. None of the studies showed effectiveness of surgical crisis training on situational awareness in open surgery, whereas one showed face validity of a 2-day non-technical skills training course. The authors of the systematic review concluded that curriculum development was patchy and evidence of transferability of skills was lacking. This is not surprising at this stage of development in a new domain and will surely improve with time.

There are several studies that show technical skills acquired in the simulated setting improve OR performance.[1] Most of this research has focused on surgical trainees' ability to complete a particular part of procedure. The Fundamentals of Laparoscopic Surgery (FLS) programme is ubiquitous in the United States, having been validated and implemented nationally.[16] Surgical educators are now advancing the field in different and innovative ways, by concentrating on models of delivery to enhance development of psychomotor skill and studying distributed, deliberate and mental practice techniques. These allow learning

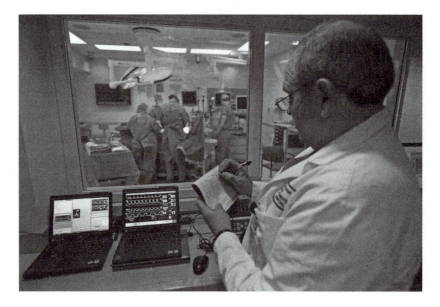

Figure 9.3 Simulation training for surgeons (note the NOTSS observer watching from control room behind the one-way glass).

of surgical skill utilizing adult learning theory and underpinning psychology, leveraging the reduced available time in the OR as a means of prompting technology out of the OR to enhance performance.

Nicolas Dedy and colleagues in Toronto, Canada, published a systematic review on training non-technical skills, providing a thorough overview of the methods of training and evaluation.[17] They reviewed 23 studies, including 4 randomized controlled trials and 19 pre- and post-observation studies. The dominant finding was that behaviour can be improved by training non-technical skills and that simulation (either high-fidelity OR or lower fidelity arenas depending on training goals) is a useful method. In fact, high-fidelity simulation followed by debriefing sessions has been found to be superior to didactic and practice alone at skill acquisition. Video analysis of self or peer performance in simulation is also commonly used to allow participants to reflect on their own skills and identify learning gaps. Evidence of effectiveness of this type of training is variable, but it is stronger for process measures like teamwork than patient safety outcomes. This is understandable as most efforts are on developing training curricula at present rather than developing sophisticated

randomized prospective trials that also take into account clinical outcomes. This represents the future of research efforts in this field.

A potential limitation to scalability is the ability of faculty to teach using this technology and to implement learner-centred skills training in place of the traditional didactic teaching. For some surgeons and other clinical faculty who are used to teaching in a real OR or lecture theatre this represents quite a challenge. Not all are comfortable or have the time or inclination to learn to teach using this modality.

9.5.2 SIMULATION TRAINING FOR SURGICAL TEAMS

Simulation training is not reserved solely for surgical trainees, however. Team training utilizing surgical simulation is increasingly common. One such example is the Harvard OR Team Training with Simulation project.[18] This is a large-scale, multi-institutional simulation training for OR teams sponsored by CRICO, a leading malpractice insurer. The programme, a collaborative of the Harvard-affiliated teaching hospitals, brings complete, mature OR teams – an attending surgeon, an attending anesthesiologist, nurses, technicians and residents – together for a full day of simulation training focusing on OR emergencies. Full-scale realistic simulation scenarios were created and executed in sophisticated high-fidelity simulation centres or, at one site (Boston Children's Hospital), in an *in situ* embedded training session in a real OR. Training sessions were coupled to post-simulation debriefing to reinforce the experiential learning.

The pilot study was conducted over an 18-month period and provided one day of training to 221 active OR staff members (58 attending surgeons, 38 attending anesthesiologists and 69 nurses and surgical technologists).[19] The programme aims to train 600 teams over 3 years to 2016. The real cost of this programme, including facility and direct costs of supplies and simulation equipment including faculty development and teaching time, runs into millions of dollars. There is abundant evidence to suggest that this investment will provide a very worthwhile return based on experiences in other medical specialties, including anesthesiology and obstetrics where simulation team training has led to measurable declines in malpractice claims and adverse patient outcomes.

This programme is leading the vanguard of simulation training for surgical teams and highlights the move to an advanced phase of training, with focus on inter-professional team training in simulated clinical environments. This new era of simulation combining individual and team-level training allows complete teams to practise their non-technical skills, including how to best communicate, share information, arrive at a differential diagnosis, co-ordinate activities and lead an OR team through a crisis or an acute episode of care. Some of this training is in professional silos, for example, surgeons receiving feedback on their communication and teamwork skills on an individual basis,[20] and other training focuses on multidisciplinary teams such as simulation-based team training for OR teams.[19] Other research utilizing simulation focuses on training very specific skills to enhance performance in a team context, such as use of OR crisis checklists.[21] Not all team training requires simulation to be effective,[6,22] but simulated learning environments allow standardization and reproducibility that ensure participants receive the same training experience.

Methods of instruction that appear to work in these environments can be rolled out on a larger scale and taught by different faculty with the same end result.

Finally, emerging work examines simulation in an integrated patient care pathway[23] or multiple team events (e.g. *code teams*, comprising surgery, emergency physician, anesthesiologists and nurses, or *transcatheter aortic valve replacement teams*, comprising cardiology and surgery teams). These take into account the interactions with the wider hospital organization that impact co-ordination of care, and ultimately the safety and quality of patient care. The drive for non-technical skills training and interventions to improve team performance is not restricted to surgery, however. There is also growing transfer of these methods to train teams on hospital wards, in trauma bays, in post-acute care, in intensive care units and in the emergency department. The challenge is to demonstrate that such team simulations reduce the likelihood of errors and improve patient outcomes.

9.5.3 CLASSROOM TEACHING

Certain types of training to improve skill do not require a high-fidelity simulated OR. For example, learning vocabulary of non-technical skills and practising language for closed-loop communication or speaking up can be taught in classroom settings. Finally, part task trainers, virtual reality, bench models and laparoscopic surgical simulators are usually limited to teaching technical or procedural skills, but they can also be used to teach decision making and other cognitive skills.

For teaching knowledge, the curriculum developed in the United States is based around a book chapter with vignettes of surgical scenarios and test questions that have been available online. The SCORE national curriculum is focused on underpinning knowledge of the four NOTSS categories and background reading, which students read before a 'flipped classroom'-style group discussion with faculty. A faculty teaching guide with learning and discussion points was developed to help facilitate this.

Other methods of training underpinning non-technical skills in classroom settings focus on small group discussions of videos. These are often surgical scenarios filmed to show specific behaviours and prompt discussion about non-technical skills in surgery. Videos of team performance and non-technical skills in other industries may also be used, highlighting the role of non-technical skill failure in aviation and other industrial accidents. Finally, it is important to mention that there is a distinction between teaching underpinning knowledge and ability to recognize/assess non-technical skills and teaching to improve the skills.

9.5.4 COACHING

To develop non-technical skills, coaching – often using simulation-based training – has been shown to be useful in other performance-based industries.[24] Regular coaching on non-technical skills based on observation of performance in simulation is one way to maintain focus on enhancing team performance and professional behaviours (Figure 9.4). Repeated coaching is done routinely in the military in what are termed 'after-action reviews'[25] and found to enhance team performance, efficiency, communication and cohesion during training sessions. Recently, after-action reviews specifically for debriefing medical scenarios have been designed,[26] so applying these systematically in surgical training is the next logical step.

Apart from teaching trainees, there is a current lack of coaching for practising surgeons and thus potential benefit in assessing performance improvement.[27,28] A study by Hu et al.[29] showed that video-based coaching was valuable for surgeons at all stages of their career. Coaching as a method of enhancing performance is not a new phenomenon and is in fact commonly encountered in many other professional fields, such as sports, music, education and business.[28,30]

Regardless of the level of expertise of the person being coached, coaching in surgery is necessary because surgeons require deliberate practice to master tasks.[31] A critical component of achieving this mastery is constructive feedback provided by an expert coach to mediate self-directed development.[32] Coaches may behave differently depending on whom they are coaching. For example, a coach may act more as a partner and a collaborator for practising surgeons and more as a teacher and an instructor for the trainees. Tailoring the style of coaching would allow trainees a smoother transition into independent practice and practising surgeons to reach and/or maintain expertise.[27]

As professional surgical societies begin to recognize the need for surgical coaching at all levels, we will need to expand beyond the traditional apprenticeship paradigm to fit today's surgical

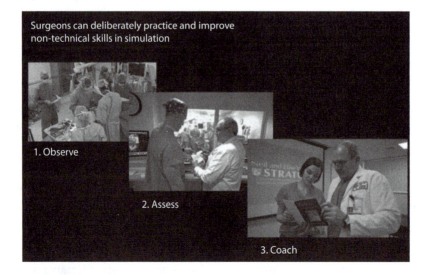

Figure 9.4 Process of coaching non-technical skills.

culture and needs. In a recent systematic review,[33] eight studies were found that focused on evaluating the impact of coaching on non-technical skills improvement.[11,12,22,34–38] All studies were team-level interventions, and 50% of these studies took place in a simulation setting.[12,35,37,39] The other half took place in ORs during real operations.[11,22,34,36] Although several studies employed non-surgeons as coaches,[11,12,22,35,36] the preference was to combine a surgeon and a social scientist to provide the full range of coaching and support.

Five of the eight studies on coaching non-technical skills demonstrated that the coaching interventions were successful as they were associated with higher NOTECHS scores and surgical situation awareness,[36] improved debriefing quality within the team,[34] improved non-technical skills and performance under stress[37] and significant improvement of team performance measured by the Trauma Team Performance Observation Tool.[35] On the other hand, three other studies showed inconclusive results.[12,22,39] Catchpole et al. attempted to measure the effect of aviation-style team training on three different surgical subspecialties focusing on non-technical skills and found that one site demonstrated an improvement after the coaching intervention, whereas the other two sites showed either no change or a worsening effect. Nurok et al. showed a significant improvement of communication and team skills immediately after coaching, but skills had returned to baseline when reassessed three months later.

The reviewed studies were appraised to have low strength of evidence according to GRADE criteria because of the risk of bias, given the lack of control groups, non-blinded observers and common methodological constraints of field research. However, scores on medical education assessment criteria (MERSQI) were more favourable, in part attributable to the use of various validated assessment tools such as the Oxford NOTECHS scoring system and the 360° evaluation of five non-technical criteria. For the evaluation of non-technical skills, it seems that non-surgeons are effective coaches who can be utilized as either an alternative to or in addition to a surgeon coach.

The long-term impact of coaching has yet to be studied in detail, and data on sustainable behaviour changes after coaching interventions are not commonly collected or reported. Most studies do not assess long-term retention of surgeons who are coached, and the one study that did showed no significant difference in non-technical skills 3 months after intervention.[12] It is also unclear whether assessing for behavioural intention instead of the actual change is particularly helpful in assessing coaching interventions.[39] Longitudinal follow-up studies of clinicians' behaviour are incredibly difficult to orchestrate in real-world settings. Current focus is on developing capacity and infrastructure to give more surgeons access to coaching.[40] As the importance of coaching in surgical performance continues to gain credibility, the prospect of larger scale longitudinal work with sufficient power to demonstrate impact on future behaviour and outcomes becomes possible.

9.6 PRACTICAL MATTERS AND FUTURE POSSIBILITIES

Assessment and teaching of non-technical skills will develop dramatically over the next 5 years, and this will become a vital area of concentration as health care moves forward. There is likely to be desire from trainees for more feedback and strategies for improvement, need from surgical trainers for more guidance and tools to help them support trainees' development and demand from practising surgeons in academic medical centres and private practice alike to improve and maintain their skills in this area.

To achieve this, training and assessment tools are required that are easy to use for faculty and trainers that help them teach and evaluate trainees in an objective manner and give specific feedback on strategies to improve skills. E-learning will grow in importance as will cloud and smart technology as methods of scaling implementation and providing access to those in rural locations and surgeons who do not work in university hospitals or academic medical centres. It is difficult to assess people without training packages for assessors and learners, so new content in advanced non-technical skills will need to be developed. Non-technical skills have so far been focused on developing professional skills, and it seems important that the focus remains on lifelong learning rather than remediation.

If your intention is to develop and implement a non-technical skills training course, then the following are some of the main questions you need to ask yourself as you plan:

1. What is the learning gap to be addressed, and what evidence makes this a training priority?
2. What are your aims and specific goals of the training programme?
3. Specifically, what change do you intend to achieve (attitude, knowledge, skill or behaviour)?
4. How will you measure the impact of the training course?
5. How will you know if your training programme has been successful in meeting the aims and goals?
6. What is the best training modality to achieve those goals (real OR, simulation, classroom, e-learning …)?
7. How are you designing the training to take into account the current level of the participants (e.g. junior trainee, senior trainee or consultant) and their current experience in non-technical skills?
8. Do you plan to train individual surgeons, or surgical teams?
9. Is it possible to integrate with existing technical/procedural training?
10. How will you recruit and train faculty to teach your course?

Of course, there are some important research questions around scalability of training, demonstrating impact on performance and outcomes in the OR, and longitudinal studies of learning curves in non-technical skills to be conducted if this is to be supported in the most efficient and effective manner. This will also require research funding and continued partnership between colleges, surgeons and research groups. Effective leadership, situation awareness, decision making, communication and teamwork will save many lives, lead to less morbidity, improve quality and result in lowering the cost of surgery. Patients will demand it, and the surgical community now has the ability to make it happen.

REFERENCES

1. Sachdeva AK. Acquiring skills in new procedures and technology: The challenge and the opportunity. *Arch Surg.* 2005 Apr;140(4):387–9.
2. Bass BL, Polk HC, Jones RS, Townsend CM, Whittemore AD, Pellegrini CA et al. Surgical privileging and credentialing: A report of a discussion and study group of the American Surgical Association. *J Am Coll Surg.* 2009 Sep;209(3):396–404.
3. American College of Surgeons DoE. ACS/APDS surgical skills curriculum for residents, phase 3: Team-based skills. [Accessed May 15, 2014.] Available from: http://www.facs.org/education/surgical-skills.html.
4. Halverson AL, Casey JT, Andersson J, Anderson K, Park C, Rademaker AW et al. Communication failure in the operating room. *Surgery.* 2011 Mar;149(3):305–10.
5. Young-Xu Y, Neily J, Mills PD, Carney BT, West P, Berger DH et al. Association between implementation of a medical team training program and surgical morbidity. *Arch Surg.* 2011 Dec;146(12):1368–73.
6. Neily J, Mills PD, Young-Xu Y, Carney BT, West P, Berger DH et al. Association between implementation of a medical team training program and surgical mortality. *JAMA.* 2010 Oct 20;304(15):1693–700.
7. Dedy NJ, Bonrath EM, Zevin B, Grantcharov TP. Teaching nontechnical skills in surgical residency: A systematic review of current approaches and outcomes. *Surgery.* 2013;154:1000–8.
8. Goldstein I, Ford J. *Training in Organizations: Needs Assessment, Development, and Evaluation* (4th ed). Belmont, California: Wadsworth; 2002.
9. Kanki B, Helmreich R, Anca J (Eds.). *Crew Resource Management* (2nd ed). San Diego, California: Academic Press; 2010.
10. Alvarez K, Salas E, Garofano C. An integrated model of training evaluation and effectiveness. *Hum Resource Dev Rev.* 2004;3:385–416.

11. Halverson AL, Andersson JL, Anderson K, Lombardo J, Park CS, Rademaker AW et al. Surgical team training: The Northwestern Memorial Hospital experience. *Arch Surg.* 2009 Feb;144(2):107–12.

12. Nurok M, Lipsitz S, Satwicz P, Kelly A, Frankel A. A novel method for reproducibly measuring the effects of interventions to improve emotional climate, indices of team skills and communication, and threat to patient outcome in a high-volume thoracic surgery center. *Arch Surg.* 2010 May;145(5):489–95.

13. Salas E, Burke C, Bowers C, Wilson K. Team training in the skies: Does Crew Resource Management (CRM) training work? *Hum Factors.* 2001;43:641–74.

14. Graffland M, Schraagen J, Boermeester M, Bemelman W, Schijven M. Training situational awareness to reduce surgical errors in the operating room. *Br J Surg.* 2015;102(1):16–23.

15. Gallagher A, Seymour N, Jordan-Black J, Bunting B, McGlade K, Satava R. Prospective, randomized assessment of transfer of training (ToT) and transfer effectiveness ratio (TER) of virtual reality simulation training for laparoscopic skill acquisition. *Ann Surg.* 2013;257:1025–31.

16. Society of American Gastrointestinal and Endoscopic Surgeons (SAGES). Fundamentals of laparoscopic surgery. 2015. [Accessed April 23, 2015.] Available from: http://www.flsprogram.org.

17. Dedy N, Bonrath E, Zevin B, Grantcharov T. Teaching nontechnical skills in surgical residency: A systematic review of current approaches and outcomes. *Surgery.* 2013;154:1000–8.

18. Bass B. Preparing for the worst: A promising step in the right direction. *Ann Surg.* 2014;259(3):411–2.

19. Arriaga A, Gawande A, Raemer D, Jones D, Smink D, Weinstock P et al. Pilot testing of a model for insurer-driven, large-scale multicenter simulation training for operating room teams. *Ann Surg.* 2014;259(9):403–10.

20. Kissane-Lee N, Fiedler A, Mazer L, Pozner C, Smink D, Yule S (Eds.). *Coaching Surgical Residents on Leadership in a Simulated Operating Room: Randomized Controlled Trial.* Chicago, IL: Amercian College of Surgeons Clinical Congress; 2013.

21. Arriaga AF, Bader AM, Wong JM, Lipsitz SR, Berry WR, Ziewacz JE et al. Simulation-based trial of surgical-crisis checklists. *N Engl J Med.* 2013 Jan 17;368(3):246–53.

22. Catchpole KR, Dale TJ, Hirst DG, Smith JP, Giddings TA. A multicenter trial of aviation-style training for surgical teams. *J Patient Saf.* 2010 Sep;6(3):180–6.

23. Arora S, Cox C, Davies S, Kassab E, Mahoney P, Sharma E et al. Towards the next frontier for simulation-based training. Full-hospital simulation across the entire patient pathway. *Ann Surg.* 2014;260:252–8.

24. Hackman JR, Wageman RA. A theory of team coaching. *Acad Manage Rev.* 2005;30:269–87.

25. Villado A, Arthur WJ. The comparative effect of subjective and objective after-action reviews on team performance in a complex task. *J Appl Psychol.* 2013;98(3):514–28.

26. Sawyer T, Deering S. Adaptation of the US Army's After-Action Review for simulation debriefing in healthcare. *Simul Healthc.* 2013;8(6):388–97.

27. Greenberg C. Surgical coaching: An idea whose idea has come. *ACS Surgery News.* 2012. [Accessed May 17, 2014.] Available from: http://www.acssurgerynews.com/opinions/editorials/single-article/surgical-coaching-an-idea-whose-time-has-come/b2e6e8e538fd87e5414c4ff9cb4f74a5.html.

28. Gawande A. 'Personal best: Top athletes and singers have coaches. Should you?' *The New Yorker.* October 3, 2011.

29. Hu YY, Peyre SE, Arriaga AF, Osteen RT, Corso KA, Weiser TG et al. Postgame analysis: Using video-based coaching for continuous professional development. *J Am Coll Surg.* 2012 Jan;214(1):115–24.

30. RN Bush. Effective staff development in making our schools more effective. *Proceedings of Three State Conferences.* San Francisco, California: Far West Laboratories; 1984.

31. Reznick RK, MacRae H. Teaching surgical skills – changes in the wind. *N Engl J Med.* 2006 Dec 21;355(25):2664–9.

32. Ericsson KA. Deliberate practice and acquisition of expert performance: A general overview. *Acad Emerg Med.* 2008 Nov;15(11):988–94.

33. Min H, Rivera Morales D, Orgill D, Smink S, Yule S. Systematic review of coaching to enhance surgeons' operative performance. *Surgery.* 2015 (in press).

34. Ahmed M, Arora S, Russ S, Darzi A, Vincent C, Sevdalis N. Operation debrief: A SHARP improvement in performance feedback in the operating room. *Ann Surg.* 2013 Dec;258(6):958–63.

35. Capella J, Smith S, Philp A, Putnam T, Gilbert C, Fry W et al. Teamwork training improves the clinical care of trauma patients. *J Surg Educ.* 2010 Nov–Dec;67(6):439–43.

36. McCulloch P, Mishra A, Handa A, Dale T, Hirst G, Catchpole K. The effects of aviation-style non-technical skills training on technical performance and outcome in the operating theatre. *Qual Saf Health Care.* 2009 Apr;18(2):109–15.

37. Mueller G, Hunt B, Wall V, Rush R, Jr., Molof A, Schoeff J et al. Intensive skills week for military medical students increases technical proficiency, confidence, and skills to minimize negative stress. *J Spec Oper Med.* 2012 (Winter);12(4):45–53.

38. Reed DA, Cook DA, Beckman TJ, Levine RB, Kern DE, Wright SM. Association between funding and quality of published medical education research. *JAMA.* 2007 Sep 5;298(9):1002–9.

39. Peckler B, Prewett MS, Campbell T, Brannick M. Teamwork in the trauma room evaluation of a multimodal team training program. *J Emerg Trauma Shock.* 2012 Jan;5(1):23–7.

40. Greenberg C, Ghousseini H, Pavuluri Quamme S, Beasley H, Wiegmann D. Surgical coaching for individual performance improvement. *Ann Surg.* 2015 Jan;261(1):32–4.

10

Assessing non-technical skills in the operating room

SIMON PATERSON-BROWN, STEPHEN TOBIN AND STEVEN YULE

10.1 INTRODUCTION

The assessment of clinical skills is ingrained in all areas of medical practice, irrespective of the sub-specialty, from medical students through specialist training and culminating in a summative assessment before obtaining a completion certificate to practise independently. Each medical specialty has developed their own methods of assessment, but all share the aim of using techniques that are fair, reproducible and reliable. They must of course be reliable between assessors, specific and have construct validity – in other words, test what they are supposed to test. In this chapter, we will review the criteria for assessment tools in surgery, focus on how to assess non-technical skills with behaviour marker tools, consider how behaviour assessment fits with current models of assessment in surgery and then attempt to give advice on possible courses of action when ratings are less than acceptable in the form of remediation and retraining.

10.2 EMERGENCE OF NON-TECHNICAL SKILLS ASSESSMENT

In surgery, it is not enough just to test clinical skills and knowledge; technical skills must also be examined, and this has resulted in the Objective Structured Assessment of Technical Skill (OSATS), which was developed and presented by Professor Richard Reznick and his team in Toronto, Canada.[1] However, as this book outlines in great depth, the surgical community is now well aware that surgical proficiency and good outcomes cannot be guaranteed without accompanying non-technical skills. However, this has posed several problems: first they are often present, but tacit, and neither the trainer nor the trainee may be aware of exactly what they are. Second, this makes observation, teaching and assessment of them nearly impossible. The first attempt to identify these skills came from Edinburgh, Scotland, in 1999, when the late Dr Pamela Baldwin, a clinical psychologist, carried out an anonymous postal survey of 68 consultant surgeons from all specialties in the southeast of Scotland and identified 70 separate skills that were considered important in a successful surgical trainee.[2] Of these, only 19 (27%) were technical and 22 (31%) clinical, with 29 (41%) related to communication, teamwork and application of knowledge. Shortly after this, Professor Sir Alfred Cuschieri from Dundee, Scotland, and a group of experienced senior surgeons from around the world carried out a study to identify what skills should be looked for when selecting and assessing surgical trainees.[3] They came to a similar conclusion and recommended that assessment during training should be based on clinical judgement, operative skills and cognitive ability, with standardized checklists (such as OSATS) being used to assess technical ability. These studies certainly assisted in identifying what factors were important in making one surgeon better than another when their technical skills were similar.

Following on from the initial southeast of Scotland study, a surgical assessment form was developed to assess basic surgical trainees in the 70 tasks previously identified.[4] This form scored trainees according to their performance in five key areas:

1. Patients and relatives
2. Application of knowledge
3. Teamwork
4. Clinical skills
5. Technical skills

Each trainee was assessed by someone from each of the following groups: consultant surgeons, specialist registrars, surgical secretaries, ward nurses, theatre nurses and outpatient clinic nurses. The form was shown to be feasible, reliable and valid. Furthermore, when trainees were asked their opinions of the skills required for surgeons they were in agreement with all these skills already identified.[5]

However, it was not until the Non-Technical Skills for Surgeons (NOTSS) project was completed[6] (see also Chapter 3) that the cognitive and social skills that underpin good surgical performance were really understood and described. The production of the taxonomy and associated rating system then allowed these non-technical skills to be identified and rated. The NOTSS system was produced 'by surgeons for surgeons' and was assessed by 44 consultant surgeons and 26 trainees using filmed scenarios of simulated operations that demonstrated good and bad behaviours. The group first underwent a short training workshop to understand the taxonomy. The NOTSS taxonomy and rating system was shown to be reliable,[7] although more so for the social skills (communication and teamwork and leadership) than the cognitive skills (situation awareness and decision making). Further work using the NOTSS taxonomy to assess trainees during a 6-month period of training demonstrated that there was good construct validity, in that the taxonomy assessed what it was supposed to assess.[8] The next step was to examine both technical and non-technical skills performances at the same time, as they should both complement and support each other. This was carried out by a group in Sheffield, UK, led by Professor Jonathan Beard, who demonstrated that using OSATS for the assessment of technical performance[1] and a workplace-based assessment using the NOTSS taxonomy provided a reliable and generalizable assessment of trainees' operative performances.[9] This has now been incorporated into the UK surgical assessment process for the Intercollegiate Surgical Curriculum Project (ISCP) and is described in more detail later. In 2014, in the United States the Surgical Council on Resident Education also incorporated modules on non-technical skills based on the categories in NOTSS,[10] but the American Board of Surgery has not yet incorporated non-technical skills into their final assessment. In fact, they only started mandating operative performance assessments for trainees completing residency in the 2012–2013 academic year.

10.3 PRINCIPLES OF ASSESSMENT

There are two distinct forms of assessment: formative and summative. Formative assessment provides an opportunity for the assessor to give narrative feedback to the trainee. 'Formative assessment is seen as taking place when teachers and learners seek to respond to student work, making judgements about what is good learning'.[11] The nature of formative study enables the collection of outcomes before and throughout assessment. This, in turn, allows students to adjust learning strategies and promotes self-directed learning. Summative assessment requires the trainee to reach a specific goal, and the various examinations represent summative assessment at different stages of the training programme. Both assessments, however, must be objective and be shown to be fair, reliable and valid. In other words, that they assess the skills they are supposed to be assessing over time and as part of the assessments, subjectivity on the part of the assessor should be minimized. More recently, it has become easier to assess some of the required surgical skills by the introduction of simulated technologies. In addition to being valid and reliable, assessment tools themselves should be able to differentiate between levels of performance; identify poor performers for remediation training; and, above all, be used to enhance the safety and quality of surgery for patients. There are several forms of validity and reliability that are of interest when selecting an assessment system (Table 10.1). The behavioural assessment tools used in surgery have been evaluated against many of these criteria during development and refinement as part of psychometric testing. The concepts of validity and reliability will also be of particular interest to practitioners who are selecting a behavioural marker system for implementation.

Table 10.1 Reliability and validity criteria of assessment tools

Reliability/ validity test	Definition	Application to surgical behavioural assessment tools
Inter-rater reliability	Relationship between two or more raters' assessments for the same behaviour category or element over multiple rating occasions.	The degree to which a group of raters agree on ratings of the surgeons depicted in micro-scenarios, measured by intra-class correlations and within-group agreement (r_{WG}).
Inter-rater agreement	Degree to which raters agree on absolute assessments or are consistent in their pattern of assessment.	Two raters assess a surgical resident in a simulation study. If both assess leadership as 3 out of 4, there is perfect agreement among raters. If they provide different assessments (e.g. 1 and 3), then the degree of absolute agreement can be calculated. Here, we are concerned about the size of the difference between raters. Bland Altman plots can be used to capture this.

(Continued)

Table 10.1 (*Continued*) Reliability and validity criteria of assessment tools

Reliability/ validity test	Definition	Application to surgical behavioural assessment tools
Factor analysis/ internal structure	Robustness and stability of multi-factorial assessment tools is measured by describing variability among observed variables and how they are grouped into factors.	For example, in NOTSS, the situation awareness factor can be measured by three variables (elements): gathering, understanding and predicting. Exploratory factor analysis can be used to identify latent factors and how individual assessment items correlate as factors. Confirmatory factor analysis can be used to test an existing factor structure with a new data set to see how robust the structure is.
Internal consistency	Measures whether several items that propose to measure the same general construct produce similar scores.	Usually used for surveys to test the reliability of individual items that make up factors (e.g. using Cronbach's alpha).
Test–retest reliability	Stability of assessment by individual raters over time.	The same residents are assessed during the same surgical operation 2 months apart. Ideally, if all things are equal there should be no significant difference between assessments. This would indicate that the assessment tool acts in the same way in different assessment opportunities. Reliability in this sense is not about differences in level but about stability over time, based on a correlation model.
Spilt-half reliability	When it is not possible to repeat the test as in test–retest, this performs a similar function with cross-sectional data. The test is split into two parts and an individual's scores on both halves are compared.	About 20 trainees are assessed using the 12 elements of NOTSS. For each resident, the total score is recorded along with the sum of the scores for the even-numbered elements and the odd-numbered elements. A correlation coefficient between even- and odd-numbered questions is calculated. As this tends to 1, the test is more reliable.
Generalizability	Generalizability theory is not easy to summarize briefly, but it estimates the proportion of ratings that vary systematically and the proportion of ratings that are due to measurement error. It is important to determine what factors might impact performance, measure them and add to the analysis.	Crossley et al.[9] identified the degree of measurement error in NOTSS assessments and concluded that six assessments need to be conducted per trainee to establish a generalizable picture of their non-technical skills.
Face validity	Extent to which the whole test is subjectively viewed as covering the concept it purports to measure. It refers to the transparency or relevance of a test.	When reviewing an assessment tool, ask yourself the following questions from the points of view of the assessor and the assessed: does it look like an assessment tool of non-technical skills? Does it make sense? How easily could I use this tool?

Table 10.1 (*Continued*) Reliability and validity criteria of assessment tools

Reliability/ validity test	Definition	Application to surgical behavioural assessment tools
Content validity	Content validity examines whether the measure reflects the construct in both content and scope. It is the extent to which items of a measurement instrument are important and relevant to performance.	This is tested by user evaluation or expert panel. They would decide if the behaviour assessment tool is complete, determine if any major skills thought to be important to non-technical skills are not present and ensure that there is sufficient conceptual breadth.
Observability	Extent to which behaviours can actually be observed in the OR or simulation sufficiently to be rated.	This applies to all behaviour rating tools: the social skills such as communication, teamwork and leadership are generally observable. However, to what extent is it possible to actually observe the cognitive skills of decision making and situation awareness? Tools need to have behaviours that are observable to make an inference of those cognitive skills.
Convergent/ concurrent validity	Degree to which an assessment tool is correlated with other assessment tools that measure the same underpinning construct.	For example, leadership is a category in NOTSS and NOTECHS. Gather data using these two tools together when observing the same participants, and determine the degree of correlation between assessments. It should be high for there to be good concurrent validity. This test is ideally used when comparing scores on a newly developed tool with those from an already established validated one.
Criterion-related validity	Degree to which behaviour assessments predict an external performance criterion.	How well do NOTSS scores assessed at time 1 predict patient outcomes assessed at time 2?
Sensitivity and specificity	Extent to which participants can detect non-technical skills and discriminate between good and poor performances.	A perfect predictor would be described as 100% sensitive (e.g. all poor performers fail a NOTSS assessment) and 100% specific (e.g. all competent trainee surgeons pass a NOTSS assessment). There is usually a trade-off between sensitivity and specificity. For instance, when using a non-technical skills assessment for pilots, airlines may set a high threshold, which triggers detection of low-consequence behaviours that are unlikely to cause adverse events (low specificity), to reduce the risk of passing candidates who have potential to engage in occasional risky behaviours such as poor delegation under pressure, which may pose a threat to aircraft safety (high sensitivity).

10.4 BEHAVIOURAL MARKER SYSTEMS

10.4.1 WHAT ARE BEHAVIOURAL MARKER SYSTEMS AND WHY ASSESS NON-TECHNICAL SKILLS?

Non-technical skills are at the centre of surgical performance. It is not sufficient simply to be technically excellent if your goal is to ensure high-quality and safe procedures for patients. Analyses of surgical adverse events often cite failures of awareness, communication and teamwork in the operating room (OR), so it is important to focus on these and how surgeons can be supported to improve these skills if required. The benefits of having a team with members who are better able to share information, lead and delegate tasks, be on the same page as others, detect errors early (or even before they occur) and speak up about them are undeniable. The best way of assessing these skills is by using behavioural assessment (marker) tools using observation methods to assess behavioural competencies and teamwork. The premise is that a third-party observer who is not involved in the operation uses a validated framework to assess the behaviour of individuals or teams for a defined period of time (e.g. one case or the operative list). The observer is trained to assess specific behaviours, be they overt as in the case of social skills (leadership, teamwork and communication)

or more implied and implicit as in the case of cognitive skills (situation awareness, situation assessment and decision making). Observers are trained to use a specific framework, and the aim is to enhance objectivity of judgements regarding effectiveness and appropriateness of team skill. Behavioural assessment (marker) tools tend to comprise three components:

1. A skills taxonomy
2. Behavioural indicators of levels of performance for each skill
3. A rating scale

Table 10.2 demonstrates an example of a behavioural marker system from the Royal Australasian College of Surgeons (RACS),[12] with levels from the newly graduated doctor to the experienced surgeon.

Behavioural marker systems allow assessors to identify, categorize and assess behaviours that contribute to superior or substandard performance. As discussed in Chapter 2, in non-health care industries there have been many investigations highlighting the central role of non-technical skills in performance failures,[13] which have given rise to behavioural rating tools like NOTECHS for use in aviation[14] and systems developed for professionals working in the energy sector and transportation. In health care, the rise of behavioural marker systems has tracked a similar trajectory. They were developed in response to observational research and closed claims analysis that highlighted the role of non-technical skills and

Table 10.2 An example of a behavioural marker system from RACS

Communication level	Illustrative behaviours
Pre-vocational	Provides accurate and concise information when communicating with patients, their relatives and the team
Novice	Ensures patients are fully informed, and that they fully understand, prior to giving consent
Intermediate	Recognizes and adapts communication to potential bad news situations
Competent	Appropriately identifies and addresses unspoken concerns.
Proficient	Informs patient, family and relevant staff about the expected clinical course for each patient

Source: Royal Australasian College of Surgeons (RACS), Becoming a competent and proficient surgeon: Training standards for the nine RACS competencies, 2012, Accessed September 2014, Available from: http://www.surgeons.org/media/18726523/mnl_2012-02-24_training_standards_final_1.pdf.

behaviour of operative performance and patient safety. The first behavioural assessment tools were developed in anaesthesia,[15] and the Anaesthetists' Non-Technical Skills system has been used widely to support training and assessment in that field, giving rise to other behavioural rating systems for anaesthetic assistants[16] and blazing the trail for the development of assessment tools for scrub practitioners[17,18] and surgeons.[6]

Development of these tools has continued in parallel with many observational studies that have identified the individual, team and organizational factors that appear to underpin safe performance in the OR.[19-27] The results of these studies have been used to drive development and adoption of behavioural rating tools in surgery,[28-35] with the explicit goal of developing training and assessment techniques to translate the findings of primary research into methods to improve performance and safety in the OR.

These skills can now be assessed, and there is a range of validated assessment tools for surgeons that have all emerged in the past 10 years or so. The dominant tools are NOTSS, Objective Teamwork Assessment in Surgery (OTAS) and surgical versions of NOTECHS (non-technical skills), as described in Table 10.3.

These tools all differ on how they were developed, for whom they were developed, the level of analysis used and for what purpose they were developed. However, all are marker systems and rely on being context specific and must be developed for the situation in which they are to be used. For example, the NOTECHS system was originally developed and evaluated with pilots from civil aviation,[14] but then it was applied to the OR where it showed good levels of reliability.[32,34] This tool has been critiqued for not being developed specifically for surgeons or surgical teams but rather by taking the general principles of non-technical skills from the cockpit and applying them in the OR. The OTAS system took a different approach and is a behaviour rating system developed from a theoretical model of teamwork.[31] By applying teamwork theory to the OR, this gives the system grounding in what should happen from a conceptual standpoint. Systems have also been developed for neurosurgery.[36] In the past couple of years, a host of behavioural marker systems have also been developed to assess behaviours of individuals or teams in health care but outside the OR, including the post-operative phase of surgery,[37] trauma,[35] resuscitation,[38] critical care[39] and in the emergency department.[40] A forthcoming project is extending this work to emergency surgical wards.

Table 10.3 Major behavioural marker (assessment) tools to assess surgeons in the OR

Behavioural marker tool	Scope and applications
NOTSS	Developed using cognitive task analysis with panels of SMEs (surgeons). To observe and assess individual surgeons in simulation or real OR. Forms basis for training workshops and national curricula in surgical training.
	NOTSS (Europe, Australia and North America)[6,28]
	NOTSS dk (Denmark)[29]
	jNOTSS (Japan)
	NOTSS-RW (limited-resource settings)
OTAS	A teamwork assessment tool for three OR sub-teams.
	Based on theoretical model of teamwork[30]
	OTAS (England)[31]
NOTECHS	A teamwork assessment tool based on the NOTECHS system developed in aviation and used to assess individual pilots.
	Oxford NOTECHS[32]
	Oxford NOTECHS II[33]
	Revised NOTECHS[34]
	T-NOTECHS[35]

OR, operating room; SMEs, subject matter experts; OTAS, Objective Teamwork Assessment in Surgery.

10.4.2 HOW TO USE BEHAVIOUR ASSESSMENT TOOLS AND THE ACCURACY OF ASSESSMENTS

Behavioural markers are a prescribed set of behaviours indicative of some aspect of performance. If designed properly, they are developed with the end user in mind according to a set of design criteria to allow observers to identify, categorize and rate the quality of observed behaviours that are thought to illustrate those competencies. For example criteria, see Chapter 3 in this book and Klampfer et al.[41] for more detail. The end point is that these observations allow the assessor to make a valued judgement regarding the competence of the individual. The focus of these is for formative assessment, but the same model could be applied to summative assessment. Usability of behaviour assessment tools is also important for widespread adoption, and this was tested during the development of the NOTSS system in a usability trial in the OR[42] (see Chapter 3 for a complete description of usability testing).

The best way of assessing these skills is direct observation by a trained observer during a real or simulated operative case using a validated assessment tool, either in simulation or the real OR. For example, using NOTSS to observe specific behaviours in the OR, categorizing them according to the four categories and then rating how well the surgeon performed in each category can be very insightful. We finally have tools and vocabulary to focus on the full range of behaviours in the OR that make for high-performing teams and successful surgery. Furthermore, we can now measure and improve these skills in surgeons and trainees using tools like NOTSS. Assessments are becoming more and more objective as these skills taxonomies are refined and used more regularly.

However, there are a range of options available and questions still to be answered, such as how many observers are required? Should they be surgeons or social scientists? How much training do raters require? Which tool should be selected? Should they assess 'live' or from video? There is now a consensus for training faculty assessors that can help with these decisions.[43]

10.4.3 WHO SHOULD BE AN OBSERVER?

The observer is often a subject matter expert (SME) themselves on the technical task being undertaken, although this is not always the case. For example, pilots are commonly assessed by other pilots who for a period of time are employed by airlines or the regulator as an observational assessor.[44] There are several reasons why being a SME helps assessment; often, the context is appropriate to determine judgement of behaviour (especially for situation awareness) and experts implicitly understand those, often subtle, features that lay observers cannot detect or understand. SMEs are more credible as observers for those receiving feedback, whether formative or as part of dialogue around a summative assessment process. However, lay observers such as psychologists have been utilized in behaviour assessment and the advice from the recent consensus document[43] is to utilize a combination of surgeons and psychologists for certain types of assessment. In a related topic, research studies often combine clinical and non-clinical observers with implicit understanding that the latter, often psychologists, are experts in identifying, coding and interpreting behaviours. This is particularly the case for more overt behaviours such as leadership, communication and teamwork where keystone behaviours can be identified and described without requiring technical knowledge of the operative procedure. Clinical observers can also be consumed by minor technical details of the case that can be distracting when the aim is to apply a behaviour skills taxonomy. Other members of the OR team such as nurses and perfusionists are also experienced in observing surgeons' behaviour in close quarters, so they may also be valid observers for certain purposes.

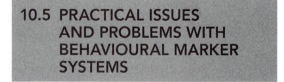

10.5 PRACTICAL ISSUES AND PROBLEMS WITH BEHAVIOURAL MARKER SYSTEMS

One challenging issue in determining surgical proficiency is the presence of a senior surgical trainee (in the United States, a chief resident) with good technical skills but poor non-technical skills. Should they be allowed to become a consultant/attending surgeon and enter independent practice? In reality, this will be a rare situation, but the answer would be a firm 'no'. No hospital, health board or university should allow someone to proceed to become a consultant if there is knowledge that their non-technical skills are substandard. With the current availability of reliable and reproducible assessments of these non-technical skills, training programmes must develop surgeons who are fit for purpose. In the future, it will become increasingly likely that surgical trainees will be assessed on their non-technical skills, not only during their training (formative) but also as part of their final 'certifying/board' examinations (summative). This will provide focus on non-technical skills throughout training, as we know that assessment drives learning (and is actually better than repeated study in some cases for long-term retention). No surgeon knowingly wishes to be an ineffective communicator, a poor leader or incapable of making effective decisions.

It is interesting that in the United Kingdom, no specialty currently has either technical or non-technical skills assessment as part of summative assessment. In fact, technical skills are thought to be best assessed in situ in the workplace as part of a formative assessment program. This is driven mainly by the feeling among surgeons that summative assessments do not sufficiently reflect competence.

10.6 CURRENT METHODS FOR ASSESSING SURGEONS

In assessing clinical skills, Miller's pyramid provides a four-stage framework, which progresses from cognition to behaviour.[45] 'Knows' forms the basis of the pyramid, whereas 'Does' is at the apex (Figure 10.1).

The pyramid demonstrates how assessment eventually translates into clinical behaviours. In the pyramid, 'Knows' (the trainee is cognizant of information) is at the base of the triangle and is considered the foundation for the development of clinical

competence. 'Knows how' is where the knowledge that is acquired can be used to analyse and interpret information and data. 'Shows how' (the trainee is able to transition thinking to behaviour) is applicable when the trainee is able to demonstrate and translate learned information to a clinical environment. Finally, 'Does' is where the trainee is able to perform clinical duties on a daily basis.

Surgeons need to be assessed in a number of domains and ideally by a wide group of assessors from different professional groups. All countries have their own methods, but increasingly they are using standardized and well-recognized techniques, which are summarized here. The methods used in both the United Kingdom and Australasia will be used as examples. From the perspective of the RACS, a competency framework underpins the Surgical Education and Training (SET) program and comprises three technical skills (medical expertise, technical expertise and judgement (i.e. clinical decision making) and six non-technical skills (professionalism and ethics, communication, health advocacy, collaboration and teamwork, management and leadership and scholar and teacher). The level and frequency of assessment corresponds with their level within the SET program. This program is run by the RACS in partnership with the specialty societies (cardiovascular surgery, general surgery, neurosurgery, orthopaedic surgery, otolaryngology, paediatric surgery, plastic and reconstructive surgery, vascular surgery and urology), with the typical time period for training – varies with specialty – being 4–7 years. In the United Kingdom, trainees are assessed using similar methods to the RACS according to the guidelines produced by ISCP. The principles behind the various assessment methods available are outlined in Sections 10.6.1–10.6.7.

10.6.1 IN-TRAINING ASSESSMENT: AUSTRALASIA

'Authentic assessment' is the terminology used to describe medical assessment that focuses on direct performance assessment. This has given rise to the authenticity movement, whereby assessments are now given where the student is in an 'authentic' situation.

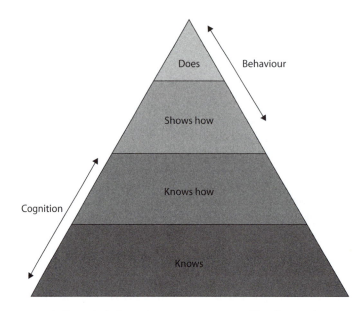

Figure 10.1 Miller's pyramid. 'Does': daily patient care – assessed by direct observation in clinical settings (performance). 'Shows how': demonstration of clinical skills – tested by objective structured clinical examination (OSCE), standardized patients, clinical exams and so on (competence). 'Knows how': application of knowledge – tested by clinical problem solving and so on. 'Knows': knowledge – tested by written exams. (Adapted from Ramani S and S Leinster, *Med Teach*, 30(4), 347–64, 2008.)

Assessment in authentic situations can focus on how students combine knowledge and skills, judgements and attitudes in dealing with realistic problems of professional practice. Moreover, ongoing assessment of performance in day-to-day practice enables assessment of a range of essential competencies, some of which cannot be validly assessed otherwise, such as professional behaviour, efficient organization of work, communication in teamwork, and continuous learning skills.[46]

The in-training assessment (ITA) tool is a valuable measure of clinical performance and can be defined as an assessment that has multiple observations within the workplace setting. All trainees should be assessed regularly during each training position and have a formal review ideally by each training unit and then the training programme. Apart from day-to-day clinical interactions, RACS assesses all trainees midterm and at the completion of each rotation. This form of assessment will allow the trainee to receive structured feedback regarding their performance and provide an opportunity to discuss possible areas to focus on in the next part of the rotation. The ITA should lead to increased trainee confidence in the clinical setting

and should complement the formative assessment and feedback that occurs during each rotation. Indeed, without the ITA, the formal end of rotation assessment will not have adequate information to provide feedback and any opportunities to address potential areas of concern during the rotation will be missed.

10.6.2 PROCEDURE-BASED ASSESSMENTS

Procedure-based assessments (PBAs) have been designed to provide structure in assessing competency-based clinical skills in the OR.[47] The supervisor is required to directly observe the trainee carrying out a specific procedure, provide feedback and then assess (usually online). PBAs are expected to be used as frequently as possible to assist the trainee in the learning process and be used as an overall performance review and evidence of progression.[48] Depending on how they are set up, this particular method of assessment is effective in monitoring the trainee's performance during a specific procedure but can also include clinical knowledge and communication skills.

PBAs have been shown to be a reliable method of assessing trainees' technical competence in the OR,[47] with typically three to six observations required for each trainee. Using this particular assessment tool enables continuous data on trainee performances during actual operations to be recorded. It also assists in enhancing the supervision process for both supervisors and medical educators. Direct observations of procedures are similar but refer to procedures performed outside the OR. These methods of assessment are also a useful platform for supervisors to provide feedback and to discuss possible improvements for training.

10.6.3 MULTI-SOURCE FEEDBACK

As was shown in the early work from Scotland,[4] using a large variety of assessors from different domains including the trainees themselves and patients, where possible, results in a reliable and valid assessment of the trainee. This form of assessment is now part of many surgical training programmes' routine assessment, and trainees are asked to identify people with whom they work to provide an assessment. The areas assessed usually focus on communication and teamwork skills, professionalism and clinical skills rather than operative skills, depending on how they are designed. Increasingly, 360° appraisals involving all members of the OR and peri-operative teams are being used to assess and rate surgeons. Harvard hospitals in particular use 360° assessments of surgeons on a range of behaviours in and out of the OR, including some non-technical skills.

A part of this process involves self-assessment, but self-judgements are not always accurate for a variety of reasons and self-assessment of non-technical skills has been shown to be less reliable than that of technical skills using currently available assessment tools. However, these methods are becoming very popular and link the workplace assessment model to more general characteristics or traits of the surgeon. There are also knowledge and attitude scales for teamwork and communication. These methods all provide different and often complementary data. However, direct observation using a validated assessment tool is the most favoured method.

10.6.4 WORKPLACE-BASED ASSESSMENT IN NON-TECHNICAL SKILLS

As mentioned in Section 10.2, workplace assessment using the NOTSS taxonomy has been developed by surgeons in Sheffield and has now been incorporated into ISCP so that surgical trainees can have their non-technical skills assessed during a specifically identified procedure. This is the first time that UK trainees have had their non-technical skills formally assessed, and the concept is obviously new to both trainees and trainers. As a result, it is an absolute requirement for all trainers to undergo a short web-based training programme – 'NOTSS-in-a-Box' – before they are permitted to assess and score the trainees (only accessible through ISCP-recognized trainers or fellows of RCSEd). Trainees are also encouraged to use this training programme, so that they can understand what skills will be assessed and the science behind the taxonomy.

10.6.5 DEALING WITH POOR PERFORMANCE

With trainees, poor performance usually triggers a need of additional training or remediation, whereas for established surgeons, degradation of skills is likely to contribute to poor outcomes for patients. Trainee surgeons who underperform can create a significant burden for peers, colleagues and supervisors. They create extra workloads particularly when there is misunderstanding in communication that can cause conflict and needless error. Such conflict can result in the cost of litigation; costs of management productivity; training new staff; individuals feeling unwell due to stress (sick time); compensation claims; and, depending on the outcomes of the conflict, increased care for patients harmed.[49] One major way that assessment can help is by identifying trainees who are struggling or underperforming early. This allows for more tailored training or, in some cases, transfer to another area of specialism more suited to the trainees' skill set. However, this does not always happen and one concern is when supervisors do not fail trainees who are underperforming or who are problematical. Barriers include lack of good documentation or evidence, anticipating an appeal process and lack of remediation options to help those who fail.[50]

10.6.6 DEGRADATION AND REMEDIATION OF SKILLS

The negative effects of 'burnout' including depression and clinical performance[51,52] affect trainees and established surgeons alike. Help is available, though, for example, the RACS has a well-developed remediation programme for surgeons covering technical and social factors related to surgical performance.[53] These wider issues that affect the performance and health of surgeons are discussed more in Chapter 11.

10.6.7 AGE AND SURGICAL PERFORMANCE

Although there is undoubtedly a relationship between experience and better outcomes,[54] there will come a time when the deteriorating functions associated with age make it difficult for surgeons to maintain their performance.[55] In a study examining correlations between mortality and the older surgeon, surgeons over the age of 60 years were more likely to have higher mortality rates in pancreatectomy, coronary artery bypass surgery and carotid endarterectomy.[56] Furthermore, inexperienced older surgeons are often less proficient than younger surgeons, especially with laparoscopic technique[57] (see Chapter 11 for a wider discussion of the impact of age on non-technical skills and surgical performance, which will be particularly relevant to surgeons who are towards the end of their careers).

10.7 SUMMARY

It is now clear that recognition, understanding and assessment of the non-technical skills that support good surgical performance are essential for both surgical training and ongoing professional development. There are a wide range of methods for surgical assessment, and with formal courses in NOTSS and team training now being available it will become easier for these non-technical skills to be understood, taught and assessed. This will also help in the recognition and support of the under-performing surgeon and may also become part of the remediation process. Technical and cognitive skills invariably deteriorate with age, and while experience might protect or slow this deterioration better teamwork and communication within surgical teams will identify and support the failing surgeon, allowing appropriate action to be taken before outcomes can be affected.

ACKNOWLEDGEMENT

Stephen Tobin acknowledges the assistance of Ms Rachel Lennon in developing Chapter 10.

REFERENCES

1. Martin JA, Regehr G, Reznick R, Macrae H, Murhaghan J, Hutchison C et al. Objective structured assessment of technical skill (OSATS) for surgical residents. *Brit J Surg.* 1997;84:273–8.
2. Baldwin P, Paisley AM, Paterson-Brown S. Consultant surgeons' opinions of the skills required of basic surgical trainees. *Brit J Surg.* 1999;86:1078–82.
3. Cuschieri A, Francis N, Crosby J, Hanna GB. What do master surgeons think of surgical competence and revalidation? *Am J Surg.* 2001;182:110–6.
4. Paisley A, Baldwin P, Paterson-Brown S. Feasibility, reliability and validity of a new assessment form for use with basic surgical trainees. *Am J Surg.* 2001;182:24–9.
5. Driscoll PJ, Paisley AM, Paterson-Brown S. Trainees' opinions of the skills required of basic surgical trainees. *Am J Surg.* 2003;186:77–80.
6. Yule S, Flin R, Paterson-Brown S, Maran N, Rowley D. Development of a rating system for surgeons' non-technical skills. *Med Educ.* 2006 Nov;40(11):1098–104.

7. Yule S, Flin R, Maran N, Rowley DR, Youngson GG, Paterson-Brown S. Surgeons' non-technical skills in the operating room: Reliability testing of the NOTSS behaviour rating system. *World J Surg.* 2006;32:548–556.

8. Yule S, Flin R, Rowley D, Mitchell A, Youngson GG, Maran N et al. Debriefing surgical trainees on non-technical skills (NOTSS). *Cogn Tech Work.* 2008:10:265–74.

9. Crossley J, Marriott J, Purdie H, Beard J. Prospective observational study to evaluate NOTSS (Non-Technical Skills for Surgeons) for assessing trainees' non-technical performance in the operating theatre. *Brit J Surg.* 2011;98:1010–20.

10. Surgical Council on Resident Education. [Accessed July 27, 2014.] Available from: www.score.org.

11. Pryor J, Crossouard B. A socio-cultural theorisation of formative assessment. *Oxford Rev Educ.* 2008;34(1):1–20.

12. Royal Australasian College of Surgeons (RACS). Becoming a competent and proficient surgeon: Training standards for the nine RACS competencies. 2012. [Accessed September 2014]. Available from: http://www.surgeons.org/media/18726523/mnl_2012-02-24_training_standards_final_1.pdf.

13. Weick K. The vulnerable system: An analysis of the Tenerife air disaster. *J Manage.* 1990;16(3):571–93.

14. Flin R, Martin L, Goeters K, Hormann H, Amalberti R, Valot C et al. Development of the NOTECHS (non-technical skills) system for assessing pilots' CRM skills. *Human Factors and Aerospace Safety.* 2003;3(2):95–117.

15. Fletcher G, Flin R, McGeorge P, Glavin R, Maran N, Patey R. Anaesthetists' non-technical skills (ANTS): Evaluation of a behavioural marker system. *Br J Anaesth.* 2003;90:580–8.

16. Rutherford J, Flin R, Irwin A, McFadyen A. Evaluation of the prototype Anaesthetic Non-Technical Skills for Anaesthetic Practitioners (ANTS-AP) system: a behavioural rating system to assess the non-technical skills used by staff assisting the anaesthetist. *Anaesthesia.* 2015 (in press).

17. Mitchell L, Flin R, Yule S, Mitchell J, Coutts K, Youngson G. Evaluation of the Scrub Practitioners' List of Intraoperative Non-Technical Skills (SPLINTS) system. *Int J Nurs Stud.* 2012;49:201–11.

18. Mitchell L, Flin R, Yule S, Mitchell J, Coutts K, Youngson G. Development of a behavioural marker system for scrub practitioners' non-technical skills (SPLINTS system). *J Eval Clin Pract.* 2013 Apr;19(2):317–23.

19. Catchpole K, Mishra A, Handa A, McCulloch P. Teamwork and error in the operating room: Analysis of skills and roles. *Ann Surg.* 2008 Apr;247(4):699–706.

20. Anderson O, Davis R, Hanna GB, Vincent CA. Surgical adverse events: A systematic review. *Am J Surg.* 2013;206:253–260.

21. Christian CK, Gustafson ML, Roth EM, Sheridan TB, Gandhi TK, Dwyer K et al. A prospective study of patient safety in the operating room. *Surgery.* 2006 Feb;139(2):159–73.

22. Greenberg CC, Regenbogen SE, Studdert DM, Lipsitz SR, Rogers SO, Zinner MJ et al. Patterns of communication breakdowns resulting in injury to surgical patients. *J Am Coll Surg.* 2007 Apr;204(4):533–40.

23. Henrickson Parker S, Yule S, Flin R, McKinley A. Towards a model of surgeons' leadership in the operating room. *BMJ Qual Saf.* 2011 Jul;20(7):570–9.

24. Lingard L, Espin S, Whyte S, Regehr G, Baker G, Reznick R. Communication failures in the operating room: An observational classification of recurrent types and effects. *Qual Saf Health Care.* 2004;13:330–4.

25. Regenbogen S, Greenberg CC, Studdert D, Lipsitz S, Zinner MJ, Gawande AA. Patterns of technical error among surgical malpractice claims: An analysis of strategies to prevent injury to surgical patients. *Ann Surg.* 2007;246(5):705–11.

26. Roth E, Christian C, Gustafson M, Sheridan T, Dwyer K, Gandhi T et al. Using field observations as a tool for discovery: Analysing cognitive and collaborative demands in the operating room. *Cogn Tech Work*. 2004;6:148–57.

27. Way LW, Stewart L, Gantert W, Liu K, Lee CM, Whang K et al. Causes and prevention of laparoscopic bile duct injuries: Analysis of 252 cases from a human factors and cognitive psychology perspective. *Ann Surg*. 2003 Apr;237(4):460–9.

28. Dickinson I, Watters D, Graham I, Montgomery P, Collins J. Guide to the assessment of competence and performance in practicing surgeons. *ANZ J Surg*. 2009;79:198–204.

29. Spanager L, Lyk-Jensen H, Dieckmann P, Wettergren A, Rosenberg J, Østergaard D. Customization of a tool to assess Danish surgeons' non-technical skills in the operating room. *Dan Med J*. 2012;59(11):1–6.

30. Dickinson T, McIntyre R. A conceptual framework for teamwork measurement. In Brannick MT, Salas E, Prince C (Eds.), *Team Performance Assessment and Measurement: Theory, Methods, and Applications* [Internet]. Mahwah, New Jersey: Lawrence Earlbaum Associates Series in Applied Psychology; 1997. pp. 19–43.

31. Russ S, Hull L, Rout S, Vincent C, Darzi A, Sevdalis N. Observational teamwork assessment for surgery: Feasibility of clinical and nonclinical assessor calibration with short-term training. *Ann Surg*. 2012 Apr;255(4):804–9.

32. Mishra A, Catchpole K, McCulloch P. The Oxford NOTECHS system: Reliability and validity of a tool for measuring teamwork behaviour in the operating theatre. *Qual Saf Health Care*. 2009;18:104–8.

33. Robertson E, Hadi M, Morgan J, Pickering S, Collins G, New S et al. Oxford NOTECHS II: A modified theatre team non-technical skills scoring system. *PLOS One*. 2014;9(3):1–8.

34. Sevdalis N, Davis R, Koutantji M, Undre S, Darzi A, Vincent C. Reliability of a revised NOTECHS scale for use in surgical teams. *Am J Surg*. 2008;196:184–90.

35. Steinemann S, Berg B, DiTullio A, Skinner A, Terada K, Anzelon K et al. Assessing teamwork in the trauma bay: Introduction of a modified 'NOTECHS' scale for trauma. *Am J Surg*. 2012;203:69–75.

36. Michinov E, Jamet E, Dodeler V, Haegelen C, Jannin P. Assessing neurosurgical non-technical skills: An exploratory study of a new behavioural marker system. *J Eval Clin Pract*. 2014; Oct;20(5):582–8.

37. Nagpal K, Abboudi M, Fischler L. Evaluation of postoperative handover using a tool to assess information transfer and teamwork. *Ann Surg*. 2011;253(4):831–7.

38. Andersen P, Jensen M, Lippert A, Ostergaard D, Klausen T. Development of a formative assessment tool for measurement of performance in multi-professional resuscitation teams. *Resuscitation*. 2010;81(6):703–11.

39. Frengley R, Weller J, Torrie J. The effect of simulation-based training intervention on the performance of established critical care unit teams. *Crit Care Med*. 2011;39(12):2605–11.

40. Flowerdew L, Gaunt A, Spedding J, Bhargava A, Briwn R, Vincent C et al. A multicenter observational study to evaluate a new tool to assess emergency physicians' non-technical skills. *Emerg Med J*. 2013;30:437–43.

41. Klampfer B, Flin R, Helmreich R. *Enhancing Performance in High Risk Environments: Recommendations for the Use of Behavioural Markers*. Zurich, Switzerland: Swiss Federal Institute of Technology (ETH); 2001.

42. Yule S, Paterson-Brown S. Surgeons' non-technical skills. In J.A. Sanchez (Ed.). *Surg Clin North Am*. 2012;92(1):37–50. Philadelphia, Pennsylvania.

43. Hull L, Arora S, Symons NR, Jalil R, Darzi A, Vincent C et al. Training faculty in nontechnical skill assessment: National guidelines on program requirements. *Ann Surg*. 2012;258:370–375.

44. Musson D. Putting behavioural markers to work: Developing and evaluating safety training in healthcare settings. In Flin R, Mitchell L (Eds.), *Safer Surgery: Analysing Behaviour in the Operating Theatre*. Farnham, England: Ashgate; 2009. pp. 423–36.

45. Ramani S, Leinster S, AMEE guide no 34: Teaching in the clinical environment. *Med Teach*. 2008;30(4):347–64.

46. Govaerts MJB, Van Der Vleuten CPM, Schuwirth LWT, Muijtjens AMM. Broadening perspectives on clinical performance assessment: Rethinking the nature of in-training assessment. *Adv Health Sci Educ*. 2007;12:239–60.

47. Kogan JR, Holmboe ES, Hauer KE. Tools for direct observation and assessment of clinical skills of medical trainees. *JAMA*. 2009;302(12):1316–26.

48. Norcini JJ, McKinley DW. Assessment methods in medical education. *Teach Teach Educ*. 2007;23:239–50.

49. Marshall P, Robson R. The nature of conflict and some common myths. RCPSC Website. 2013. [Accessed March 2013]. Available from: http://www.royalcollege.ca/portal/page/portal/rc/resources/bioethics/primers/conflict_resolution#references.

50. Dudeck NL, Marks MB, Regehr G. Failure to fail: The perspectives of clinical supervisors. *Acad Med*. 2005;80(10):S84–7.

51. Thomas EJ. Resident burnout. *JAMA*. 2004;292:2880–9.

52. Insull P, Kejriwal R, Segar A, Blyth P. Surgical inclination in senior medical students from the University of Auckland: Results of the 2005 Senior Students Survey. *N Z Med J*. 2006;119(1234):1–7.

53. Quinn J. RACS approach to remediation. Presentation. 2014. [Accessed May 2014.] Available from: http://www.surgeons.org/media/20748284/quinn_revalidation_melbourne_march_2014.pdf.

54. Neumayer LA, Gawande AA, Wang J, Giobbe-Hurder A, Itani KMF, Fitzgibbons RJ et al. Proficiency of surgeons in inguinal hernia repair: Effect of experience and age. *Ann Surg*. 2005;242(3):345–52.

55. Blaiser RB. The problem of the ageing surgeon. *Clin Orthop*. 2009;467(2):402–11.

56. Waljee JF, Greenfield LJ, Dimick JB, Birkmeyer JD. Surgeon age and operative mortality in the United States. *Ann Surg*. 2006;244:353–62.

57. Peisah C, Wilhem K. In the public eye: The impaired ageing doctor. *Int Med J*. 2002;32:457–9.

11

What next? Development of non-technical skills

GEORGE G YOUNGSON AND THORALF M SUNDT III

The widespread recognition and acceptance of the importance of non-technical skills for surgical performance and their impact on surgical outcome is relatively recent, but the skills themselves are not new. This chapter looks forward to how non-technical skills may be further developed and enhanced and how their new-found place in the surgical curriculum can be consolidated. The next stages of the development and use of non-technical skills in surgery all receive comment, including their place in patient safety management systems, their relationship with other initiatives in patient safety programmes, their role in the analysis of routine performance and specific adverse incidents and the legal consequences. Preserving high levels of competence and performance is a requirement for surgeons at every stage of their career, and the importance of non-technical skills in coping with that challenge is discussed.

Attainment of clinical skills, whether technical or non-technical, like many other learning experiences, involves a degree of trial and error with the provision that patients are protected as much as possible from the potential for harm while trainees are on their learning curve. Experiential learning in operative surgery in the clinical setting (as opposed to simulation) is therefore traditionally heavily and expertly supervised. Graduated withdrawal of that supervision as competence is acquired and demonstrated by the trainee encourages independent responsibility to develop. Tacit evaluation of the competence of the learner as part of that delegation process is an implicit part of surgical education and training and is expected by the trainee as a matter of course. Although sometimes subtle, the assessment, rating and calibration of the learner's technical skills is part of the process that allows delegation of duties and tasks with the confidence that patients will remain safe during the training process. This same process of evaluation is far less conspicuous when it relates to non-technical skills, and a number of challenges surround establishing the same level of confidence in relation to the patient's safety and the assessment of a surgeon's judgement, decision-making, risk evaluation and interpersonal skills.

Grading and evaluating these aspects of intra-operative performance is particularly important as they contribute to the understanding and definition of non-technical skills, a concept that still has to be embedded throughout many areas of the surgical profession. Although early acceptance of the relevance and importance of non-technical skills has occurred in many centres, other surgical institutions and agencies remain less informed. Moreover, although the importance of teaching of judgement and evaluation of risk has been long accepted, there is a gap in the appreciation of the impact of interpersonal skills. This vacancy provides an opportunity to identify how non-technical skills can feature in surgical education and how they might be rated and assessed, as well as developed to be further utilized in the future. This chapter brings together the perceived and actual benefits of effective training in non-technical skills and their utility as part of the intra-operative surgical repertoire. It also explores their possible application and development in the decade to come.

11.1 ACQUISITION: EDUCATION IN PATIENT SAFETY AND NON-TECHNICAL SKILLS

11.1.1 WORKPLACE-BASED ACQUISITION

Presentation of the failure of technical skills is usually immediate and apparent to all, often taking the form of a post-operative complication, such as sepsis, which may follow an anastomotic leak. By contradistinction, failures of non-technical skills are less conspicuous and often less directly attributable to the individual surgeon. One of the challenges inherent in acquiring surgical non-technical skills is that their application is heavily dependent on having had exposure to appropriate past experience in the setting of operative surgery with skilled role models providing informed feedback. While the principles of non-technical skills can be discussed and read about, the identification, relevance and importance of these skills and attributes will not be completely appreciated unless there has been prior exposure to operative surgery. Furthermore, these skills may be subtle in their execution and lessons learned from the consequences of their implementation may be missed unless the teacher is explicit in calling attention to them or the learner is primed to recognize their execution. Furthermore, if the student is adequately prepared he or she will learn from bad examples as well as good.

However, if non-technical skills are only introduced into consideration of surgical performance late in the surgical learning programme, the opportunity for formative development of these skills is reduced. There is, therefore, real value in exploring the underlying principles of patient safety early in the clinical years of medical school training, with increasing subsequent emphasis on non-technical skills being provided incrementally throughout the surgical training programme.

An early step in addressing learning in non-technical skills is to outline the generic area of patient safety and quality improvement within the training curriculum with the importance of an understanding of human factors science being identified and emphasized. This serves to underline the relevance of this aspect of delivery of care and also promotes the recognition of non-technical skills as an essential component of professional performance of a surgeon.

Thus, in the absence of any specifically identified time at which the learning process on the content of non-technical skills training should be started, there is some merit in setting out the nature, the basic categories involved and their value at an early stage in medical education, as some medical schools have realized. It is acknowledged that much of the learning experience will be vicarious and for surgeons an appreciation of the significance of non-technical skills may be limited by a lack of exposure to the operating theatre environment and a restricted understanding of the challenges posed by operative surgery. Nonetheless, there are generic aspects to the display and use of non-technical skills, which are common to complex teams in general and can be appreciated by learners in their early years by observing their presence or absence and deployment by the members of various clinical teams. The principles of teamwork and communication, as well as the value of good surgical leadership at the operating table, will be evident to the students from the outset and these social skills, along with an exposure to factors affecting decision making, and the understanding and management of information flow during surgery, are important learning opportunities for senior medical students and young doctors irrespective of their specialty career ambitions.

11.1.2 PATIENT SAFETY IN MEDICAL SCHOOL CURRICULA

To ensure that the next generation of doctors is aware of and sensitive to the potential for harm during clinical care delivery, many medical schools around the world are including patient safety teaching into the undergraduate curricula. The World Health Organization (WHO) has formulated such a curriculum through the World Alliance for Patient Safety.[1] Much of this work was based on the Australian Patient Safety Education Framework, where 11 topics were set out.[2] Both curricula emphasize the fundamental importance of human factors being taught in the undergraduate curriculum and the

interactions of humans with humans, humans with equipment and technology, human–environment interaction and dependency of high-quality clinical care on the interaction of the multi-professional team. The delivery of a curriculum in patient safety is achieved through different formats ranging from taught courses through to e-learning modules, ward rounds, tutorials and small group working. Each of these allows for different areas of the patient safety curriculum to be explored. In keeping with sound educational methodology, there is progression from 'knowing' to 'knowing how' and to 'showing' and 'doing', as outlined in Chapter 9. Feedback during these stages is crucial to efficient learning of elements of the curriculum and should emphasize on not only an understanding of the causes of adverse events but also how to manage them.

11.1.3 METHODS OF UNDERGRADUATE TEACHING

The use of video material from aviation in particular has allowed introduction of the concepts of Crew Resource Management (CRM) and, with that, the value of non-technical skills in managing all types of clinical situations. Follow-up studies of medical school curricular content[3] have confirmed the effectiveness of this style of delivery, but they emphasize the importance of a sufficiently expert and sizeable faculty of teachers for this type of learning. This teaching template provides a suitable basis for introducing the contents of non-technical skills into the final phase of undergraduate and early years of surgical training and encourages the students to make observations of surgical performance during their attendance in the operating theatre. Although there has been a tradition of the senior clinician being placed in the teacher role, many non-technical skills can be well taught to medical students by graduate students and residents, in itself an early introduction to leadership as it underlines the fact that leadership is not entirely predicated on or related to seniority. It also serves to underline that while management is a positional role and confined to a few individuals, leadership responsibilities are ubiquitous and leadership/followership behaviours are identifiable throughout clinical practice and in the operating room in particular and can be identified and rated as good or bad and effective or ineffective.

11.2 USING, DEVELOPING AND ENHANCING NON-TECHNICAL SKILLS

11.2.1 HOW OTHERS DO IT

Once surgeons are established in independent practice, the opportunity to observe and work alongside other surgical experts is limited. However, the trend towards surgeons working together in teams is becoming more commonplace than was the case a few decades ago. This practice is especially applicable to and is of particular value in protracted and complex procedures. The NOTSS classification provides a good basis for planning the procedure during such pairings, and assigning roles through mutual consent is aided by reference to the taxonomy. Similarly, the analysis of the procedure can be carried out by reference to the non-technical skills elements of teamwork. This allows both planning before the procedure and self-reflection and performance review in a non-judgemental fashion after the procedure and provides a shared perspective for the surgeons involved, as well as being a positive reinforcement for future co-working.

11.2.2 WHO IS QUALIFIED TO TEACH AND ASSESS?

Accreditation of approved trainers in non-technical skills is still a distant prospect in medicine. Most teaching in non-technical skills arises from enthusiasts who have awareness, insight and background experience and knowledge of the literature or have been actively involved in the development of non-technical skills programmes. Accreditation of the non-technical skills teaching processes in most other industries tends to focus more on accreditation of the individual student/trainee rather than accreditation of the teacher, process or content. In aviation, however, there are now specific requirements and standards that relate to becoming a

CRM instructor/examiner, as outlined in the Flight Operations Inspectorate of the UK's Civil Aviation Authority.[4] There is thus a need for a similar accreditation framework in surgery, which would be best organized at the global/international level but be applied at the local level. Differences in international standards for surgeons' non-technical skills (if they exist at all) have not as yet been published; but empirical observations suggest that in spite of different cultures possibly influencing attitudes and behaviours in operating rooms throughout the world the central principles of the NOTSS taxonomy are applicable to all venues, all countries and all continents. Countries classified as low- and middle-resource settings in particular perhaps require surgeons with proportionately more creative decision-making ability and a more innovative approach as a consequence of the dearth of resources available to them during and after surgery. And their relative inability to rescue the clinical situations following development of complications as a consequence of limited facilities places an even greater emphasis on the intra-operative competence of the individual surgeon. However, the identification of an underpinning non-technical skill set has been an important first step in the development of the NOTSS curriculum and the apparent acceptability of this on the international stage is an endorsement of its relevance to and importance in surgical practice from the global perspective.

11.3 COACHING AND DEBRIEFING USING NON-TECHNICAL SKILLS FOR SURGEONS

The utilization of non-technical skills is influenced by a wide range of factors that change with the different stages of career development. The surgical novice has learning and skill acquisition as a primary place for non-technical skills, whereas the established or senior surgeon may wish to readjust current practice by using self-evaluation of non-technical skills. Both may be in need of coaching to produce such a change in clinical practice and, yet, coaching as an aspect of professional development for operative performance is in its infancy. It is still underused and is possibly unwelcome in many operating theatres. Nevertheless, progress through the scale of learning to proficiency and then through to excellence requires as much assistance as is available, particularly when in pursuit of the mastery of complex tasks that are a feature of some complex major procedures. Incremental progression in the use of non-technical skills is similarly challenging for a range of reasons. The novice (and others) will tend to concentrate simply on the actions involved in completing a step within the operation – the mechanics of the task – rather than necessarily how well or the manner in which it is performed. Perception and comprehension (levels 1 and 2 of situation awareness, and the first two elements of the category in the NOTSS taxonomy) may thus be at a substantially lower level in the novice who will be focusing on completion of the technical task. In comparison, the expert is likely to place more emphasis and focus on those two levels of situation awareness and attempt to make precise predictions for the next stages of the procedure (level 3 situation awareness) and the ultimate recovery of the patient.

Do all surgeons use their non-technical skills in the same way, and does the impact of non-technical skills produce the same effect for all surgeons? For some, awareness of non-technical skills will be about their contribution to the learning curve of operative surgery, for many, it will be more about enhancing existing skills and for a few, it will be about remedying deficient skills. Atul Gawande has been persuasive when writing about the use of coaches by elite athletes, musicians and tennis players.[5] If the best of these professionals, each accustomed to high-demand situations, get benefit and become better still from coaching, then why not surgeons at various stages of their careers[6]? One answer may be to identify the value of non-technical skills in all assessment modalities, be that formative assessment in training or in the recertification and revalidation processes of established surgeons. The greatest challenge here is the intensity of resources required to assess these skills on a national scale. However, the first step is to introduce the use of non-technical skills into personal reflection and self-assessment, with their place in summative assessment being a possible future contribution.

Debriefing is being increasingly valued as a method of commenting on individuals or the team in a positive fashion, and provided the debriefing tool is used effectively feedback is of educational value and provides a basis for performance enhancement and improvement. It can be used in other ways, for example, for recording and documenting, and therefore may be of historic value. If formally accepted, then it is also useful as a way of minimizing subjective and sometimes destructive commentary following critical or adverse events. Building it into a routine process confers the advantage that it is not only utilized during exceptional circumstances and removes it from the role of being perceived as only a tool for remediation.

The NOTSS taxonomy provides an effective denominator and context for debriefing on those critical areas of decision making and situation awareness. It also allows the dynamics of the operating team to be reviewed and any changes required for similar future events to be discussed in a non-adversarial fashion.[7] Too often today, a debrief does not go far beyond a few cursory comments regarding availability of equipment and the like and there is not enough discussion about the non-technical aspects including the nature and quality of interactions. This represents a particular opportunity to 'repair' relationships that may have been bruised during the interactions that occurred 'in the heat of battle' during particularly stressful or anxious moments.

11.4 NON-TECHNICAL SKILLS AND QUALITY IMPROVEMENT

11.4.1 PATIENT SAFETY ORGANISATIONS

A wide range of agencies and institutions have emerged in response to a need for better quality assurance, safety and improvement in care, if harm associated with health care is to be reduced and the safety of care increased. The Institute of Healthcare Improvement, which was established in Boston, Massachusetts, in 1991, is one such institution. The methodology used in their educational programme is based on consistent, evidence-based practice methods promulgated in the form of 'bundles of care' to emphasize the importance of reducing variation in practice, encouraging all clinicians to practice routinely in a consistent if not an identical fashion, so that even minor improvements in care can be measured and identified. Within Europe, Scotland is one of the first countries to institute a countrywide approach to improving patient safety through implementation of a national programme – the Scottish Patient Safety Programme[8] – which introduces quality improvement into a range of different clinical communities ranging from adult acute care, maternity and child health to mental health and primary care.

11.4.2 QUALITY IMPROVEMENT AND NON-TECHNICAL SKILLS

Non-technical skills are identified to be relevant in many of these areas; but it is in the peri-operative care section where complexity is high, decision making must be rapid despite ambiguity and consequences are profound, that one of the primary drivers is the creation of a team culture attuned to detecting and rectifying intra-operative errors. Although the care bundle identifies the use of briefings, team training, standardizing intra-operative policy and 'readiness responses', prepared for adverse situations as appropriate measures, all these, along with the maintenance of the teams' focus, are dependent on the suite of non-technical skills contained by the NOTSS taxonomy.

The importance of non-technical skills in promoting an understanding and underpinning of the effectiveness of quality improvement programmes is essential, and the NOTSS components all feature in an integral fashion in those programmes. Examples include the importance of vigilance as a part of 'situation awareness' as a key ingredient of early detection of change to physiological parameters during monitoring (e.g. early warning systems). 'Decision making' is aided and abetted by having approved policies, rules and guidance implemented in a non-discretional fashion, ensuring that high compliance produces consistency in performance and high and measurable success rates. This 'rule-based' approach to decision making also liberates thinking capacity for more challenging clinical

situations (see Chapter 5). 'Teamworking', supporting and 'leading' are contingent on precise, effective and reliable 'communication', which are all features of improvement programmes and all parts of the non-technical skill set. These quality improvement programmes, dependent as they are on the application of previously approved protocols and policies, have found high levels of acceptance, engagement and utilization by nursing staff. However, there has been a slower commitment to the same level of uptake by medical staff (perhaps because they are less of a challenge to diagnostic skills), but these programmes merit the same attention by doctors if they are to achieve a safer environment for clinical care.

11.5 SAFETY MANAGEMENT SYSTEMS

11.5.1 SAFETY MANAGEMENT SYSTEMS (SMS) IN HEALTH CARE

Safety management systems are systematic and comprehensive processes for the proactive management of safety risks.[9] They integrate operational aspects of the service with technical aspects and financial and human resource management. They are designed to deal with adverse events so that valuable lessons are applied to improve safety and efficiency, and they build capacity into their systems to anticipate and address safety issues before they result in incidents or accidents. In health care, this requires a significant commitment from hospital managers to develop an overall safety strategy and a framework to put responsibilities in place as part of a system where hazards are identified, risks are determined and analysed, solutions are recorded and tasks and responsibilities are allocated with clarity and commensurate with the abilities of the recipient.

11.5.2 SMS IN OTHER INDUSTRIES

Other industries have combined tools used for implementing quality improvement techniques and human factors principles with systems for recording adverse and near miss incidents and introduced these into the development of their safety management systems. This allows exemplary practice of safe performance and is contingent on a positive attitude of the organization towards safety. Industries such as the maritime and oil and gas industries have moved away from a situation where accidents, adverse events and complications can be accepted as an obligate by-product of the interventions used in high-risk situations into the development of an attitude that safety, efficiency and effectiveness are to be expected in all circumstances. Safety management systems are thus the application of organizational and management processes directed at safety as part of the regulatory framework in that industry. Risks and hazards are identified as part of the system, and there is an explicit outline of the defences and mitigating steps to be applied to protect against those hazards. Attention to human factors in accident analysis and the non-technical skills/CRM training programs are part of that process.

11.5.3 SMS AND NON-TECHNICAL SKILLS

In health care, the fusion of improvement methodology in combination with non-technical skills and human factors application to safer practice offers the best prospect of producing an embryonic form of safety management system for reduction of harm as a consequence of care. Risk management in health care is more often reactive than strategic and challenges surround, ensuring complete and accurate reporting of adverse and near miss events. Investigation of medical error is still opportunistic, and there is no 'industry standard' developed as yet for evaluating all surgical errors. Although there is a large body of knowledge about the particular risks of any given surgical procedure and all surgeons should be able to quote that operative risk to patients as part of the informed consent process, there is a paucity of knowledge and insight into the magnitude of risk facing a patient as a consequence of the effect of the health care system as a whole. There is an increasing appreciation of non-technical skills and their contribution to the safety of the health care system, particularly while the patient is in the operating theatre. This goes some way to having a more informed picture of the total risk of

harm complicating the treatment of any individual and allowing the possible development of a safety management system for surgery.

11.5.4 NON-TECHNICAL SKILLS AND THE WHO SURGICAL CHECKLIST

The WHO surgical checklist may be perceived as one step towards the development of the safety management system in operating theatres even if this process has many inherent restrictions and limitations that prevent it from in itself constituting such a system. As has been outlined in previous chapters (Chapters 6 and 7), its imperfect application not just represents a deficit in the practice but actually poses a risk.[10] This risk works on the basis that assumptions are made that barriers to harm are in place when, in fact, this is not the case. Use of the checklist possibly preconditions against the possibility of adverse intra-operative events and potentially compromises situation awareness. Indeed, the proliferation in number and expansion of checklists runs the danger of disengagement among surgical staff. The use of multiple checklists may itself constitute a distraction from the true goals of effective teamwork of bidirectional communication, shared situation awareness, shared mental models and resilient high-reliability performance. The ensuing cynicism among surgical staff may give rise to the unintended prospect of prejudicing this shift in safety culture, and caution must be exercised in equating safety to the use of the safety checklist.

The effect, benefit and indeed the success of the WHO surgical checklist, however, relate closely to the fact that it utilizes many, if not all, of the categories of non-technical skills, and Figure 11.1 outlines that synergy between the checklist and the component parts of the NOTSS taxonomy.

11.6 SAFETY CULTURE AND NON-TECHNICAL SKILLS

Behavioural norms are influenced by those working around you, but the past acceptance of morbidity as an obligate part of the landscape of health care

Situation awareness

Teamwork

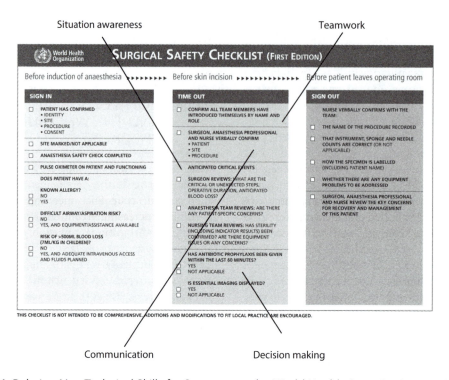

Communication

Decision making

Figure 11.1 Relating Non-Technical Skills for Surgeons to the World Health Organization surgical checklist.

in general and surgery in particular has changed in the last two decades (albeit slowly). What was once tolerated as 'the way it is', given the vulnerable nature of some patients and the increasingly potent characteristic of new interventions for diseases previously considered resistant to treatment, is being replaced with a more aspirational zero tolerance approach to error and adverse events. A new scrutiny of standards, of conduct, process and commitment to care, has to be welcomed.

Safe practice does not need to be translated into risk-aversive behaviour. Identifying the perilous status of some patients and providing optimal care to a recognized standard of safety is a practice that needs to be spread evenly across all clinical groups and venues. The need for prominence and the importance of a culture of safety are becoming progressively more accepted by a clinical community that is accepting of its limitations and increasingly recognizing the associated hazards of care. For some, the scale and complexity of health care delivery may be used as a reason for a reluctance to accept that there is a preventable aspect to much

of the morbidity that surrounds surgical care and this is manifesting in huge variations in outcomes for the same conditions of the same range of severity, thus indicating that some institutions and individuals perform well and others do not.

The application of non-technical skills has given a glimpse into the reasons behind that variation, and their application has contributed to an appreciation of the fundamental importance of human factors in the safe execution of clinical duties. As surgeons practise and encourage the safer ways of working taught in non-technical skills courses, the norms of behaviour shift accordingly and the safety culture strengthens.

11.7 LIABILITY, INDEMNITY AND NON-TECHNICAL SKILLS

Although the principal goal of developing non-technical skills is optimizing clinical outcomes, there are also important medicolegal implications of being able to explicitly identify failures in explicitly identify failures in non-technical skills. Breakdowns in communication among caregivers are commonly and specifically cited as complaints in lawsuits, as are breakdowns in effective communication between caregivers and patients.[11] Furthermore, beyond specific information transfer, the overall relationship between patient, family and care provider has a clear impact on the likelihood of litigation in the event of an adverse outcome. Finally, the cohesiveness of the care providers as a team may have an impact on the evolution of a lawsuit, with the testimony of disaffected providers unlikely to be of much help – and perhaps even creating harm – in a court of law. These legal implications have been recognized by insurers, with some offering reductions in payments for premiums for physicians who undertake specific training in safety, teamwork and non-technical skills.[12]

Conversely, the threat of legal action may represent an obstacle to optimizing performance, as concerns about liability inhibit open sharing of errors. But there is more standing in the way of disclosure including personal reluctance to risk the loss of prestige. It is, therefore, important that students come to view open disclosure itself as a fundamental aspect of the continuous learning of non-technical skills. Skills should be learned for appropriate confession, and apology with expressions of contrition (including what will be done differently in future to prevent recurrence) and offer of compensation if appropriate. Note that disclosure itself is a skill, as the aim is open sharing of factual information without raising uncertainty and suspicion that will undermine faith in the dedication and good intentions of the care team. Conducted inappropriately, disclosure may raise more doubt and actually do more harm than good, particularly when the ultimate outcome is ambiguous.[13]

11.8 ADVERSE EVENT ANALYSIS AND NON-TECHNICAL SKILLS

Methodologies for adverse event analysis need to be directed specifically to capture the impact and influence of non-technical contributors to adverse events.[14] Team debriefing in an open and psychologically safe setting should be facilitated by specialists in adverse event analysis. It is equally important that a true systems approach is adopted, with recognition that there is seldom if ever truly one single 'root cause'. A focus on resilient teams demands a multifaceted understanding of error capture and recovery, as well as error prevention. Currently, there is no accepted best practice for conduct of mortality and morbidity conferences nor is there a universal mandate that such should occur. Such meetings are, however, becoming increasingly common and are spreading from the traditional review of surgical cases to now include all patients who die in hospital at some institutions (Mayo Clinic and Massachusetts General Hospital, among others). Perhaps, the most comprehensive approach is one that has been introduced in the state of Michigan by its statewide cardiothoracic surgical society quality collaborative.[15] By adopting a tool for the analysis of all peri-operative deaths that requires attribution of mortality 'triggers' to a particular phase of care, including preoperative, intra-operative, intensive care (therapy) unit, floor or post-discharge phase, they were able to draw attention to some of the non-technical aspects of care. Specifically, scrutiny was brought to the preoperative decision-making phase. This stimulated caregivers to consider a more structured mortality review. Although the impact of the manner and tone of specific interpersonal communications cannot necessarily be captured, generic breakdowns in communication are identified in a structured manner using this tool. This could serve as a starting point for further refinement of breakdowns using the NOTSS taxonomy.

11.9 DEMONSTRATING AND RETAINING COMPETENCE IN NON-TECHNICAL SKILLS

The United Kingdom implemented its first statutory change to the medical regulatory requirements to demonstrate ongoing competence as part of the process of retention of a licence for doctors to practise in December 2012.[16] This process is termed revalidation, and annual appraisals of a surgeon's performance across the entire scope of practice accumulate over a 5-year period to result in an endorsement and re-provision of the licence. That cycle repeats on a 5-yearly basis. This system is in its early stages, and the complexity of application across the entire medical profession has possibly blunted the potential customization for individual surgical specialties. With maturation and refinement of the process, however, there is an opportunity for a demonstration of safe practice to become a required field in that accountability process. There is an expectation that summative presentation of surgical outcomes will soon become a prerequisite and, as part of that, an accountability of non-technical skills (perhaps carried out through a multi-source feedback method) may provide further evidence of sufficiency if not proficiency in the standard of surgery being practised.

Other countries have alternative requirements for recertification. In the United States, requirements for maintenance of medical certification are still very much in their infancy. Requirements vary from specialty to specialty and focus primarily on documentation of participation in educational programmes and on clinical outcomes. There is certainly interest in aspects of patient safety and teamwork; however, there are no direct assessments of non-technical skills. Means to do so may evolve over time, although direct measurement remains a challenge.

Surgical education and its associated agencies (colleges such as the Royal College of Surgeons of Edinburgh, Royal Australian College of Surgeons or American College of Surgeons and specialty associations such as Association of Surgeons of Great Britain and Ireland) have placed primacy on acquisition of surgical skills through training and maintenance of skills through continuous professional development; but there is little, if any, attention paid to the prospect of skill degradation in the latter phases of surgical career. This, as yet an under-researched aspect of surgical performance, is likely to apply as much to non-technical skills as it does to technical skills, and the authority for continuation of surgical practice is currently unregulated and defers to the individual practitioner. It is unsurprising that with the vested interests in this community of surgeons, that the characteristics of skill degradation remain obscure; this is in no small part due to the fact that there is a trade-off in past experiences compensating for any emerging deficiency in technical skills and non-technical skills.

However, a number of studies have found that patient mortality rates increase with increasing years of practice in procedures such as carotid endarterectomy, pancreatectomy and coronary artery bypass.[17] Rates of recurrence following laparoscopic inguinal herniorrhaphy are higher when performed by older surgeons compared to younger surgeons.[18] And although age alone is not an accurate predictor of decline,[19] reviews of changes in cognitive and physical faculties show an inexorable decline of these faculties with age.[20,21] Indeed, some industries have approved fixed retirement ages (US commercial airline pilots, 65 years; Federal Bureau of Investigation officers, 57 years; and air traffic controllers, 56 years), but there is no mandatory retirement age for surgeons in many countries. The ageing surgeon programme developed at Sinai Hospital in Baltimore, Maryland, is a creative approach designed to protect senior surgeons from unreliable assessment and also to assess potentially treatable reversible disorders and improve functional capacity, as well as assisting in the decision to withdraw from clinical care.[22] The NOTSS taxonomy may provide another opportunity and a metric for self-reflection for the community of surgical seniors to evaluate their continuing proficiency.

Until recently, it was difficult, if not impossible, to either recognize an underperforming surgeon or, more importantly, do much about underperformance in surgeons if suspected. This has begun to change, although there is still much to be done. Whereas the United Kingdom has introduced revalidation, Australasia is introducing similar requirements for continued professional development and multi-source feedback.[23] However, there still remain significant problems for both individual surgeons and hospitals in providing reliable and adequate surgeon-specific data.

In England, surgeon-related outcomes for cardiac surgeons have been in the public domain for many years but were only published for other surgical specialties in 2013, and now they are being made mandatory across all surgical disciplines. However, data are taken from national databases, all of which required voluntary contributions. What is becoming increasingly clear is that the majority of surgeons who are referred to higher authorities for poor performance are more often referred because of failures in their non-technical skills than in their technical skills.[24] Furthermore, they are usually older surgeons, who perhaps have not been able to keep up with technological developments or have found the changes in clinical practice difficult to accommodate. Either way, their response tends to become apparent in their behaviours to colleagues, trainees, nurses and patients. At present, periods of 're-training', often in other hospitals, is usually suggested. Although this might address technical and clinical deficiencies, it will not necessarily address non-technical deficiencies. Hopefully, the wider implementation of NOTSS workshops and other team-training courses[25] will improve both insight and teamworking skills so that (1) poorly performing individuals can recognize when they might be starting to fail and (2) others can recognize the early signs and take steps to support and help them.

11.10 LIMITS AND BOUNDARIES

The duty of care of surgeons for their patients includes a requirement for any practitioner to identify the situations where, either because of the complexity of the case in hand or because of the relative infrequency of performing such treatments, the patient would be better served by onward referral to another practitioner who has more expertise in that particular area. For surgical practice, an important consideration is the technical complexity of the operation under consideration and onward referral is common practice and usually attracts commendable comment.

By contradistinction, the situations where a surgeon's non-technical skills are stretched to the limit, or indeed are overstretched, are less apparent and may not be identified by the individual concerned but may be quite obvious to those working with him or her. Decay of non-technical skills seems to be tolerated in a way that poor technical skill may not be. For example, inappropriate levels of indecision may be passively accepted rather than actively challenged. Poor teamwork, communication and leadership are more often tolerated than to be in receipt of critical comment, and a lack of awareness of the circumstances and information surrounding a procedure may often be deflected onto inadequacies of others rather than accepted as a limitation of self.

By emphasizing the relevance of non-technical skills to operative performance, deficiencies in any one of the categories of non-technical skills can be recognized and should prompt a surgeon to review their own practice and attempt self-remediation. This review could include getting assistance and advice from a colleague, thereby putting patient safety at the centre of all actions and for meeting the needs for future practice. Ideally, the surgeon may adopt a different role, for example, as an assistant surgeon, or may choose to routinely ask another surgeon to assist him or her while remediation takes place. Conversely, one with outstanding teamwork skills may be able to leverage the collective input of the entire team more effectively and in such a manner compensate for individual limitations.

11.11 CONCLUSIONS

The preceding chapters clearly demonstrate that the quest for excellence in operative surgery is constituted by achieving technical proficiency complemented by a full suite of non-technical skills. This repertoire, which has the safety of patients at its heart, involves more than the performance of just the individual surgeon. The engagement, support and cooperation of the entire surgical team has to be secure, and the surgeon has an important role to fulfil in achieving that.

Examples have been taken and lessons learned from other high-risk environments. These have been analysed and, where appropriate, modified for use in the operating room. Surgeon-specific non-technical skills have been developed into the NOTSS framework and evaluated, allowing the creation of a classification and vocabulary that have performance in the operating room as its context. The distinctive characteristics of that environment have created specific risks and threats, and how the surgeon is able to absorb these and manage them to good effect has important implications for the behaviour of the surgeon and awareness and decision-making processes. All these aspects of non-technical skills have been set out, defined and illustrated in Part II. This was followed by a discussion on how those skills might be assessed, evaluated, taught and maintained in Part III.

The contributions and importance of each of the cognitive and social categories contained in the NOTSS taxonomy have been amplified and the effects of external influences including limitations to performance imposed by fatigue and stress have been discussed, as have some of the techniques that can be used to mitigate these deleterious effects.

The latter chapters in this book have focused on how non-technical skills can be acquired and the implications of their evaluation for training, recurrent training and endorsement of continuing practice.

Non-technical skills have emerged as an integral feature of operative performance of surgeons of every specialty. This new-found recognition has provided due cause and justification for this book. It was designed to stimulate its readers to give further thought to how such skills can be deployed and utilized at the operating table and how they can be enhanced and developed to promote safe, effective and skilful surgery.

REFERENCES

1. World Health Organization. WHO Patient Safety Curriculum. 2009. [Accessed March 26, 2015.] Available from: http://whqlibdoc.who.int/publications/2009/9789241598316_eng.pdf.

2. The Australian Council for Safety and Quality in Health Care. Australian Patient Safety Education Framework. 2005. [Accessed March 26, 2015.] Available from: http://www.safetyandquality.gov.au/wp-content/uploads/2012/06/National-Patient-Safety-Education-Framework-2005.pdf.

3. Patey R, Flin R, Ross S, Parker S, Cleland J, Jackson J et al. WHO Patient Safety Curriculum Guide for Medical Schools. Evaluation Study. Report to WHO Patient Safety Programme. August 2011. http://www.who.int/patientsafety/education/curriculum/EN_PSP_Education_Medical_Curriculum/en/index.html. [Accessed March 26, 2015.]

4. Civil Aviation Authority. The Crew Resource Management Structure (CRMI) and Crew Resource Management Structure Examiner (CRMIE.) Accreditation Framework. March 2013. [Accessed March 26, 2015.] Available from: http://www.caa.co.uk/application.aspx?catid=33&pagetype=65&appid=11&mode=list&type=sercat&id=22. Standards document number 29 version 5.

5. Gawande A. 'Personal best: Top athletes and singers have coaches. Should you?' *The New Yorker*. October 3, 2011. [Accessed March 26, 2015.] Available from: http://www.newyorker.com/magazine/2011/10/03/personal-best.

6. Hu YY, Peyre SE, Arriaga AF, Osteen RT, Corso KA, Weiser TG et al. Postgame analysis: Using video-based coaching for continuous professional development. *J Am Coll Surg*. 2012 Jan;214(1):115–24.

7. Yule S, Flin R, Maran N, Youngson G, Mitchell A, Rowley D et al. Debriefing surgeons on non-technical skills. *Cogn Tech Work*. 2008;10:265–74.

8. Healthcare Improvement Scotland. Scottish Patient Safety Programme. 2008. [Accessed March 26, 2015.] Available from: http://www.scottishpatientsafetyprogramme.scot.nhs.uk.

9. Hale AR, Heming BH, Carthey J, Kirwan B. Modelling of safety management systems. *Saf Sci*. 1997;26:121–40.

10. Rydenfalt C, Ek A, Larsson PA. Safety checklist compliance and a false sense of safety: New directions for research. *BMJ Qual Saf*. 2014;23:183–6.

11. Gawande AA, Zinner MJ, Studdert DM, Brennan TA. Analysis of errors reported by surgeons at three teaching hospitals. *Surgery*. 2003 Jun;133(6):614–21. PMID:12796727.

12. Arriaga AF, Gawande AA, Raemer DB, Jones DB, Smink DS, Weinstock P et al. Pilot testing of a model for insurer-driven, large-scale multicenter simulation training for operating room teams. Harvard Surgical Safety Collaborative. *Ann Surg*. 2014 Mar;259(3):403–10.

13. Youngson GG. Medical error and disclosure – a view from the UK. *Surgeon*. 2014;12;68–72.

14. Flin R, Fioratou E, Frerk C, Trotter C, Cook TM. Human factors in the development of complications of the airway management: Preliminary evaluation of an interview tool. *Anaesthesia*. 2013;68:1817–25.

15. Shannon FL, Fazzalari FL, Theurer PF, Bell GF, Sutcliffe KM, Prager RL. A method to evaluate cardiac surgery mortality: Phase of care mortality analysis. *Ann Thorac Surg*. 2012 Jan;93(1):36–43; discussion 43.

16. Youngson GG, Knight P, Hamilton L, Taylor I, Tanner A, Steers J., et al. The UK Proposals for Revalidation of Doctors: Implications for the recertification of surgeons. *Arch Surg*. 2010:145:93–6.

17. Waljee JF, Greenfield LJ, Dimick JB, Birkmeyer JD. Surgeon age and operative mortality in the United States. *Ann Surg*. 2006;244:353–62.

18. Neumayer LA, Gawande AA, Wang J, Giobbie-Hurder A, Itani KMF, Fitzgibbons RJ et al. Proficiency of surgeons in inguinal hernia repair: Effect of experience and age. *Ann Surg*. 2005;242:343–8; discussion 348–52.

19. Eva KW. The aging physician: Changes in cognitive processing and their impact on medical practice. *Acad Med*. 2002;77:S1–6.

20. Bieliauskas LA, Langenacker S, Graver C, Lee HJ, O'Neill J, Greenfield LJ. Cognitive changes and retirement amongst senior surgeons (CCRASS): Results from the CCRASS Study. *J Am Coll Surg*. 2008;207:69–78.

21. Greenfield LJ. Farewell to surgery. *J Vasc Surg*. 1994;19:6–14.

22. Katlic MR, Coleman JA. The ageing surgeon. *Ann Surg*. 2014;260:199–201.

23. Breen KJ. Revalidation – what is the problem and what are the solutions? *Med J Australia*. 2014;3:153–6.

24. NHS Clinical Assessment Service. NCAS casework. The first eight years. September 2009. [Accessed March 26, 2015.] Available from: http://www.ncas.nhs.uk/publications/.

25. Neily J, Mills PD, Zu YY, Carney BT, West P, Berger DH et al. Association between implementation of a medical team training program and surgical mortality. *JAMA*. 2010;304:1693–700.

Index